Contents

HEALTH
SERVICES

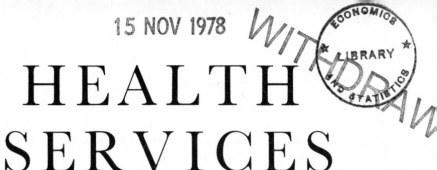

HEALTH SERVICES

Their nature and organization,
and the role of patients, doctors, nurses,
and the complementary professions

Editor: Elliott Jaques

with members of the Brunel Health Services
Organization Research Unit

Heinemann · London

Heinemann Educational Books

LONDON   EDINBURGH   MELBOURNE   AUCKLAND
TORONTO   HONG KONG   SINGAPORE   KUALA LUMPUR
NEW DELHI   NAIROBI   JOHANNESBURG   LUSAKA
IBADAN   KINGSTON

ISBN 0 435 82474 0

First published 1978

Published by
Heinemann Educational Books Ltd
48 Charles Street, London W1X 8AH

Printed in Great Britain by
Butler & Tanner Ltd, Frome and London

Preface

Outline of the Book and the Role of the HSORU

Elliott Jaques

This book presents some of the main findings arising from the work of the Brunel Health Services Organization Research Unit (HSORU) in connection with the National Health Service in England and Wales. The work of the Unit began in 1966 and is currently financed until 1984. During this period the total service underwent a radical reorganization. Implemented on 1st April 1974, this reorganization was planned between 1971 and 1974. The Unit has thus had a once-in-a-lifetime opportunity to be involved in the design of a very large-scale and complex social change, and to follow through the consequences of that change for at least ten years.

The Structure of the Book
The Unit's experience to the time of writing will be presented in the book in the following way.

First of all the Unit's mode of work – that of social analysis – will be described, with illustrations of the specially deep access to the inner workings of the organization which this method achieves. In addition, the means will be demonstrated by which analysis (rather than recommendations) can facilitate social change and lead to eventual evaluation of change.

The provision of health services is a particularly delicate human activity. The design of health services organization encounters all the problems of how to give highly personalized services by means of large-scale bureaucratic systems. Some of these very general social issues are presented in Chapter 1.

The rest of Part One is devoted to a series of chapters which outline some of the main concepts used in the Unit's analysis of the NHS. These concepts are general in the sense of being applicable in many different types of social institution, and as such may contribute to social science theory in general, as well as to the development of social administration. They include the notion of the natural health care community – a notion which links to the fundamental question of how to analyse community organization. The question of 'clinical autonomy' and of the doctor–patient relationship are then considered: the latter is a dyadic relationship which has long been of interest to sociologists. Of equal interest is the issue of professions, professionals, and professionalization – a question considered in detail as a foundation for the analysis of the many disciplines incorporated within health services organization.

There then follow two chapters on organizational structure – in particular the stratification of the work systems. The application of a general structure of work-strata and grading is described, and the generalized work content of the various work-strata is outlined. This stratification system is linked to human capacity and the significance of various levels of professional work.

The final chapter in Part One considers questions of leadership and the functioning of teams, including the vexed question of multi-disciplinary clinical teams. These questions are of crucial importance in a service in which the growth of teams of all kinds has become rampant.

In Part Two a series of particular issues is dealt with: organization of physiotherapy and occupational therapy; the future of child guidance; full-time and part-time patients in relation to domiciliary care; geriatric departments; assessment of mental handicap; and the organization of care for the severely mentally handicapped.

These particular issues are not intended to give a comprehensive review of the reorganization. They have been selected because they have been studied intensively by members of the Unit, and have been analysed in sufficient depth to illustrate many general points relevant throughout the Service: professional independence; prime responsibility for patient care; functioning of teams; levels of professional practice and recruitment, education and qualification standards; inter-professional relations, including doctors and other professions; the conditions for home care as against hospitalization; problems of the so-called Cinderella services such as those for old people and for the mentally ill and handicapped; questions of what are health services as against welfare or social services; the emergence of the various services likely to combine into one field of psychotherapy including some parts of clinical psychology, occupational therapy, speech therapy, psychiatric social work, psychiatric nursing, etc.

Part Three considers some more general issues of collaboration between health and other services, along with the equally general questions of public and employee participation.

Some Issues Not Dealt With

A number of major services have not been considered in the book. Their omission is in no way a reflection upon their importance; it is simply that the Unit's follow-up studies in these areas are not sufficiently advanced.

Nursing organization has not been included. There are, for example, many new developments in specialized nursing, both in hospitals and in work with general practitioners, and these are in process of being analysed. Some of the material on upgrading in clinical practitioner work without need to take on administrative duties, described in Chapter 9 on PT and OT, will be recognized as having application in the nursing field.

Administration and Community Medicine are frequently referred to in the context of other services. They are in the process of re-analysis by the Unit, however, in connection especially with the meaning of the 'professionalization' of administration and the meaning of the 'consultant' status of specialists in community medicine.

In the area of finance the vexed question of who should have control of budgets is currently under analysis, including the question of consultants and medical department heads as budget holders.

One very large area, in which too little analysis has been done so far and many problems remain, is that of the scientific and technical services: radiology, chemical pathology, microbiology, immunology, histopathology, haematology, physics, radiotherapy, EEG, ECG, clinical measurement, audiometry, etc. A complex set of relationships between consultants,

graduate scientists, and technicians remains to be clarified and is
the subject of active study by the Unit.

Finally, there is little reference to the major issue of the organization of the representative committee structure by means of
which doctors can participate in the development of service
policies. Here again the Unit is involved in field studies – but
many features remain to be clarified.

The Mode of Work of the HSORU: Social Analysis

The view of the NHS obtained by members of the HSORU,
and used as the focus for the observations presented here, is a
special one. It calls for brief comment, since it helps to explain
the particular nature of the content of the book. The Research
Unit's method of work may be thought to lead in some ways
to a limited view, a sketchy and uneven one. It is in other ways
a deep view, a view of how things really work at the heart of
the Service. In effect, complete coverage at the surface has been
sacrificed to deep penetration at certain points. There is good
reason to believe that systematic coverage of the whole and
analysis in depth are not readily consistent with each other. Different types of relationships with the field are required by each.
The Unit has opted for the latter.

The Unit has been in the field since 1966, when it began as
the Hospital Organization Research Unit.[1]

Its mode of work from the beginning has been that of *social
analysis*.[2] The point of this approach is that it is specifically
designed to provide the social research worker with access in
depth to important questions which people have about what
is going on within the organization. For example, what is really
happening in working relationships between given professional
groups and individuals? What are the current personal feelings
about the Service? What are people's real thoughts about what
ought to be done? What are the personally experienced frustra-
tions and satisfactions? How do things actually work as distinct

[1] Under the direction at that time of Maurice Kogan (now Professor and
Head of the Department of Government Studies at Brunel).

[2] This method has been outlined in: Elliott Jaques (1965), 'Social-Analysis
and the glacier Project'; Wilfred Brown and Elliott Jaques, *Glacier Project
Papers*; R. W. Rowbottom *et al.* (1973), *Hospital Organization*, Appendix B;
and is comprehensively described in R. W. Rowbottom (1977), *Social Analysis*.

from how they are supposed to work or what the regulations say? What are the feelings about career prospects and rewards? What are the rivalries and conflicts? What are the procedures which work well and could be extended? Who is actually accountable for what? What authority do professional workers have? What ought the working relationships to be between doctors and nurses, doctors and other professionals, various groups of professionals? Who really runs a particular laboratory or service? Where do administrators fit in, and what do they think their role ought to be?

The aim in gaining access in depth is twofold: first, to be able to make first-hand contact with what is really going on; second, to help to resolve problems by working them through with those immediately concerned, in the hope that generalizable solutions might be generated by the thorough-going resolution of particular cases. Let us comment briefly on both these processes.

In its simplest terms, the Unit's mode of work is as follows. Research is carried out only as a result of requests from specific groups or individuals for help with particular problems which they are experiencing. A confidential relationship is established. The Unit members help to analyse and thus to clarify the nature of the problem, and do not advise on actions. It is for those concerned to decide what to do, aided if possible by the analysis and clarification provided by the research. It is not for the research worker to arrogate the power to decide and recommend what ought to be done – that would undermine and weaken the resolve and competence of those involved in the problem.

Reporting of results takes place only in collaboration with those with whom work is done. It is for them to decide when the work has proceeded sufficiently far to be of possible interest to others; or perhaps to decide to report preliminary findings or formulations to others in order to share experience or to seek comment or to test ideas in other settings against the experience of others.

In order to achieve eventual communication of results on a wide basis and to obtain the wide testing which makes for generalization or reveals the need for revision of concepts, a wider sanctioning structure is maintained. One of the conditions of the Unit's work is that the Department (DHSS) shall provide a Steering Committee to consider the Unit's work, to set priorities, and to clear results for wider dissemination. Equally, attempts are made to have Steering Committees for local projects, as well as at intermediate levels. By these means the Unit's on-going work can be continually subject to practical scrutiny and evaluation, and cleared material from project work has a route through from the local situation to dissemination and testing on a wide scale. During the aftermath of NHS reorganization the working of this Steering Committee structure has suffered from some of the difficulties in NHS organization structure which will be discussed.

Another condition is that the Unit conducts a regular series of working conferences, organized nationally, in which newly emerging formulations can be presented for discussion and criticism. Working notes from these conferences have been combined with the results from field-work in the preparation of a special series of Working Papers, edited versions of which have been included in this book.

As far as the working through of difficulties is concerned, it is a matter of policy for members of the Unit to stay with a project development so long as those concerned wish them to do so. In many cases this leads to periods of collaboration extending over periods of years – with more and less active phases – during which analysis may lead to the adoption of new arrangements. These new arrangements can then be tested in practice. As difficulties and shortcomings are discovered, further analysis is carried out, and further modifications tested. By this means, novel formulations and procedures may be developed by successive approximation with careful field testing at every stage.

It is the accumulation of these tested experiences, worked with through time, which provides the material from which more general formulations may be developed.

In short, the main steps in social analysis may be summarized as follows:

  (*a*) development of rigorously defined concepts with which to describe and communicate patterns of organization (presented in Appendix B);

(*b*) the construction of ranges of alternative models of organization to be tried and tested under varying circumstances in relation to particular problems;

(*c*) follow-up testing of the application of particular models in specific cases, and modification as necessary both of concepts and models using the concepts;

(*d*) testing of given models under other circumstances – sometimes by others on their own and sometimes in collaboration with them – with ensuing generalization of results;

(*e*) discussion and checking of results with steering committees;

(*f*) communication of results in writing and in conferences to provide for further testing and modification as well as for dissemination of findings.

Is This Method Scientific?

It may be noted that one of the limitations of this mode of working is that the research worker cannot choose and determine what problems he will work on, nor can he approach people and ask to be allowed to carry out particular studies, or to collect systematic data, or to establish control groups.

For these reasons no significant statistical data can be collected; no control studies can be conducted; no systematic comparisons can be made between different methods, with quantitatively significant correlations. Some distinguished colleagues would deny that such a method is worthy of the name of scientific research. Experience with social analysis would suggest a very different view.

It is true that there is a need for social research in which social trends are studied, and various methods compared under control conditions, and that such studies require detailed statistical data and analysis. Unfortunately, however, in Britain today there is a tendency to consider that statistical studies of this kind constitute the whole field of social research – that they are the only method of 'true' research. That narrow view reduces the field of research to an unnecessarily limited and arid preoccupation. One of the problems in any science has always been to get deeper and more detailed access to the field of study – by means, for example, of microscopes, telescopes, cloud chambers, moon shots. Moreover, studies of particular eclipses and other so-called experiments of opportunity are all a part of the general equipment of any mature science – alongside its controlled and statistically analysed surveys and experiments. All these methods are necessary, and in this spirit we claim unequivocally that the results to be described in this book make a rigorous scientific contribution to an understanding of the organization and functioning of the NHS.[3] They do so not only by presenting the results of field studies in depth, but by their use of a system of rigorously defined working concepts.

Conceptual Clarification

An appreciation of this latter point is relevant to an understanding of the objectives and the meaning of the book – and to an intelligent consideration of its content. For one of several crucial problems in the social sciences is to develop sets of well-defined working concepts which can enable even the simplest beginning to be made to describe in objectively understandable ways what is going on. Nowhere is this need more urgent than in the study of our social institutions.

This problem can, unfortunately, readily be illustrated with respect to the organization of the NHS, where it is absolutely critical. There is hardly one concept available to the NHS (or to any other enterprise) which can be used in describing reorganization, which it can be confidently expected will be widely understood, and which can therefore be used for formulating and communicating organizational structures and procedures. The list of utter confusion is a long one: grading; management; administration; manager; supervisor; team; coordination; monitoring; job evaluation; secondment; responsibility; reporting to; matrix organization; participative management; consultation; participation; authority, accountability; representative; committee; collaboration; prescribing; profession and professional; technician; technologist; scientist; department head; to be in charge of; chief executive officer; chairman; working with; piece work; incentive bonus; productivity bargain; autonomous work groups; job enrichment; job; task; assignment; the organization; clinical freedom; patient

[3] The scientific argument is pursued in detail in R. W. Rowbottom, *Social Analysis*, op. cit.

responsibility; independent practitioner; medical administration; financial accountability; budget holder; and so on and on. Not a single one of these concepts has a clear, unequivocal, and generally established meaning.

Confusion over these issues is universal. It is profound. It is true not just of the Health Service, but of every single employment system – whether in government departments, in social services, in education, in industry, in commerce – and not only in this country, but in every other industrial nation, and in the business schools, and the management textbooks, and the sociology of institutions and organization as well.

But does it matter? Is there any need for disquiet? Is is not just 'a question of semantics'? To which the answer is a firm and unequivocal 'no'! The mismanagement of employment systems has become one of the major tragedies of modern times in all industrial societies. We suffer particularly in the United Kingdom because we are still the most advanced industrial nation in the world in the sense of employing a larger proportion of our working population in these employment systems than any other nation (over 90 per cent – 23 million men and women). And among this massive organizational confusion sits the NHS, nearly a million strong, one of the largest and certainly by far the most complex employment system in the world.

What, if any, are the negative consequences? They are legion. It is impossible to devise adequate formulations to establish various possible patterns of working relationships between doctors and other ancillary services such as nursing, the remedial therapies, or scientific and technical staffs – with the result that stress and tension are widespread, strike action is perennially nascent, and patients suffer; the non-medical ancillary staffs – porters, engineers, telephonists, cleaners and others – are in many places in states of chronic ferment; overstaffing and over-complex organization result from emphasis upon professional career structures rather than upon the work to be done; many professional groups are seeking equivalent status to doctors, especially in such fields as the scientific services, and psychotherapy for adults and children, with intense rivalries growing between the Colleges and Professional Associations; there has been chronic unclarity in relationships between RHAs and AHAs, between RTOs, ATOs, and DMTs;

stresses arise in the plethora of various types of 'team' because of uncertainty about which members have what authority and who is accountable if something goes wrong; fair differential payment is practically impossible to achieve when there are forty-eight Whitley Councils working on payment structures.

These and a wide range of similar problems will be familiar enough. They are probably no better, and no worse, in the NHS than in any other large-scale employment system. But they are serious nonetheless – just as they are serious in these other systems.

It is precisely with problems of these kinds that the members of the Unit have been invited to become involved in collaboration with members of the NHS who are individually involved in them. And here is where the absence of agreed concepts shows up from the very start as an enormous obstacle. It is impossible to formulate the current situation – who is related to whom, in terms of what authority, accountable for what, and so on. It takes painstaking effort to establish what is the extant situation; different people make their own assumptions about what is happening or what should be happening; and it is impossible to know at first whether the same assumptions are being made but expressed in different terms, or whether different assumptions lie concealed under the same words which are being used, or whether any of the assumptions, however expressed, are within shooting distance of expressing the real situation.

Many examples of this type of problem will be illustrated in the practical studies described in detail in the book. The main concepts used are set out and defined in Appendix B at the end of the book. The preoccupation of the Unit with clear conceptual definition, and their insistence on the using of one term, and that term only, for any particular concept, has often been impatiently referred to as 'Brunelerie' by those who feel that this approach verges perhaps upon the pedantic. The clarification of language and concepts and the introduction of new terms in medical and other sciences is accepted as a normal and necessary part of scientific growth; by contrast, the same process in the social sciences is seen as the creation of jargon, the general taste still being for the illusory common sense of Babel. Our experience, however, leads us to take these criticisms in good spirit – for the only alternative is to contribute further to the already ghastly muddle and confusion which exists.

The Role of the HSORU in the NHS Reorganization – 1974

The Unit members are aware that many of the difficulties in organization experienced since April 1974, when the reorganization of the NHS was implemented, have been laid at the door of the Unit and its work with the Management Steering Committee of the DHSS and the Grey Book which that committee prepared. Such criticism is wide of the mark, since it does not take into account that the Unit's role was an analytical one. It was no part of the Unit's responsibility to press for any particular solutions, but rather to present alternatives and to identify any inconsistencies or non-requisite ideas.

We are, however, aware of many areas of incomplete analysis in our work at that time. A noteworthy example was our lack of a satisfactorily worked-through analysis of paramedical and scientific and technical services to put forward to the Committee. We were, of course, not alone in lacking the necessary concepts for such an analysis (but it is our hope that the necessary concepts are now emerging as illustrated in the essay – Chapter 9 – on PTs and OTs). At the same time, we did contribute certain critical analyses such as the analysis of why consultants and GPs cannot have managers.

In general terms, without attempting to review in detail the pros and cons of various analyses, and the contributions of various groups, it is perhaps useful to keep the following broad issues in mind. The problem of designing a new organization for the NHS faced those concerned with certain out of the ordinary difficulties. First, an enormously complex organization was involved – a whole quantum leap different in complexity from any other employment system. Second, there was the exceedingly tight time schedule, dictated by the Parliamentary timetable of the government's term of office. Third, there was the fact that certain major Cabinet decisions had already been made setting the framework within which the organization had to be fitted: there were to be both Regional and Area Authorities; Area Authorities were to be conterminous with local authorities (except for the special problem of Inner London); health care was to be organized at District level, and therefore there would be many multi-district Areas; the DHSS was to have a major role in NHS administration.

Some of the consequences of these irreversible decisions could readily enough be foreseen – such, for example, as the probable uncertainty of relationship between the Regional and the Area tiers, and of both in relation to the Department.[4]

On the other hand, by contrast, many of the severe difficulties arising out of the problem of relating AHAs to multi-district Areas were not sharply enough perceived. Whether those concerned, within the constraints of government policy, of time, and of the acute professional sensitivities which were also at work, did all that might be expected in the circumstances, is a judgment of Solomon. The point the Research Unit would wish to argue, however, is that to the extent that it did succeed in contributing to conceptual clarity for the analysis, then such a contribution could only be positive. This argument is made not as an apologia for the Unit or its work, but to emphasize still further the urgency of the need to forward conceptual clarification and conceptual rigour in the social sciences.

Some Difficulties Foreseen

Finally, three issues which were not adequately catered for in the reorganization, and which are the source of growing difficulty, need to be mentioned.

The first of these issues is that the range of health care services is steadily widening – as a result of scientific development, of social understanding, of economic advance, of education, and of professionalization. It would appear that the role of the doctor may be changing in certain fields, and that the relationships between doctor, patient, and other professionals may be changing as a result.

---

[4] Thus, for example, a very detailed critical evaluation of this arrangement was prepared for the Management Steering Committee by Sir Richard Meyjes and Professor Elliott Jaques. This analysis examined the question of how far a National Health Services Commission might achieve a radical simplification of organization through a direct single relationship with the Secretary of State, and leaving much greater freedom of action for Area Health Authorities. This analysis was discussed with the Secretary of State, but the political timetable, among other considerations, ruled out the possibility of a full development and discussion of this analysis, or of other possible alternatives.

Such fields in which services are extending and change is occurring include, for example, geriatric care, mental illness and mental handicap, general psychotherapy and psychological guidance and care, and educational procedures and provision of aids to enable the physical and mentally handicapped to use their abilities as fully as possible. There appears to be a growing number of circumstances in such areas in which prime responsibility for patient care passes by default from medically qualified to non-medically qualified practitioners – psychotherapists, psychologists of various kinds, physiotherapists and occupational therapists, speech therapists, nurses and so on – a doctor being called in if such a person in care becomes 'physically' ill, just as the family would call upon the doctor when necessary.

These changing situations are often encountered under circumstances where so-called multi-disciplinary clinical teams are brought into being. It is not necessarily always clear which members of the team are accountable for what, and which member of the team is accountable in the final analysis for what happens to the patient. In such a setting the patient or the patient's family are certainly concerned and certainly entitled to know just who is responsible for the treatment he or she is receiving.

These issues are considered in a number of chapters – those concerned with the definition of teams and leadership, with professionals, with stratification, and with special services. It is when issues of this kind arise that the argument about the need for clarity of conceptual definition and the construction of ranges of alternative models for trial and testing takes on its greatest force.

The second issue is connected with the fact that there is a strong tendency to create organization to provide for the career aspirations of employees, rather than to provide the necessary roles to get the required work done. The two modes of organization may not necessarily be consistent. Indeed, it is rarely if ever the case that the two requirements are entirely consistent with each other; and, paradoxically, if the career consideration predominates in determining organization, it usually turns out to be to the detriment of both the patients and the members concerned.

Organization for careers rather than for work is an

increasingly common feature of many large-scale institutions.[5] The major difficulty with this career-oriented organization planning is that it tends to put a premium upon: the creation of higher-level career-peak roles with impoverished and unsatisfactory work content, where incumbents come to feel, and are felt as being, in the way; and the creation of an increase in the number of grading levels – these grades then coming to be used as managerial levels and creating too many levels of organization. The result is that professional practitioners, for example, tend rapidly to be pushed up out of clinical work into unrealistic and unnecessary administrative grades: they get slightly increased pay and status related to the number of subordinates they can collect and count, but vastly increased feelings of dissatisfaction from lack of interesting work to replace the clinical work which they have had to leave behind and which many of them prefer.

How some of these problems may be overcome will be discussed in the general chapters on work stratification and on professionalism (Chapters 5 and 6), and illustrated in the chapters on such services as PT and OT (Chapter 9).

Third, it may be noted that there is no explicit allocation of responsibility for the monitoring of the organization structure itself. This lack of specialist attention to organization is still a feature of most large-scale social institutions, and the resulting cost in social stress and inefficiency is high. In the NHS, many groups are variously involved, including administration, personnel, Whitley Councils, special committees and commissions, planners, heads of service. But no one function can be held accountable for having specialist knowledge of organization and for anticipating organization difficulties and helping to sort them out.

In a service as large and as complex as the NHS, the lack of a specialist function concerned with organization can have serious consequences. Organizational disjunctions tend to persist; administrative training programmes are less on the mark

[5] The Fulton Report in the British Civil Service, for example, proposed the merging of the clerical, executive, and administrative classes for the explicit purpose of providing for an improvement in career progress flow, and made no reference to how this reorganization might improve the possibilities of allocating duties and managerial accountability in a more efficient and humanly satisfying way.

than they could be; inadequate solutions to organization problems lead to trial after trial of new models with the disheartening experience of repeated failure.

The definition and design of organization structure is a serious matter. It determines the context of working relationships between members of the Service, and the mode of deployment of the human resource. Both these factors are of great importance in the provision of satisfactory care for patients.

Acknowledgments

Our main acknowledgment is to those in the Department of Health and Social Security and in the National Health Service who have actively supported our work during the past twelve years by involving us in collaboration with them in the endeavour to cut through the great difficulties inherent in understanding the complexities in organizing health services in the interests of the individual patient.

We appreciate the help of our colleagues in the Brunel Social Services Organization Research Unit – David Billis, Geoffrey Bromley and Anthea Hey – who have contributed material, as co-authors, to this book.

In our work over the years we have been fortunate in having the loyal and impeccable support of the able administrative team of Mrs Lynn Drummond, Miss Jayne Baker, Mrs Pat Frankish and Mrs Betty Whiteley. They have all been involved in the typing and checking of the various drafts of this manuscript, and Mrs Frankish has maintained the master copy through all its amendments and changes.

Part One
Basic Conceptions

1

Complex Organization and Individual Freedom

Elliott Jaques

The development of an effective organization for the National Health service throws up one of the major problems of modern society – that of providing certain large-scale services for individuals while preserving the personal touch and concern for each individual as a unique human being. For it seems to be a paradox of industrial societies that as they provide increasingly humane social services to the individual – schools, hospitals and doctors, social services, housing, parks and recreational facilities, and many other vital services besides – they seem inevitably to take away from his freedom and individuality. This dilemma of giving benefits with one hand and taking away individuality with the other arises from the increases in service being provided via governmental agencies leading to an extension of bureaucratic machinery under whose social mass the individuality of the citizen readily becomes more and more submerged.

The potential conflict between on the one hand the freedom of the individual, his personal dignity, his existence as a singular human being with his own particular and special personality, needs and idiosyncrasies, his self-respect and intactness of self, and on the other hand the requirements of bureaucratic rationalization to ensure that adequate services are available for everyone, the maintenance of standards and uniformity of service and of administrative tidiness and efficiency, are epitomized with painful sharpness in governmentally provided health and medical services.

Over the past thirty years it has become increasingly the case in industrial societies that the medical care of the sick person will be provided by some form of local or central government health service or health insurance scheme, to such an extent that now and in the foreseeable future such services will be almost exclusively provided in that way. As a result, being ill in an industrial society is now a human condition which may throw up a complex pattern of apparently conflicting forces.

On the one hand, there is the sick person, debilitated, more or less helpless, unable to work and earn a living, anxious about his future capacity to live, fearful of death – and in need of care and reassurance from family and from a doctor, a nurse, or other medical person whom he knows personally, likes and believes in, and trusts in terms both of personal character and of scientific and technical competence.

On the other hand, there are what appear to be the overwhelming forces of the impersonal – the great bureaucratic systems by means of which health care is organized and provided, and the scientific technology by means of which medicine is now practised. Each of these forces, bureaucratic and technological, seems to vitiate the efforts and concern of doctors, nurses, and other staff to provide personal care and attention for each individual patient.

The view is widely held that this depersonalization of what ought to be humanly sensitive, delicate, and personal services is an inevitable accompaniment of large-scale organization – not only in health, but all governmentally organized personal and social services, education, welfare, and housing. Growing impersonality is thought to be one of the costs to be paid for whatever advantages are to be gained from such organization – in fairer distribution of service, economies of scale, democratization of social policy, and in research and the development of new services.

There is some experience to show that this view of inevitable inconsistency and conflict of interest is unnecessarily pessimistic. So long as organization is designed with the proper objectives in view, it is possible to arrange for highly personalized services through large-scale organization systems. Nowhere is the search for this possibility more sharply and dramatically called for than in the case of a health service. Certainly not just any organization structure will do. It must be a requisite structure which can serve the needs of a very large number of individuals. The overriding issue is how can responsibility for health provision be organized as closely as possible to those who are working together to give the care, and to those who are living together as a community receiving the care?

The Basis of Requisite Health Organization

It is a frequent criticism of the work of those concerned with health services organization that they are concerned with organization problems rather than with patients. Such criticism ought not to be tenable, for all health services organization has inevitably to do with patients. It is through organization that the human and other resources for patient care are provided. The nature of organization affects the type of care received, and how that care will be given, in the most profound and dramatic ways. That is why in any sound organizational work it is essential to be utterly clear in the first place about the social objectives of a service. A poor law charity service in which a patient is on sufferance and ought to be grateful for whatever care he gets will be organized very differently from one in which as a matter of entitlement he is receiving the care due to a free citizen.[1]

The goal of organization study must be the achievement of requisite organization. Requisite organization may be defined as that form of organization required by the situation. For our purposes we shall assume a two-fold dimension to this concept. The first is the obvious one: efficiency and effectiveness – the provision of the best quality of service, properly distributed, within the resources available. That dimension may be taken for granted as an object of organizational design.

It is the other dimension which is less often taken for granted, less obvious, less often noted and taken into account. It has to do with the provision of a service based upon the rights of the individual patient to remain a free citizen even when in the role of patient, and not to be absorbed into a paternalistic social

---

[1] A good example of this issue is the turmoil which was caused in some hospitals in the early days of the introduction of the policy allowing mothers to stay as much as possible with their babies and small children in hospital. The upset to established ward routines was sometimes felt to outweigh the importance of the maintenance of emotional bonds between child and family.

system in which individual gratitude for care received may be transformed into an episode of subservience. It is this type of issue which has led many countries to opt for health insurance schemes in which the individual is free to seek his health service care when and where he wishes. Competition in the provision of service can have constructively stimulating effects upon those who are in the field of providing those services. On the other side of the argument, however, are such difficulties as avoiding gross differences between regions and localities in the quality of service available, and pressures towards the over-prescribing of service so as to increase professional incomes.

The preservation of the dignity of the individual in illness, and the maintenance of ties as close as possible with family can, however, readily be a fundamental tenet of the policy of a national health service. It most certainly must be a cornerstone of the approach to health service organization adopted in social analytical work if requisite organization is being sought. Thus, for example, the aim of the NHS to provide a thoroughly human and personalized service has been expressed most unequivocally in the flexibility of approach, regard for individual feelings, concern for the patient and family, outlined in *The Organization of the In-Patient's Day*, the Report of a Committee of the Central Health Services Council of the DHSS.[2]

If the assumption is adopted that the requisite organization of a national health service will be the one which will best recognize the individuality of the patient, that assumption leads to emphasis upon how to organize thoroughly professional development in various parts of the service; upon how to protect organizationally the rights of patients to a personal confidential relationship with a doctor who has clinical freedom; upon how to ensure the growth of preventive services and the establishment of appropriate rehabilitation and handicap services, all in line with NHS policies, so that the umbrella of health care can extend more fully to restoration of the individual to satisfactory functioning, both physically and mentally, and not be limited solely to the important but nevertheless insufficient goal of providing for medical emergencies and the overcoming of the acute phases of illness.

[2] DHSS (1976).

The Constitution of Liberty

The problem of finding a requisite organization for the National Health Service is thus part of the much larger theme of individual liberty, of individual humanity, of the intactness of the person and his family, of the intactness of human and intimate and personal community, in the context of the advantages to be gained from the types of service which can become available through large-scale planning in industrial nations.

The dangers have been repeatedly pointed out. Once large-scale governmental services are established they tend to take over. The person, his family, and the community disappear from view, and individuality becomes too costly a luxury. Out of such consequences has come the bad name given to many large-scale public services of all kinds, especially governmental services, with their imputed facelessness. And yet the general experience is that most members of services such as the National Health Service are individually doing their best to provide personal and individualized service with a human touch. Employment in a large-scale bureaucratic system does not provoke profound changes in the depth of people's characters and personalities. Such changes are far more difficult to achieve than can be produced by a mere employment system, even though employment may strongly influence the way people behave.

What then of the criticisms? Are we all at heart impersonal and unconcerned about others? Are we all autocrats under the surface? Are we all like lemmings, to become part of one great corporate mass moving out to sea never to regain our individual freedom?

This negative outcome is far from inevitable if we can get our organizational relationships right; that is to say, if we can establish an institutional or organizational context whose structure of relationships is such as to enable people to take up constructive roles in which they can have constructive working relationships with others, working to fulfil social policies determined by democratic means.

Professor F. A. Hayek[3] is one of those who argue most strongly that there must be an inevitable loss of individual freedom as a consequence of monopoly governmental services. One

[3] F. A. Hayek (1960), *The Constitution of Liberty*.

example which he uses to bolster his argument is precisely the National Health Service in Britain. His argument – one of the more sophisticated and thoughtful of this liberal individualist school of thought – is worth considering as a yardstick against which to measure any particular organizational arrangement, to ensure that it is not in fact supporting the extreme anti-libertarian view against which Hayek and others such as Professor Karl Popper and Milton Friedman have been waging their vigorous campaign.

As Hayek puts it:

> There is little doubt that the growth of health insurance is a desirable development. And perhaps there is also a case for making it compulsory since many who could thus provide for themselves might otherwise become a public charge. But there are strong arguments against a single scheme of state insurance; and there seems to be an overwhelming case against a free health service for all. From what we have seen of such schemes, it is probable that their inexpediency will become evident in the countries that have adopted them, although political circumstances make it unlikely that they can ever be abandoned, now that they have been adopted. One of the strongest arguments against them is, indeed, that their introduction is the kind of politically irrevocable measure that will have to be continued, whether it proves a mistake or not.[4]

He argues further:

> The case for a free health service is usually based on two fundamental misconceptions. They are, first, the belief that medical needs are usually of an objectively ascertainable character and such that they can and ought to be fully met in every case without regard to economic considerations and, second, that this is economically possible because an improved medical service normally results in a restoration of economic effectiveness or earning power and so pays for itself.

On these two counts the British experience shows that this view is not necessarily correct. It was only in the very early

[4] Op. cit., p. 298.

days of the NHS that medical needs were thought by some to be objectively ascertainable, or that they could be fully met in all circumstances. Experience soon taught that there was not simply a limited amount of illness in the population which could be brought under control and budgeted for. The medical need changes and is readily expandable as resources become more freely available. The planning of service was therefore found to be essential.

The point about planning has been to create institutions which give a reasonable chance of making good *judgments* about medical needs and priorities and of making good *judgments* about how much resource should go towards fulfilling those needs as compared with other needs. The fact that medical need is a financially bottomless pit has become familiar to every doctor, planner, and health service worker. Nor has health service planning been related to any conception of 'paying for itself'. The scale of service has been determined by financial provision argued in terms of national social priority as compared with other social needs.

But there is a further argument which Professor Hayek produces which gets much nearer to the heart of the democratic issue and which warrants the most thoughtful consideration. He states:

There are so many serious problems raised by the nationalization of medicine that we cannot mention even all the more important ones. But there is one the gravity of which the public has scarcely yet perceived and which is likely to be of the greatest importance. This is the inevitable transformation of doctors, who have been members of a free profession primarily responsible to their patients, into paid servants of the state, officials who are necessarily subject to instruction by authority and who must be released from the duty of secrecy so far as authority is concerned. The most dangerous aspect of the new development may well prove to be that, at a time when the increase in medical knowledge tends to confer more and more power over the minds of men upon those who possess it, they should be made dependent on a unified organization under single direction and be guided by the same reasons of state that generally govern policy. A system that gives the indispensable helper of the individual, who is at the same time an agent of the state, an insight into the other's most intimate concerns and creates conditions in which he must reveal this knowledge to a superior and use it for the purposes determined by authority opens frightening prospects. The manner in which state medicine has been used in Russia as an instrument of industrial discipline gives us a foretaste of the uses to which such a system can be put.[5]

This type of criticism, along with the more general import of the criticism of those like Professor Hayek who see an inevitable grey mediocre uniformity that must inevitably spread over national governmental monopoly services, must be answered. These are serious issues, and point to problems that are not easily avoided.

A number of conditions must be established if these criticisms are to be satisfactorily answered. What is required is the opportunity for patient choice of doctor (and the reciprocal right of the doctor not to have a particular patient); a private and confidential relationship between doctor and patient; the right of the doctor (and of specified other professionals as well) to independent practitioner status; and the avoidance of written records on patients which are unknown or unavailable to the patient and over which the patient has no control.

These conditions are not matters only for a governmentally provided national health service. They apply to any kind of health service whatever. In addition, in the case of a national health service there is required opportunity for participation in the making and control of policy by the public served and by employees of the service. How each of these conditions is provided for in the National Health Service may be briefly outlined. Whether these developments will succeed in retaining an individual and personalized feel to the services, and in ensuring quality and variety of service, will be a major matter of social policy to be evaluated during the coming years.

Clinical Autonomy and Personalized Service
A first and crucial feature of the NHS is that it provides for a personal confidential relationship between doctor and

[5] Op. cit., p. 300.

patient. This relationship is built into the service in the form of the explicit retention of what is commonly referred to as the clinical freedom or clinical autonomy of the doctor. As is shown in Chapter 3, full clinical autonomy contains a number of elements, all of importance to the patient, namely: independent practitioner status and the carrying of prime responsibility by the doctor; and mutual patient–doctor choice.

In short, the establishment of clinical autonomy ensures that doctors can work as independent practitioners – free to diagnose, treat, and give prognoses in accord with their own best clinical judgment. This freedom is clinical freedom, a freedom whereby society places confidence in the individual clinical judgments of a highly trained and selected group of people, relied upon as professionals. But it is a genuine freedom, and not absolute licence. That is to say, it is freedom which is given within appropriate limits: namely, those fixed by law, which include explicit NHS policies; the requirements of professional conduct established by the General Medical Council; and the dictates of what would be accepted as gross incompetence or grossly unacceptable behaviour as judged by professional colleagues.

It will be self-evident that this independent practitioner status precludes general practitioners and consultants from having a managerial superior. They are managerially free-standing, working within the very broad terms of reference established by their contracts with a Health Authority. The quality of their clinical decisions is not subject to managerial scrutiny or review (in contrast to junior medical staff who are in a manager-subordinate relationship with a consultant or GP).

The *'medical audit'*, or peer group review, is sometimes thought to supplant clinical autonomy. It does not really do so. What it can do is help to ensure that a doctor stays within policy limits, including, for example, total financial limits on prescriptions if such limits have been set, but it can never dictate his clinical judgment in particular cases, within those limits, nor determine how good that judgment is. It also provides for mutual information and education, but without managerial authority.

This independent practitioner status for doctors tends unfortunately to be argued in terms of some inherent right of the doctor *qua* doctor to be endowed with an enhanced or special status in society. In fact this independent status arises primarily to provide the patient with the personal confidential doctor–patient relationship so essential for the adequate treatment of the anxiety-bound circumstance of illness.

Thus, great concern was expressed by consultants and GPs during the reorganization planning, that they would be organized into managerial hierarchies and so lose their clinical freedom as professional practitioners. The arguments surrounding this issue became very heated, a heat that was fanned by the wide range of meanings which were attached (and still are attached and still generate heat) to concepts such as chairman, manager, chief executive officer, co-ordinator, monitor, which were bandied about in exploratory discussions about the organization. Some of this argument was stilled only when it was recognized and agreed that the prime reason for the retention of clinical freedom for consultants and general practitioners was that patients were to have the continuing right to a confidential, personal relationship with their own particular named doctor – in the first place being on the register of a specific GP.

Thus it is that the current organization pattern of the NHS maintains the independence of discretion of each GP and consultant – within the law and within public rules of professional conduct. His is the responsibility and the personal judgment which creates the diagnosis, the treatment, and the prognosis for the individual patient, so long as the patient decides to remain with him. Furthermore, primacy also remains with the doctor, added to by the possibility of transfer, at his discretion, of prime responsibility for patient care to members of other professions – professions which must develop, establish, maintain, and guard the same standards of professional freedom and independence, as has been the characteristic at their best of such professions as medicine, the law, and the priesthood.

The preservation of clinical autonomy, including freedom of choice of doctor within the resources available, can ensure for the patient the same degree of personal quality and confidentiality of care under a national service as under other types of service. The patient has his personal doctor – and it is for his doctor to arrange, by means of his prescribing authority, for the provision of the wide range of diagnostic and treatment services made available by the Service as a whole. The patient has his personal doctor – it is for that doctor to handle the bureaucracy on his patient's behalf.

A connected issue which currently requires attention might also be mentioned; namely, the issue of public records kept about individuals. Its implication for the NHS is that it points in the direction of patients having full access to their own clinical records. Is there anything that should be on record – and available to be passed on to others – which the patient as an independent citizen must not as of right be able to see and, if he wishes, have deleted? If a practitioner has private thoughts about a patient which he would not want the patient to know about, then should he not keep them in his own private mind – and not put them on record for others to see but for the patient not even to know about?

This issue is catered for in principle by the normal code of ethical practice established by the General Medical Council, the main principle being that:

> It is a doctor's duty ... strictly to observe the rule of professional secrecy by refraining from disclosing voluntarily to any third party information which he has learned directly or indirectly in his professional relationship with the patient. The death of the patient does not absolve the doctor from the obligation to maintain secrecy.[6]

The full implementation of this code is not specially a problem of a national health service. It applies to all types of medical and hospital practice, and requires to be considered as one part of the growing problem of the increasing mass of information held by government agencies about individual citizens.[7]

Growing Independence for Other Professional Groups
Further supporting the provision of personalized services in a national health service is the strengthening of the independent

[6] General Medical Council (1977), 'Professional Conduct and Discipline', pp. 16 and 17.

[7] A related issue is that of the treatment of patients who are detained in hospital under official order. Whether or not doctors should take part in such procedures is an issue outside the scope of this analysis, the point being that it is a problem which is neither created by nor limited to national health services.

practitioner role which may be provided on a wider scale if the analysis of work-strata and grading set out in Chapter 6 is accepted and implemented. The outstanding feature of the analysis is that it provides for clinical practitioner work for non-medical professionals at a variety of levels – including clinical work and independent practitioner status at higher levels of work. It would no longer be inevitable that professionals of higher clinical competence who sought promotion would automatically be absorbed into administrative posts and so be forced to leave behind their clinical competence and indeed their clinical interests and aspirations.

Furthermore, the separation of those areas of health service activity in which the standard medical model applies – that of physical treatment of physical disease – from other areas such as psychotherapy for emotional disturbances, or the education and provision of aids and appropriate environment for the handicapped, can help to add to individual freedom in the Service, in a number of ways.

First of all there would be the opportunities for various professional groups not only to take on independent practitioner status, but also to be able to assume prime responsibility for individual cases when it is clear that there are no immediate active physical illnesses requiring treatment and prognostication, or at the bottom of whatever disturbances in behaviour may be manifesting as symptoms of physical illness.

Such a development would, for example, extend the number of professions which could be independently engaged in helping to cope with emotional disturbance and mental handicap in the population, in collaboration with those in the social services, and in education, who are working in the overlapping areas of social and family distress and educational difficulties which so frequently are the counterparts of emotional disturbance and interwoven with it. And as indicated in the essay on domiciliary services, the implications extend to physical illness and its treatment as well.

Indeed, a major question which arises is whether emotional disturbance, mental and physical handicap, old age, should be treated exclusively within the health and illness frame of reference, or partly within a social or educational frame. That is one of the current controversies in modern society. The growth of professional independence of professions other than medicine can facilitate the movement away from too exclusive dependence upon the NHS for some of these services.

Our argument, therefore, is that it may be possible for the National Health Service to move in exactly the opposite direction to that predicted by Professor Hayek. Not only has the clinical autonomy of both consultants and general practitioners been preserved in the NHS, but professional independence in the form of independent practitioner status is being steadily granted to a wider and wider range of professions in the service. The issue of liberty thus reappears not only in the retention of clinical autonomy for doctors but also in the possible extension of prime responsibility to professions other than medicine.

Community-based Organization and Public and Employee Participation
In addition to the foregoing NHS policies, there could be other developments in the NHS which might point the way to the preservation of diversity and individuality in large-scale government services. One of these would be the creation of natural health care communities each with its own Authority as described in the following chapter. The organization of services in relation to such communities can help to bring about local diversity and freedom in the context of overall standards. Overall standards set base-lines – they do not inevitably imply uniformity, and need not do so. That depends upon the will of the community.

To these community forces in the direction of professional freedom must be added the creation and extension of institutions for public participation and for employee participation in policy-making. The Community Health Councils, and the growth of employee representation, which can make such participation possible, are analysed in Chapters 17 and 18. Participative procedures on this scale have not until recently been envisaged in connection with governmentally provided services.

The import of participation for staff (the argument does not require repeating here) is that the nation as the community-at-large in effect agrees not to impose a narrow uniformity upon everyone, nor to impose unacceptable employment conditions upon its employees in the name of democracy. Local rights and local differences are not only recognized but welcomed, and their expression is organizationally catered for. So too are the rights of employees safeguarded, so that the national community can avoid assuming by default the role of autocratic employer – a role which has a gradual stultifying effect upon democratic enlightment and liveliness.

In summary, then, locally controlled health services, closely related to community and local idiosyncrasy, plus the reinforcement of clinical autonomy of doctors, plus the extension of the principle of independent practitioner status and responsibility to other emerging professions, plus the removal of many non-medical conditions from the physical illness setting, plus the extension of opportunity for public and employee participation in policy-making, are the features of the present analysis which are the organizational expressions of an NHS which can ensure a reasonable standard of health care nationally within what the nation can afford to pay, while at the same time avoiding the serious perils of adding to governmental corporatism. Time will tell how far it will be possible to achieve these outcomes.

2

The Natural Health Care Community

Elliott Jaques

The reorganization of the NHS was implemented on 1st April 1974. At the time of writing some three-and-a-half years of experience of the new organization structure have accumulated. The time is too short so far for a definitive evaluation to be made.[1] Nonetheless, certain broad conclusions can be drawn about some features of the reorganization where particularly sound consequences appear to have occurred or where particularly obvious mistakes seem to have been made.

Many of the continuing problems – or indeed newly emerging problems, since organization is never static – will be considered in the following chapters. One major issue will be dealt with first, however, since it concerns the overall structure of the Service. It has to do with the structure of Regions, Areas, and Districts, and the organization of the appointed controlling authorities. Its central focus is upon the Districts through which health services are organized, and the Area Authorities which control those Districts.

We shall consider in this chapter some of the difficulties which have arisen in the working relationships between Area Health Authorities (AHAs), Area Teams of Officers (ATOs), and District Management Teams (DMTs) in multi-district Areas. Some of these working relationships rapidly became very stressful. These stresses were exacerbated by the unclarity in relationship between the Regional Health Authority (RHA) and the AHA, and therefore also between the Regional Team of Officers (RTO) and the ATO. The evidence was that too much organization had been established.

Having considered some of the symptoms of difficulty, we

[1] See the concept of the seven-year test of organization change in the Preface to Jaques (1976), *A General Theory of Bureaucracy*.

shall consider a solution which may be requisite. It is concerned with the establishment of natural health care communities, each with its own appointed Authority. These communities do not necessarily conform to the principle of conterminosity with local government organization.

AHA, ATO, and DMT

As described in Appendix A, the NHS reorganization had to be worked out within a number of major constraints. Among these constraints were the principles that: there would be an Area Health Authority conterminous (except for certain conurbations) with Local Government Councils; and that health services would be organized within Districts sufficiently large as to warrant the general run of health service facilities including a District general hospital, and yet small enough to feel local – a population of 200,000 to 250,000 was considered optimum.

Application of these two principles led to the establishment of some 90 AHAs in England. Many of these AHAs were much too large, however, for District organization, and so had to be subdivided into Districts. There were 171 of these multi-district Areas, each with two to six Districts, making some 205 Districts in all.

From the beginning, uncertainty developed in the relationships between the AHA, the ATO, and the DMTs. The AHA Chairman and members, understandably, were inclined to work through their ATOs, since it was difficult to maintain effective first-hand contact with an ATO (of four members) and two, three, or more DMTs (each with six members).

The DMT members, however, felt out of contact with the Authority. It was for them, they felt, to organize the actual provision of health services – to propose policies and plans, and to monitor and co-ordinate their implementation. But they had little on-going contact with the Chairman and members of the accountable Authority. They felt the ATO as an obstacle – a barrier – between themselves and the Authority.

The ATO members, on their part, felt too heavy a burden of responsibility placed on their shoulders by the AHA Chairman and members, when compared with the authority they possessed. They seemed to be held accountable for all that went on, yet were limited to monitoring and co-ordinative action.

At the same time, the AHA Chairman and members felt they could not readily control what was going on in the Districts. Without regular contact with the DMTs they were forced to rely upon their ATO, and were thus always working at one remove from the real field of action.

Some quite strained working relationships developed. Thus, for example, there was opportunity for considerable rivalry between members of ATOs and DMTs in the same disciplines – the nurses, the administrators, the finance officers, the community physicians. DMT members wanted their own direct contact with AHAs, and if they got it then the ATO members often felt by-passed. Or, it would have been useful for the AHA Chairman to meet regularly with the DMTs – but any such activity would have been heavily over-taxing for him.

These difficulties were exacerbated by the existence of the RHA and the RTO. Lines of communications were extremely extended: if the Department of Health had to deal with a complaint or problem about some local service, it had to contact a Regional Officer, who contacted an Area Officer, who contacted a DMT member, who contacted the relevant persons within the District, and then the whole process had to be repeated in reverse as the return communication was passed upwards. Area jealously guarded its right to be in the chain of communication, and District and Department felt miles removed from each other.

One other factor, finally, added fuel to the fire. The ATO Chief Officer roles had been established at the same organizational level as the DMT Officer roles – a correct decision reflecting the fact that the ATO was to do staff work for the AHA and was in no sense managerially superior to the DMT. But – and this was a big 'but – the Area Officer roles were established at one grade higher than the District Officer. The explicit reason for this higher grading was to provide a 'career peak' for each discipline.

The ATO members were thus at a grade one higher than their DMT colleagues, even though their level of work might not necessarily be higher. These career-based differences in status – independent of responsibility carried – were a source of festering trouble. The design of organization to cater for professional careers rather than for work always causes trouble.

District Boundaries

At the same time as these organizational difficulties emerged it became apparent that District boundaries were often badly drawn because of the constraints of conterminosity. Thus, for example, there were some single-district Areas, which had been established simply because they conformed to a particular county or borough. Natural health districts readily overflowed these boundaries with impunity, leading to the need to make complex overlap arrangements. If local authority boundaries could have been disregarded, different parts of such an Area might well have fitted in better with adjacent parts of neighbouring counties or boroughs.

There were other difficulties as well at District level. General hospitals were, as often as not, situated in inconvenient places for District organization and planning and for being a focus for the network of general practice. Hospitals for the mentally ill and the mentally handicapped were often concentrated in one particular District while their facilities had to be shared between several Districts. Teaching hospitals and special hospitals with regional facilities added to the complications. So did those services which were being provided for several Districts at once because this appeared to effect possible economies of scale, such as pharmacy, ambulance services, central sterile supply departments, large-scale building projects.

Such problems as these will always exist. Populations shift and change. The pattern of urban and rural life is in flux. The centres of large cities are crowded with commuters by day and left with a tenth of that population in the evening. The chance that a well-situated large general hospital will be as well situated in the community in fifteen years' time is not very high. Such are the vicissitudes of social existence which make difficult the planning of organization for health care services, or indeed for any other service.

The Natural Health Care Community

In considering how to overcome some of these difficulties we shall take as our starting point a dominant conception which we assume to be widely agreed as of fundamental social and democratic value in the provision of government services to the public. This conception is that there should be an interaction between central government and local community, in which the local community – however that community is defined – would have a major hand in the control of its local services under an umbrella of centrally established policies which would ensure acceptable minimal standards and a reasonable spread in the sharing of nationally financed resources.

As far as the NHS is concerned the national element exists. The service is a national taxation financed service. The Secretary of State is in a position to re-allocate resources so as to raise standards of care in parts of the nation as required. He can, moreover, establish general priorities so as to ensure that particular services are developed in relation to changing community needs – such as medical care needed for an ageing population – where such changes might otherwise not occur, at a rate or on a wide enough scale to match the rate of growth of the problem as seen in terms of national social need and social policy.

At the local level, however, despite the best of intentions and strivings, it has not been easy for the AHA members and Chairmen to develop that kind of close working tie and personal relationship with the members of DMTs in multi-district Areas – much less with the large number of heads of services within the District – which is necessary for effective working relationships. Even in a two-District Area, the AHA Chairman must divide his attention between four members of the ATO and six members of each of the DMTs (plus, in the background, some sixty heads of the various services in the two Districts). It is a humanly impossible situation.

The problem is compounded as the number of Districts increases, so that in a four- or five-District Area there is little that the AHA members can do other than work almost completely through the ATO. It is always possible, of course, for AHA members to have a regular rota of visits to the various Districts, but, as we shall try to establish, there is a big psychological difference between a visiting relationship – even a regular one – and a close and involved working relationship with a strong leadership component.

What seems to be required is the setting up of health care Districts based upon existing real communities, and not necessarily within Areas conterminous with local authorities. The existing Districts do not always match these communities. We shall outline the characteristics of such communities, which seem to be regarded as desirable as far as the public, the health service, and the country are concerned, and shall then turn to analyse how such health care communities might be established, indicating difficulties which might also be expected.

By a Natural Health Care Community is meant a community with recognizable homogeneous characteristics. It is this type of community which is sometimes referred to by planners as the natural district or human zone: it is that minimum-sized community which can provide the full range of work, recreation, and leisure facilities, shopping centres, primary and secondary education, and social and health services (but excluding the special provisions associated with the largest urban centres). Such communities range in population from about 100,000 to 500,000 – but in some few cases of large cities may still be found with populations nearing the million mark.

The reorganization of local government was intended to establish separate local authorities for each of these natural districts or human zones. Experience since this reorganization suggests that the urban borough boundaries may have been not too badly drawn up, but that the counties which were created may have been too large in the sense of encompassing more than one natural district or human zone.

From the health services point of view, the optimum situation would be for there to be unitary health care districts conterminous with realistically bounded natural districts or human zones. Discovery of the Natural Health Care Communities could help to point to the boundaries of the existing natural districts or human zones.[2]

Hospital facilities in such a community will comprise at least one DGH – in some cases a teaching hospital – with often several small hospitals, and comprehensive clinic services. The GPs will form naturally into one Local Medical Committee

[2] This problem of finding natural communities in modern industrial society is, of course, a very general one. It is similar in some respects, for example, to the problem of the Church of England finding its natural diocesan and deanery boundaries under present-day conditions. The type of community sought for the deanery has many features in common with the natural health care community.

(LMC); and the consultants are readily organized, or could be organized, into a realistic system of Cogwheel committees in which they would have a natural affinity personally and from the point of view of arguing out priorities for planning and development. There might be anywhere from 200 to 500 doctors and dentists in all.

The scale of the community would warrant a reasonable range of diagnostic and treatment services. There would be a full panoply of pathology laboratory services, radiology and radiography, remedial therapies, EEG, ECG, speech therapy and psychological services, dental and other technicians, orthoptists and audiometricians, and so on. In short, the full range of everyday medical services, commonly referred to as comprehensive services, would be economically warranted by full usage.

Organization of the Natural Health Care Community

Given the assumption that reasonably definable Natural Health Care Communities in fact exist and can be discovered, experience of the reorganized Service thus far suggests that the organization pattern might not be too difficult to analyse. The following is an example of one possible model.

The first requirement would be the application of the principle of one single Authority appointed by the Secretary of State for each and every health community. It is likely that something over 200 such Authorities might be required.

These Authorities would be composed only of members appointed by the Secretary of State. They would contain no elected representatives either of local authorities or of any other bodies, but would be entirely accountable to the Health Service – and thus free to negotiate from the NHS and local health point of view with any and all other relevant bodies, including the local authority, Community Health Councils (CHCs), Staff Associations, trade unions and professional bodies.

The members could be appointed from anywhere, from any occupation, from any background. Only one condition needs to be noted. This openness of selection could include doctors, or nurses, or members of other professions, trade unions or occupational groups from within the NHS, or, indeed, local authority councillors. But one general principle would have to obtain: any such members would be there as individuals joining a corporate body and willing to join in corporate accountability for the health care service of that community.

To emphasize the issue, it needs to be put the other way around. Individual members with NHS or local authority association membership would not be on the Health Authority as elected representatives of their association and with accountability to their association. They would have definitely and explicitly to eschew any such elected representative role – including refusing to act as a back-door route to the AHA for such local groups as they might fortuitously be connected with. This problem is a familiar one, and there is plenty of experience to demonstrate that with explicit understanding and openness of attitude, secretive manipulation can be avoided and Authorities can have the benefit of being able to choose strong members including those who might have local NHS professional or trade union ties.

The point about Health Authorities not containing elected representatives from local authorities can be sharpened and made analytically more self-evident when it is realized that only in a minority of cases is it likely at the present time that the boundary of the Natural Health Care Community would coincide with the local authority boundary. In most cases each Health Authority would be involved in joint planning and negotiation with perhaps several local authorities – including their social service, education, and housing departments. And conversely, each of the local authority departments would be in negotiation and joint planning discussions with several Health Authorities and their officers.

The question is, could such a model work? To begin with, it is worth noting that the negotiations would be no more complex than at present. In a multi-district Area, local authority services have to deal with several Districts. They have to do so through an AHA and an ATO who are concerned with the area as a whole, but who cannot readily assume an effective leadership role in the development of health services within the Districts.

The fact is that the complexity of Health Service and local authority interaction would be about the same either way. The potential gains in the Natural Health Care Community with its own Health Care Authority would lie elsewhere.

The gain would be in the direct working contact and living relationship between public authority (the Health Authority) and the co-ordinative team for the community. We shall refer to this team as the HSCT (Health Services Co-ordinative Team) to emphasize its co-ordinative role, and to eliminate the kind of misunderstandings which could still arise from the title of 'District Management Team' which suggests that the DMT has managerial authority which it in fact does not and could not have.

The Unit's experience suggests that the composition of the Health Service Co-ordinative Team (HSCT) need not be changed from that of the DMT, although the level of work carried by some officers might be higher and thus provide the opportunity fully to occupy high-level people in those roles. (This point is elaborated later in this chapter.) The structure of the DMT has turned out to be a reasonably requisite one.[3] Moreover, the so-called consensus mode of functioning – with unanimous or veto voting – also appears to be requisite. It is a procedure which can in most cases force discussion through to the point where minimally acceptable solutions can be discovered.

What has generally been agreed to be missing, however, is a strong co-ordinative force within the team itself, especially – and here is the rub – in circumstances where one member of the team may be felt by the others to be a weak link. These judgments, particularly in the early stages of growing doubts or up to the point where some major difficulty is likely to burst out, leave the other members feeling disturbed and powerless. They are all colleagues, and except for extreme incompetency which undermines them all, are not accountable for assessing one another's performance.

Given, however, a situation in which a Chairman of the Health Authority can give his undivided interest and attention to one HSCT and one HSCT only, the whole picture changes. He would be able to meet regularly with the HCST; to have a clear picture of its work; personally to review and assess the

[3] It would be useful if a responsible officer from the nearest matching social services organization could also be regularly in attendance.

individual strengths and weaknesses of the officers; and to be in a position quite readily to speak directly to each of them about his assessment, praising strengths and criticizing weaknesses, and more, to keep his colleagues on the Authority informed as to how he believes the team and its members are functioning.

Further possibilities also open. Individual members of the Authority can assist the Chairman in many ways, by involvement in monitoring particular services and assessing the competence of the various service heads; by close and particular attention to the services provided in their own community; by taking on special negotiating responsibilities in relation to other local services fields and in geographical localities which they know best.

In short, the major gain would be in the achievement of a unified approach to a Natural Health Care Community, with a single close interaction between Authority, Co-ordinative Team, and Heads of therapeutic and diagnostic Services.

Higher-Level Services and Organization
Given the type of Natural Health Care Community described, with its own Health Authority, what organization might be required between it and the DHSS? This question is raised in terms of the current situation, namely one in which, apart from Wales, no established or recognized regional political or community entities exist in the sense of having a political and social being or essence. Without such integrative regions, it is likely to prove most effective for the Community Health Authority to be the sole authority directly accountable to the Secretary of State.

Political arguments are raised against such an arrangement. One of the main arguments is that health is a politically sensitive service, with large numbers of individual complaints reaching Parliament and the Secretary of State directly, and a Regional Authority as filter is held to be necessary. A related argument is that the Secretary of State and the Department could not cope directly with as many as 200 or more separate Health Authorities.

These arguments may be balanced, however, by several factors. The first is the power which could be exercised by a Health

Authority working directly with a Health Services Co-ordinative Team. A model here would be the type of independence it was possible for Boards of Governors to exercise in relation to teaching hospitals. The standard to be set for each Health Authority would be that it should be able to accept direct responsibility for its health community. Additionally, the community would be spoken for by its Community Health Council. Large-scale industrial nations simply have to learn to use local mechanisms of this kind to the full – and to keep local problems as local problems, to be resolved locally. That is where the future emphasis must lie if state corporatism is to be avoided.

In effect then, one of the fundamental principles of organizing a national service such as a health service is that management of service must be able to be given to local communities and to be handled by local communities. Here is one of the major socio-political problems of the day, and there are many opportunities in the development of health and other services for strengthening local community ties: these opportunities need to be grasped. The concept of the Natural Health Care Community and Authority needs to be evaluated within this frame of reference. The aim is to avoid monolithic institutions.

Another question is concerned with services which are scarce, or large-scale, or which otherwise do not fit readily within each Health Care Community but are better shared among several. Currently such services can be organized within large Areas or by Region. An alternative model is to organize them on the basis of consortia of Health Care Communities – one community taking on service provision for the others. Consortium arrangements of this kind are not unfamiliar, and appear to be as workable as common services provided by a higher authority: there are well-known difficulties in both types of arrangement, the balance of advantages and disadvantages being about equal.

Finally, the role of the Secretary of State and the Department remains in principle as at present. The setting of general policies of standards of service and differential budgetary allocation, as envisaged in the currently developing planning process, would be much the same. The regional consolidation of plans would be lost. But the consortia of Health Care Communities could carry this function, as well as acting to some extent as filters between each Authority and the Secretary of State. And

in addition, a directness of communication between Health
Care Community and Department would be gained – and that
gain would be likely to prove of major importance in giving
the Department a first-hand awareness of what the actual
health services were like.

With respect to the existing regional facilities at the Department, there are at least two alternative organizational possibilities. The first is that these facilities would be maintained.
They are currently divided into some five sections covering the
country as a whole. These five sections would be needed for
a range of co-ordinative and monitoring activities, covering
some thirty to fifty Health Care Communities each. The potential feasibility of such an arrangement lies in the greater independence of the Appointed Health Authorities and in the radical reduction in the number of communication links.

In this last connection is is important to note that the communication linkage from Department to Health Care Community would be reduced as follows: first, the Secretary of State
direct to Health Care Authority – with no intermediate authority; second, Department Civil Servants direct to Health Care
Co-ordinative Teams – with *two* intermediate steps removed,
those of RTO and ATO – it is this long line of communication
which is commonly recognized as a prime difficulty in which
all officers and teams have found themselves enmeshed.

A second possibility would be radically to reduce the Departmental involvement and to substitute a National Health Services Commission appointed by the Secretary of State. One
mode of organization of such a commission, providing the foregoing regional facilities, was presented to the Secretary of State
and Permanent Secretary at the time of the planning of the
NHS Reorganization.[4]

Level of Work of Health Services Co-ordinative Team
Whatever pattern of organization at national level were
arranged, it is crucial that the level of work of officers on the

[4] Richard Meyjes and Elliott Jaques (1972), 'Models of Organisation at
Department and Regional Levels of the NHS'. There was no possibility of
considering such alternatives at the time, however, as the main political
structure of Region, Area and District had already been decided by the
government of the day. See footnote on p. xviii.

HSCT (Health Services Co-ordinative Team) should be established at a realistically high level. The general principle would be that the status and level of each officer role would be determined by the level of the executive role which he or she occupied; that is to say, the level of work in the Administrator, Medical Administrator, Nursing, and Finance roles. It could thus happen that there could be officers of different status and grading levels on the team.

Such an arrangement of officer members of teams would be workable so long as at least some of the officer roles were at a sufficiently high level of work to call for the employment of senior people. By such a level of work is meant work which carries responsibilities at the equivalent level of current Regional Officers in the NHS or Directors of Social Services or Education in Local Authorities.

Analysis of the situation currently in single-District Areas suggests that such levels of work would certainly be thrown up for at least one or two of the roles of HSCT officer members. The HSCT as a whole would thus be enabled to function at the level of planning and foresight required to interact with the Authority and its Chairman, and with local authority and other services.

Boundary of the Natural Health Care Community
It is the Unit's experience so far that those concerned with District service – and they are after all the ones in the direct front line, the firing line, giving actual health care services to the people – have developed a fairly coherent picture of just where the boundaries of optimum Health Care Communities are – the Natural Health Care Community. These boundaries are not always administratively tidy, nor are they sharp, thin, and clean boundaries. Sometimes, especially in some county Areas, they match the county, making for a very useful and convenient single District conterminous with a local authority. More often than not, however, they overlap county and borough boundaries, breaking the principle of conterminosity.

Many existing single-District Areas have the characteristics of the Natural Health Care Community. But there are many which do not. These latter are usually composed of two communities which have little working relationship, are sometimes geographically quite separate, and sometimes with one or both of the communities being natural parts of one whole community which has been split asunder by a county or borough boundary, one part being the 'overlap' cousin of the other.

It is clear that there will inevitably be some difficulties, and that some community boundaries may have to be artificially stretched on way or another to take account of the location of existing hospitals, variations in density of population, special geographical features, etc.; thus, for example, cities like Nottingham, Leicester, and Derby might be taken as Natural Health Care Communities even though very large, in order not to damage their natural homogeneity, and divided perhaps into sectors. Under such conditions the high-level roles described for officers on the HSCT would be clearly required.

Even if established, the boundaries of Natural Health Care Communities will need to be kept under periodic review – and renegotiated as necessary – because populations change, doctors change, capital service resources wear out and change, professions grow and diminish, or emerge and disappear with changing technology, knowledge and experience. Life does not stand still; nor can a national health service. Freedom from the constraints of absolute local authority conterminosity could facilitate flexibility in such arrangements and in any subsequently necessary rearrangements.

The Strong Local Community

We are aware that there are many other issues in an organization revision as complex as the one under discussion; such as, for example, what the Secretary of State could substitute for the present facility of having one regular meeting with fifteen Regional Authority Chairmen all at once; the Regional contacts with medical schools; and other issues besides. We are here, however, presenting the outline of an analysis, the gravamen of which might be considered to be of some importance; namely, how can responsibility for health service provision be organized as closely as possible to those who are working together to give the care, and to those living together as a community receiving the care. That is the overriding issue.

Our experience now suggests that the line of argument pursued would lead in the direction of local management of service within national policies and financial provision. Local variation, local initiatives, local priorities, could be argued, debated, and settled in terms of local desires, local traditions, local experience, local customs and modes, local wishes, local eccentricities, local insights, local new ideas, local imaginativeness, but all at a level above the minimum standards acceptable to the nation as expressed by the Secretary of State in terms of governmental national policies.

3

Clinical Autonomy

Heather Tolliday

Summary

This chapter deals with some of the problems associated with clinical autonomy in the NHS. Two commonly held assumptions are explored: first that doctors have clinical autonomy because the nature of medical work and of medical dignity is inconsistent with making a doctor subordinate to a manager; and second, that doctors and only doctors legitimately command clinical autonomy. An alternative view is argued that GPs and consultants have clinical autonomy in the NHS because of the nature of illness and the decision in the NHS to provide personal health care through confidential relationships between doctors and patients. It is this decision, and the need for clinical autonomy which follows from it, that makes it impossible for GPs and consultants to be subordinated to a manager. Not having a manager does not mean, however, that doctors in the NHS are free to do just as they please. Control mechanisms which set limits upon the work which GPs and consultants undertake within the NHS are described.

The assumption that doctors have a legitimate monopoly of clinical autonomy in the the NHS is analysed against the background of demands from non-medical qualified caring professions such as physiotherapy, nursing, clinical psychology, and others, for opportunities for their members to achieve consultant status in the NHS. Exploration of such demands raises at least two questions. Are they demands to share with doctors the right to fashion NHS care for individual patients within a personal and confidential one-to-one relationship? Or are they demands for unmanaged status? These questions and their relation to clinical autonomy and consultant and unmanaged status are examined to show how clinical autonomy, as it is commonly used in the NHS, has in fact four distinct and separable elements: namely, independent practice, with its associated un-managed status, patient choice, primacy, and prime responsi-bility.[1] The chapter shows how, in isolating the four elements from each other, issues of the power of doctors and the position of non-doctor qualified professionals in the NHS can be con-sidered in terms of different kinds of doctoring work and dif-ferent kinds of work done by other professionals and, therefore, organization appropriate to the work required. The various ele-ments of clinical autonomy can be allocated to roles according to whether the work to be done requires any, some, or all of them.

Towards the end of the chapter thought is given to whether the formal position remains valid today whereby doctors, rather than any other professionals, act as the gate-keepers to the NHS.[2] The traditional arrangement whereby doctors admit to the NHS, determine what NHS services are needed for each patient, and guide the patient through his involvement with the NHS, assumes that a medical qualification equips the holder to understand NHS provision in its totality better than does any other professional qualification. Such an assumption is increasingly being challenged particularly by non-medically qualified professionals in the emerging field of psycho-thera-peutic practice and in the medically neglected, 'Cinderella' ser-vices of the NHS. The possibility that NHS care today is not a single field of care but separate fields of care, each with its own distinct orientation and focus, complicates the allocation of the elements of clinical autonomy to professional roles. If doctors cannot be expected to encompass the full range of NHS activity, which established profession or professions can fill the gaps, and how are the gaps to be defined?

The chapter concludes by noting that clinical autonomy is

[1] The definition of these concepts will be given later in the chapter, but for a more general discussion of their relevance to understanding professional organization in health and welfare services see Chapter 4.

[2] Access to *all* NHS services is not through doctors. Access to primary den-tal care is not through doctors for instance. But, nonetheless, because the scope of NHS dental care at a primary level is confined within very stringent limits and because the range of resources, other than their own, on which general dental practitioners can call is so very small, the statement that formally doctors and no one else can admit to the NHS remains generally valid.

far from being a matter of concern only to doctors; it is crucial for patients, if they are to continue to have personalized care. Moreover, consideration of its allocation to professionals raises questions of the current range of NHS activity and which profession or professions should be formally sanctioned to fashion that activity both generally and for individual patients.

Clinical Autonomy and Medical Dignity

The argument is widely accepted in the NHS that doctors cannot be managed because of the damage such an arrangement would cause to medical self-respect and dignity. As recently as 1975, the Merrison Committee felt it was reasonable to argue that the medical profession as a whole should be largely self-regulated because of the need to maintain its self-respect.[3]

If all that is at stake is the dignity of the profession as a whole and of its individual members, then it is hard to see how any government can allow doctors to remain unmanaged in the NHS. The fact that doctors continue to hold on to their special position[4] suggests that there is a more important reason for it than their dignity. But a failure to make this reason explicit makes the underlying justification for doctors' clinical autonomy vulnerable.

The right to practise with clinical autonomy is a right which doctors care about passionately. It is also a right that doctors in the NHS feel they have to fight to retain. They believe it is always at risk.[5]

Much of the writing on the creation of the NHS assumes that doctors' clinical autonomy was built into the service because the medical profession wanted it and the government of the day was not strong enough to refuse it. Foot's account of Aneurin Bevan's negotiations with the medical profession in the 1940s suggests that doctors' clinical autonomy and associated un-

[3] Report of the Committee of Inquiry into the Regulation of the Medical Profession (1975), p. 5, para. 11.

[4] Many doctors feared that the reorganization of the NHS in 1974 would be taken as an opportunity to deprive them of their clinical autonomy. Clinical autonomy, however, was built into the reorganized service.

[5] Only a year after the reorganization of the NHS, the President of the Royal College of Surgeons warned in his newsletter of May 1975 that he believed 'the right of a doctor to treat his patients in accordance with standards dictated by knowledge and conscience alone' was in jeopardy.

managed status in the NHS was the price the government had to pay to get the doctors to come into the health service at all.[6] In such accounts, clinically autonomous practice is seen as being consistent with a contract for service between doctor and patient where the patient pays, but inappropriate to practice where the state, and not the patient, employs and pays the doctor. In other words, the argument runs, doctors have clinical autonomy in the NHS because they insisted on practising in a state-provided health service in an identical fashion to the way they practise privately. Clinical autonomy in the NHS is thus seen to be an anachronism and anomaly, only preserved because of the preference and power of the doctors.[7]

Doctors' sense of the vulnerability of their clinical autonomy in the NHS has been increased with the increase in the number of separately established professions in health care in the last ten years or so. The assumption in the Service that clinical autonomy is in the gift of the medical profession, and is awarded to all its members, means that if other professions reach maturity and full professional status, they too will expect their members to have clinical autonomy. Such an eventuality would appear to present the NHS with an impossible management problem. One way to avoid the problem would be to deny everyone clinical autonomy. It is that which many doctors fear.

Clinical Autonomy and the Nature of Illness
HSORU's understanding of clinical autonomy and its relation to medical and other professions' practice and organization has developed in a number of stages. Our starting point was the assumption about clinical autonomy held by many members of the NHS and described above. To the extent that such assumptions attributed clinical autonomy to membership of the medical profession they were compatible with traditional sociological thinking which justified the unmanaged status of doctors on the grounds of possession of esoteric knowledge and skills.

[6] M. Foot (1962), *Aneurin Bevan: A Biography.*

[7] Freidson is a strong opponent of doctors' special position on the grounds that it benefits the doctors and not the patients and derives from nothing other than 'the entrepreneurial and individualistic ideology of the bourgeoisie from which physicians are largely recruited and from the state of mind encouraged by the profession'. E. Freidson (1970), *Professional Dominance, The Social Structure of Medical Care,* p. 98.

But the troublesome nature of such sociological explanations is well known since they do not fit the facts.[8] If clinical autonomy is seen to be conferred automatically by the profession on all its members, why is it that doctors employed as civil servants and junior medical staff are organized in the managerial hierarchies which are claimed to be absolutely incompatible with the level of work performed by any qualified doctor? And how can the fact be explained that such doctors as consultant pathologists and clinic doctors tend not to enjoy a similar degree of autonomy as that enjoyed by colleagues in general practice, surgery, and other clinical specialties?

In the discussions concerned with establishing management arrangements for the reorganized NHS, doctors argued vehemently that they should retain their clinical autonomy because of their professional status. Exploration of some of the practical problems arising from general and sociological explanations of doctors' clinical autonomy had led us to the realization that the real reason for the NHS's retention of clinical autonomy for doctors, despite the attacks on it, was far more important than anything related to doctors' self-interest or self-esteem: that reason lay in the nature of illness and, arising from that, the form of health care most likely to benefit the patient.

When anyone falls ill, anxieties are stirred. The degree of anxiety depends on the nature and seriousness of the illness and the material and emotional circumstances of the sick person. While sickness can be experienced as an irritating interruption to the normal pattern of living, it can also cause the individual to question the assumptions that have given meaning to his life. In some instances it can lead to loss of identity and purpose.

Different individuals cope with illness in different ways, but however ably the patient deals with it, some anxiety will always occur. Questions will arise in the patient's mind concerning the likely duration of the illness, whether it will have any implications for future life style, how what is being done contributes to recovery, and whether the illness is likely to recur. The vulnerability which illness creates requires that health care be provided in a form which accommodates the very particular way

[8] See, for instance, Freidson's critique of Talcott Parsons' explanation of doctors' unmanaged status, ibid., p. 24.

in which each individual responds to different illnesses at different periods of his life.

Doctors have clinical autonomy in the NHS because, although state-provided, the policy for NHS care is that of personalized care. The patient has his own doctor in whom he can place his trust and confide the most intimate of his aspirations, fears, and secrets without anxiety that such information will become public property for use other than in the management of his illness. The patient's doctor, for his part, is charged with the responsibility of determining the nature of the patient's illness and the best means of helping the patient to recover from it given the patient's circumstances, including his response to being ill. In other words, the patient's doctor is responsible for fashioning NHS care on the basis of the patient's personal circumstances within a relationship of confidence and trust.

It is the policy of providing personal care of this kind that gives doctors their right to unmanaged status. Provisions in the reorganized Service linked clinical autonomy with work and not with membership of the medical profession as such. Thus, only those doctors providing 'personal clinical services',[9] namely GPs and consultants, were to have clinical autonomy and its associated unmanaged status. Everyone else, including doctors employed as community physicians and junior medical staff, were to be set up in managerial hierarchies.

Thus the nature of illness and a belief that professional help can be provided most effectively to patients if patients have their own personal doctors underpinned the decision in 1946 and, again, in 1974 to give GPs and consultants clinical autonomy in a state-provided service. A decision to remove clinical autonomy from the NHS or a decision to retain it must ultimately be made on the basis of what sort of care based upon what sort of doctor–patient relationship is to be provided and not because of a wish either to boost or reduce doctors' power. If the NHS is to continue to provide personal care, issues of how to deal with the power this affords doctors can be looked at and dealt with without denying patients a personal service.

[9] *Management Arrangements for the Reorganised National Health Service* (1972), p. 67.

Clinical Autonomy and its Control

The decision to provide health care on the basis of a personal doctor–patient relationship in the reorganized NHS had profound consequences for its organization structure. Because of the emphasis on accountability in the reorganized service, many were in favour of establishing chief executive officers to carry responsibility, as managing directors, for health services within districts. It can be demonstrated, however, that if the nature of health care as established in the 1946 Act was not to be changed by the reorganization, but only the means of providing it, GPs and consultants could not be subordinated to a District Chief Executive Officer or any manager.

But this did not mean that GPs and consultants could not be made accountable. In many people's minds, manager was synonymous with management. Thus, if GPs and consultants could not have managers because of the work they did, it was assumed that they could not be involved in management or made part of the accountability system of the NHS in any way. Such thinking presupposed only one kind of accountability, manager-subordinate accountability, and did not fit the facts. Clinically autonomous practice, whether private or within the NHS, is not entirely free practice. All doctors are accountable for staying within limits: limits binding on the behaviour of all citizens and the limits established by the medical profession delineating acceptable medical practice.[10]

At a minimum, then, the NHS, as employer, must ensure

[10] The differentiation of these professionally established binding standards from clinical autonomy is crucial to an understanding of professional organization. As is noted in Chapter 4, the organizational effect of binding standards is to impose certain limits on possible direction by superior officers or bodies but that in themselves they do not prohibit the establishment of managerial relationships. It is a choice to get work of certain kinds done that precludes managerial relationships. The tendency to combine binding standards with clinical autonomy in thinking on reorganization structure is reflected in Sir Keith Joseph's foreword to the White Paper: 'The professional workers will retain their clinical freedom – governed as it is by the bounds of professional knowledge and ethics and by the resources that are available – to do as they think best for their patients.' Nurses are professional workers. Does such a statement imply that they have clinical freedom? Failure to differentiate binding standards from clinical autonomy reinforces the view that it is membership of a profession that precludes organization in managerial hierarchies – a view that neither fits the facts nor the needs of the NHS.

that GPs and consultants stay within the law and within professionally established binding standards. The NHS is held liable with its doctors for negligence. But it cannot do so through managerial authority; it has to use monitoring authority. Through monitoring authority, the employer is able to keep himself informed of the work being done and to advise the practitioner where his work is judged to be in danger of contravening prevailing limits. If the practitioner persists in working in ways which are likely to fall outside acceptable limits, the employer can suspend him.

The difficulty of such monitoring is well known. The binding standards of any profession change with changing social attitudes and technology.[11] It is for this reason that the employer looks to members of the profession concerned to help in this monitoring. The employing Authorities of the NHS use the device of the three wise men drawn from among doctors to keep them informed of cases of possible contraventions of binding standards. But an officer, usually a senior administrator or medical officer, is also expected to advise the Authority.

Thus far, then, employment in the NHS curtails medical professional practice no more than it is curtailed when undertaken privately. But as a major purveyor of health care in this country and as a responsible state agency, the NHS must be instrumental in setting policies to influence the definition and direction of health care in ways which forward the nation's social, economic, and defence aims. Clinicians working in the NHS find that their scope for development and change depends on prevailing policy. Prior to reorganization, such policy had tended not to be explicit and to be manifested in decisions on resource allocation. One of the aims of the reorganization was to make

[11] Speller, in quoting Lord Justice Denning's judgment on this issue, shows how sensitively monitoring of professional limits has to be done. The boundaries of acceptable practice are shifting constantly. 'It would, I think, be putting too high a burden on a medical man to say that he has to read every article appearing in the medical press; and it would be quite wrong to suggest that a medical man is negligent because he does not at once put into operation the suggestions which some contributor or other might make in a medical journal. The time may come in a particular case where a new recommendation may be so well accepted that it should be adopted'. Speller (1971), *Law Relating to Hospitals and Kindred Institutions*, 5th Edition, pp. 150–151.

health policy more explicit and to make it more susceptible to influence by all interested parties.

The reorganized structure had, therefore, to provide for monitoring of clinically autonomous practitioners to ensure that their practice kept within not only the limits binding on all medical practitioners but also the policy and resource limits determined for the NHS as a whole and locally. But the special requirements organizationally for effective and accountable clinically autonomous practice did not end there. Policy and resource limits have to be such that GPs and consultants feel that they allow them to accept responsibility for what they do for their patients. If prevailing policies leave doctors feeling that what they are able to do for their patients is personally unacceptable, no one carries responsibility.

Ways have to be found to ensure that policies are acceptable. The governing Authorities in the NHS cannot negotiate each and every policy with all its GPs and consultants individually. Nor can they establish managers to determine what will be acceptable. The only practical way was to require GPs and consultants to get together to see if they could establish a medical view, acceptable to all of them, on what they thought of proposed policies or on what they themselves wished to propose. The reorganized Service management arrangements thus adopted the representative principle developed in the local medical committees and the old hospital medical committees and, more recently, the Cogwheel committees.

Since conditions which are experienced as necessary for accepting personal responsibility for patient care within a state-provided health service constantly change, there has to be regular negotiation between governing Authorities and their clinically autonomous practitioners. A major factor in determining the scale of Health Authorities in the reorganized Service was the maximum number of clinically autonomous practitioners that a single Authority could deal with. In the first place, if there are too many for them to effectively associate and establish a view that is acceptable to all, contact between them and the governing Authority will break down. If they are too numerous to work effectively on a representative basis, they will almost certainly be too numerous for the Authority to negotiate with each individually. Secondly, even if the representative system works effectively, the governing Authority must not be experienced as being so remote as to be inaccessible. The governing Authority must be able to talk directly with its GPs and consultants, and GPs and consultants must be able to feel free to appeal to the governing Authority if they cannot convince their colleagues of the importance of their view.[12]

The difficulties of clinically autonomous practitioners agreeing the policies which will allow each of them to accept personal responsibility for the care they provide to patients, and then of reconciling those agreements with the aspirations and requirements of others, were acknowledged in the reorganized NHS by making DMTs and AMTs veto groups. The GP and consultant representatives were thereby assured that, having achieved a clinician view, it could not merely be swept aside. They have the right, *in extremis*, to take their view and the problems of reconciling it with the views of other members of DMTs and AMTs to the AHAs.

The Elements of Clinical Autonomy

In summary, clinical autonomy arises as the consequence of the policy to provide personalized care for patients. The price of the reorganized NHS continuing to provide personal care was greater complexity than would have been required had it been decided to provide agency health care. Instead of a simple pyramid with a managing director, organizational arrangements for the clinically autonomous practitioners had to take the form of monitoring and co-ordinating mechanisms. Integrated and effective health care provision relies upon monitoring arrangements to ensure that clinicians keep within the law, binding professional standards, and NHS policy and resource limits; and upon co-ordinative arrangements to ensure that established policies and proposed changes continue to allow clinically

---

[12] There is considerable evidence, however, that some Districts and Areas have too many GPs and consultants for them either to effectively associate in representative systems or to feel in touch with their governing Authorities. Moreover, even where clinicians are not too numerous, the tendency has been to set up medical representative systems that have too many tiers. The DMC or AMC (in a single-District Area) was often superimposed on existing representative structures without any consideration being given to whether an extra tier was needed. To the extent that there are too many tiers, the system will not work effectively as a means of establishing a clinician view.

autonomous practitioners to feel that they can accept personal responsibility for the care they provide.

Membership of the medical profession does not by itself, however, entitle doctors to practise with clinical autonomy and independently of managerial control. A number of years of post-registration training is required in posts subordinated to consultants before a doctor is considered qualified, let alone entitled, to practise with clinical autonomy as a consultant. And, by the 1980s, doctors wishing to take on clinical autonomy as GPs will have to undertake some years of post-registration training in subordinate trainee roles.

Such an understanding of clinical autonomy in the reorganized service provided a more realistic basis for retaining clinical autonomy in the NHS than did appeals to medical dignity, status, and power. It also enabled organization for clinicians to be constructed which accommodated a relationship between doctor and patient which was confidential and personal but which provided control over the framework within which clinicians worked. Difficulties, however, arose in linking clinical autonomy to particular roles.

Thus, for example, the work of some consultant radiologists and pathologists did not fit the criterion agreed for clinical autonomy. Many of them did not have their own patients but always worked on problems presented by patients who already had their own doctors, usually a clinical consultant. Nonetheless the general feeling was that consultant pathologists and radiologists should be exceptions to the rule, and they were afforded clinical autonomy.

By contrast the argument that clinical autonomy was the only reason for having unmanaged status had meant that community physicians and all other personnel in the NHS, other than GPs and consultants, were managed. Stresses and strains in such an arrangement soon became apparent. Doubts arose as as to whether AMOs really managed their so-called subordinate SCMs in some instances.

Moreover, some members of established non-medical health professions began to question GPs' and consultants' monopoly of clinical autonomy. Some very senior practising members of the nursing, physiotherapy, and occupational therapy professions wished to achieve the right to practise independently of managerial control. And members of some relatively new disciplines, such as medical physicists, appeared in some instances to have *de facto* recognition of their unmanaged status, their relarelationship to AHAs being more akin to that enjoyed by consultants than that obtaining between officers of AHAs and the AHAs.

Such practice and such demands, as well as suggesting that there might be grounds for justifying unmanaged status other than the provision of personal clinical services, also suggested that the ability to practise with clinical autonomy or independently of managerial control did not necessarily require a medical qualification.

Exploration of these tensions suggested that they might not all have the same cause nor, therefore, identical solutions. What the graduate physicists seemed to be asking for and, indeed, in practice getting, was unmanaged status. They were not asking to take over from the doctors. In other words, they were not wanting the right to take on patients on behalf of the NHS. In contrast, some of the demands from clinical psychologists and physiotherapists in certain fields of practice did appear to question doctors' formal monopoly of the right in the NHS to admit patients and to see them through their involvement with the health service.[13]

The possibility thus began to emerge that clinical autonomy as it was commonly used in the NHS was not in fact a single concept but a group of concepts. Such a possibility would help to explain people's instinctive sense that some consultants in the NHS had always been more clinically autonomous than others. Analysis so far has revealed at least four components. These components are elaborated in the next chapter, but may be summarized as follows.

The first component, and the meaning most commonly attributed to clinical autonomy, is that its possession allows the practitioner to use his judgment without its being subject to scrutiny

[13] An article in *Physiotherapy* in January 1972, for instance, proposed that responsibility for the patient in the field of rehabilitation 'must be shared by the team and should not rest with the doctor.... In this context, while one person must be responsible for the patient's care at any one time, this responsibility must shift in the course of care, depending on the patient's needs.' See also, Chapter 10, 'The Future of Child Guidance', for a discussion of possible relationships between doctors and other professions in child guidance.

and modification by anyone else. Thus, what we shall identify here as the right to *independent practice* precludes management of the practitioner by a manager carrying responsibility at a higher level for the work done.

Frequently combined with this first component is a second: that clinical autonomy entails the right of the client or patient to choose his practitioner and the right of the practitioner, in his turn, to refuse an individual as his client or patient. This element of clinical autonomy is called here *patient or client choice*. Providing patient choice and care on the basis of independent practice reinforces the patient's and the practitioner's sense that their relationship is personal, freely entered into, and based on confidence and trust.

The third component of clinical autonomy is that of *prime responsibility*. Health care is very rarely within the competence of a single profession. The means of ensuring that professions which might contribute to a patient's care are made available and are all co-ordinated effectively in pursuit of an agreed end, is to allocate *prime responsibility* for each patient's care to a specified practitioner. The practitioner with prime responsibility is enabled to determine what the NHS can do for the patient and to involve all who might contribute in a co-ordinated pattern of care. Prime responsibility may be reallocated from one practitioner to another.

Finally, where one profession is held to have a more encompassing and comprehensive knowledge of all the fields of NHS care than does any other discipline or profession, such that prime responsibility automatically falls in the first instance to a member of that profession, that profession may be said to have *primacy*. It is only doctors who so far have primacy in the NHS.[14]

So long as clinical autonomy was taken to be an undifferentiated concept whose main organizational consequence was unmanaged status in a state-provided service, the power the medical profession had in the NHS could be noted but its implications not fully grasped.[15] The identification of independent

[14] The exception of primary dental care must be noted. However, dental care at a primary level is largely done by the dentist himself. The extent to which he is authorized to draw on the services of separately established professionals, such as anaesthetists and pharmacists, is strictly limited.

[15] On p. 13 of *Management Arrangements* (op. cit.) it is noted that 'consultants

practice, primacy, and prime responsibility, as separate components of clinical autonomy, however, made it possible to recognize that influence and power of GPs and consultants arose not so much from their independent practitioner status as from their primacy. They make the NHS what it is. They are sanctioned to determine who shall be patients and who shall receive the services of the NHS, and are further empowered to determine what skills other than doctoring skills are appropriate to the care of those defined as patients.

At the same time, the analysis of clinical autonomy into its four components also opened up the possibility that the right to independent practice might not just rest on the giving of personal clinical services. Other kinds of work might be discovered that required independent practitioner status, but without primacy, and which would, thereby, possibly explain the unease of, among others, SCMs with subordination to AMOs.[16]

Which Health Disciplines and Professions should have which Elements of Clinical Autonomy in the Provision of Patient Care?
The differentiation of the elements of clinical autonomy allows a number of questions to be asked, of which two are of prime importance. The first is to what extent are demands from other professions for equivalent status to that held by doctors demands for independent practitioner status and prime responsibility if not primacy? And the second is to what extent are such demands in fact demands for independent practitioner status a nothing more?

Lying behind these questions is the central question of why primacy should be limited to doctors There are those who suggest that this limitation on the allocation of primacy leads to the Health Service being limited only to what medicine can

---

and general practitioners must have clinical autonomy, so that they can be fully responsible for the treatment they prescribe for their patients'. But the full implications of this statement for the development of the NHS and of professions other than the medical profession, and its consequences for organizational relationships between doctors and others, are not spelt out.

[16] HRC (74) 35 on community medicine posts and structure expressed this unease. It noted that the structure 'will thus have features different from other disciplines: for example the manager/subordinate relationship will not generally apply in the same way.'

comprehend and encompass, and thus to its being mainly an illness service rather than a health service. Moreover, the view has been expressed that too narrow a definition of illness tends to be adopted; namely, that of faults in bio-physical functioning which can be mended. As a consequence of this definition, many patients such as the mentally ill, the physically and mentally handicapped, and the elderly, are left as virtual residents in the NHS. They become the Cinderellas of the service because they fail to respond to 'real' medicine.

It is interesting that it is precisely in these so-called Cinderella services that demands from non-medical professionals to take over from doctors are strongest. The doctors' right to primacy in such fields is often disputed and team care emphasized. Prime responsibility for each patient tends to be negotiated and is not assumed to go automatically to the doctor.

Such developments raise the question of whether NHS activity is a homogeneous field of care encompassed adequately in all its aspects by a medical qualification or whether it includes distinct fields, some of which might be better encompassed by qualifications other than a medical one. Thus, for example, the lobby concerned with getting mental handicap provision out of the NHS is based on the belief that mental handicap is not illness. The emergence of a relatively powerful social welfare field of work in local authority social service departments in recent years has sharpened the question of what is health and what welfare. Much of the work of social service departments, fashioned by social workers, is felt by some to be much more in keeping with what many so-called NHS patients need than is the provision fashioned for them by doctors.

But assuming that the NHS continues to keep its present range of services, the question can still be asked as to whether doctors need have primacy in relation to all those services. For them to do so, medical education would have to be extended to equip doctors to encompass more effectively the needs of all patients whether bio-physically ill or not. While this would provide the means whereby the NHS might continue to provide all care and access to it on a single pattern, there is evidence to suggest that doctors' persistent emphasis on bio-physical functioning may not be unrealistic. The phenomenon of multi-professionalism in 'people servicing work' suggests that there may be limits to the range of work that can be done by any one profession if it is to retain a homogeneous identity, and, thereby, a coherent recruitment and qualifying programme. In other words, doctors may not necessarily be able to be all things to all men.

There are two fields of care in particular, which are experienced by some to be outside the mainstream of medical interest and concern. These are the emerging field of psycho-therapeutic practice, and the field of care (containing the 'Cinderella services') which is concerned with creating physical and psychological environments geared to maintaining maximum independence of functioning in those whose physical and/or mental abilities are permanently impaired.

In neither of these fields is it possible to identify any single profession which should obviously be recognized as having the most appropriate skills to fashion care. Practitioners come from a variety of professional backgrounds and possibly retain their original professional identities, not so much because they continue to feel part of these professions but because there is no new profession with which they can identify.[17]

It is important to note, however, that even if it is established that there are separate fields of provision in the NHS in which different professions might take the lead, it does not necessarily follow that services to patients in each of these fields should be provided on a uniform basis. Separating the elements of clinical autonomy from each other allows choices to be made, particularly with respect to primacy and patient choice.

The patterns established for primary and specialist health care at the moment are slightly different. The sense of personal care is reinforced in principle in primary care through patients being given the right to choose their GP; and through the GP

---

[17] This is true, of course, only if there are fields of practice requiring knowledge, skills, and attitudes not previously encompassed by, and not encompassable within, any established profession. If this is so, it raises questions of whether the multi-disciplinary team approach to care claimed particularly in mental illness and mental handicap work, in work for the elderly, and in some forms of rehabilitation work is truly multi-disciplinary. The work may be based on a single discipline, not yet recognized as such. In that case the differences between members would be based on whether some are recognized as being in training for the discipline as against others who are recognized *de facto* as 'fully-fledged' practitioners of the discipline.

being able to refuse a patient a permanent place on his register if he believes that a sufficient degree of trust and confidence cannot be achieved between them. In other words, general practice allows for patient choice.

In specialist medicine, however, the principle of patient choice is not so clearly established. Such choice is limited to the practices of allowing the patient to state a preference for a particular consultant and to ask for a second specialist opinion; and to the possibility that the patient's GP may choose a particular consultant on his behalf.

If, against this background, we turn to the field of psycho-therapeutic practice and the field of care concerned with maintaining maximum independence for the permanently impaired, different patterns tend to be put forward. In the case of the possible recognition of a separate field of psycho-therapeutic practice, access to it tends to be seen as occurring through independent practitioners with primacy, and with patient choice. By contrast, in the field of maintaining maximum independence for the permanently impaired, care tends to be seen as provided by independent practitioners, not necessarily with primacy and not necessarily with patient choice.

What patterns of organization would be requisite would depend on social policy. To the extent that the trend persists to preserve as many citizen freedoms as possible for those who are permanently impaired, care for such people is likely to be modelled as closely as possible on patient choice of an independent practitioner who has prime responsibility. But a change in social policy could equally well lead to care for the permanently impaired being provided on an agency basis rather than through independent practitioners. Given such a choice, practitioners would need none of the elements of clinical autonomy. They would be set up to pursue the programmes established by the governing authority and would be organized most effectively in a managerial hierarchy under a director of services.

Another possible variation on clinical organization arises in the case of those NHS services, such as some preventive services or control of epidemics, carried out at the behest of the state, and, sometimes, against the will of the individual. In such provision, where the clinic doctor is working within statutorily based programmes of prevention and treatment, and the emphasis is not on the individual's freedom but on the good of the community, it is arguable that the practitioners should command none of the elements of clinical autonomy but should be organized as managed practitioners.[18] But because most of NHS care is provided through independent practitioners, many of whom also practise with patient choice, there is some uneasiness about setting up preventive services and compulsory treatment on a different basis.

Decisions, then, on which professions should be eligible to command which, if any, components of clinical autonomy depend on decisions establishing the fields of service, decisions on which profession has the most comprehensive knowledge base in each field, and social policy decisions on how much freedom to provide for both practitioner and patient in each field. At the moment, it is possible to say that, in the bio-physical field of practice at least, medicine is agreed to be the profession commanding primacy, and the nature of care is independent practice with some possibility of patient choice in some instances. In other fields, if they exist and are agreed not to be best encompassed by medical knowledge, attitudes, and skills, the answers are not clear. Outside the bio-physical field, there is some evidence to suggest that individuals from a variety of professions – clinical psychology, physiotherapy, nursing, social work, occupational therapy, medicine, and so on – are developing new theory and associated practices not yet recognized and not readily assimilated into any single established profession. Whether such theory and practices, if established, could be encompassed by medicine or assimilated into an existing non-medical profession is not clear. If, however, a new profession or professions were established to exploit the theory and develop the practices, members might command any of the elements

[18] The Court Report (1977, *Fit for the Future*) recommends that preventive and voluntarily initiated work should be combined in the same practitioner. Not only does such a proposal raise questions about the degree of freedom such a practitioner could command (i.e. whether the state can have enough control over the way its preventive work is done if it is done through independent practitioners who are independent practitioners because of the other aspects of their work) but also questions of whether the patient could trust his practitioner to put his interests first if conflict arose between the demands of a screening programme and the wishes of the patient.

of clinical autonomy depending on decisions on how they might most effectively provide services to patients or clients.

Which Health Disciplines and Professions should have Independent Practitioners Status in the Development of New Methods and Theories? Finally, let us consider the demands for independent practice without a manager but not for any other element of clinical autonomy, which tend to be made by those non-medical professionals who are engaged in research. These demands come from scientists employed at Stratum-4 (see Chapters 6 and 7) who are engaged in innovative work; that is to say, work which involves not only the formulation of modifications in theory and practice, but also the publication of such formulations.

Why research practitioners working at Stratum-4 inevitably seem to seek recognition as independent practitioners must remain for the time being an unanswered question; it is anticipated that further understanding of the nature of work-capacity at these various levels may illuminate this problem.

One kind of work which inevitably entails modification and development and therefore, it would seem, organization as independent practice at Stratum-4 is that work done by scientists concerned to develop their basic scientific discipline for application to health problems. Thus, for example, some physicists, micro-biologists, and biochemists are employed to develop diagnostic and therapeutic knowledge and skills which, once codified, tested, and published, may be assimilated into established practice.

It is perhaps worth noting that because the results of such work are applicable outside the particular place in which they are established, it is not necessary for every health authority to provide opportunities for such work. Indeed the conditions under which the NHS might provide for such research is a controversial issue; many believe that it is more appropriately located in university-based departments associated with clinical departments.

The second justification for setting up opportunities to innovate and develop practice stems from the fact that the NHS employs the majority of members of health care professions in this country. It therefore tends to assume responsibility for providing opportunities to the professions to modify and develop professional practice.

Many of the established professions, such as radiography, physiotherapy, and nursing, recruit members who will be competent to practise within the established body of knowledge and practice, discriminating their response to each case in terms of that knowledge and practice, and within the framework established by patients' clinicians. By and large the members are not expected to contribute published knowledge to the profession's theoretical base. The fundamental modification and development of practice has to be provided for through research practitioner work at higher strata. If such development opportunities are made available to members of such professions, rather than merely leaving developments to flow from medical developments – something which is increasingly unacceptable – then the roles set up to undertake such work have to attract occupants capable of doing genuinely innovative work at the higher strata which seem in practice to require the practitioner to work independently of hierarchical management.

As in the case of the development of scientific knowledge for health problems only a few of such development roles are required. But in this development of practice of established professions a complication arises. These opportunities have to be set up in such a way that they do not raise the general basic level of clinical work of the profession as a whole. Some of these issues are discussed in Chapter 9 on Physiotherapy and Occupational Therapy.

Conclusion

The NHS is not only a very large organization, it is also an extremely complex one. Much of its complexity arises from the provision of personalized health care, and from the multi-professional nature of modern health services. It is also a dynamic service. Changes in social policy and developments in knowledge and skills require constant monitoring to ensure that what is going on is what is wanted and, if it is wanted, to provide organizational arrangements to facilitate it.

The clarification of the function of clinical autonomy has pointed up some of the complexities of, and difficulties in, the Service. The association of clinical autonomy with the nature of work to be done rather than with the prestige of the medical profession allowed explicit recognition of the nature of illness and the NHS's response to it. Further analysis led to the sorting out of the elements of clinical autonomy and the possibility that this then gave of professionals other than doctors achieving unmanaged status and, indeed, of non-doctor qualified professionals assuming the right to practise independently with prime responsibility.

The NHS is an important service and its effectiveness depends on its having an organization structure which fully accommodates the complexity of the work it does. But such organization can be provided only if there is clarity about the full range of its work and the way in which social policy decrees that work should be done. Analysis of the meaning of clinical autonomy has raised questions about the fields of NHS activity, the nature of the boundaries of professions and their relationship to NHS activity and policy bearing on that activity. Clinical autonomy is not just about how much freedom doctors should have. Choices on who should command the various components of clinical autonomy are choices about the nature of health care, and about the degree of freedom patients as citizens should have.

4

Structural Aspects of Doctor–Patient Relationships

Stephen Cang

Doctor–patient relationships furnish an excellent example of how individual and social forces interact, and of how the development of new forms of 'delivery of health care' is creating new structures which will affect individual experience, whether as patient or as doctor. Since such structures can be, and are, altered at an administrative stroke (at least in intention), the speed of change can be high. This seems to be the position of medical work at the present time.

One consequence of rapid change in structures is usually that, because their effects on behaviour are felt but not explicitly stated, expectations proper to previous structures cannot be examined in relation to the new ones. In turn, therefore, rational choosing among new structural possibilities suffers from a lack of understanding of what might follow if any particular course were adopted. For example, if the meaning of 'a personal doctor' can be defined in boundary terms (see discussion on concepts in the preface), and if the implications of health centre group practice could also be clearly stated, it would become easier to see what might follow by the adoption of policies to encourage such practice. In this essay a preliminary attempt is made to describe, in such a way as to clarify alternative models or courses of action, particular features of doctor–patient relationships and some major structures within which they take place.[1]

Our main concern is with doctor–patient relationships from

---

[1] A comprehensive analysis of the nature of doctor–patient relationships and the implications for health service policy and organization is in preparation.

two points of view which we shall try to relate to one another: first as human relationships concerned with a very particular content, which carries strong implications for those who have to deal with it whether as doctors or as patients; and secondly as a variety of structures within which these human relationships are conducted and which can be significantly changed according to the particular structure built up around it. In other words, we shall argue that there is no such thing as one single doctor–patient relationship, but rather that in reality, because of the variety of structures within which doctor–patient relationships happen, we are confronted by a cluster of different kinds of relationship, sharing the general title but diverging from one another according to a variety of factors and circumstances. It may then become possible to discuss with more precision such differences as those between, say, doctor–patient relationships in private or single-handed general practice, health centre large group practice, Accident and Emergency Department agency practice, and hospital consultant practice with its own range of differences among specialties.

' *The*' *Doctor–Patient Relationship*

Health, sickness, and measures taken to preserve the one and treat the other are all among matters of the deepest concern to the individual. It is therefore not surprising that correspondingly deep and strong emotions surround them. Such natural emotions do however tend to make it harder to detach oneself from dearly-guarded convictions and assumptions, and instead to debate difficult questions.

There are two such assumptions to be questioned: that 'doctor–patient relationship' refers only to the 'acute emergency' experience; and that any doctor and any patient may expect the same behaviour of each other irrespective of the structure within which they work, save for differences of personality.

The first assumption is reflected in medical training, in resource allocation and in popular representations of medical work. All testify to the predominance of the acute illness episode as *the one and exclusive* model of doctoring. Status, money, and emphasis have tended to belong to the world of emergency, of powerful therapeutic intervention (commonly by surgical means, as these demonstrate most concretely this particular model of doctoring), and of rapid change in the patient's condition. Only recently has more attention been paid to the fact that for most people the larger part of their experience of illness tends to be slower, less dramatic, more long-drawn-out, and less susceptible of cure, in such conditions as arthritis or degenerative disease. Both doctors and patients, however, have over the years had to spend most of their time dealing not with sudden and rapid changes, but in slowly developing relationships with diffuse and not readily classifiable signs, or in steady discussion of diagnosis and prognosis, or in the continuous review of the progress of illness and treatment, or in the work of adapting to new and difficult situations in which limited functioning or altered ways of life are at issue.

The second assumption is that 'doctor' or 'patient' are terms describing the same set of facts whatever the working context in which they come together. Such an assumption can lead a patient to expect the same relationship with, say, a clinic doctor as with his own GP; or can lead a doctor to assume likewise whether he is acting as, say, a GP in single-handed practice or in partnership with eight others all 'sharing' a list of 27,000 patients. Such an assumption, though patently misleading, nevertheless appears to be made when for example such terms as 'general practice' are used which can only refer to the administrative setting in which the doctor works, and which says nothing about *what kind* of general practice is going on. Since the intention behind the setting up of the NHS, or indeed any health service, is presumably that certain kinds of service shall be provided, it is as well to be clear about just what services different contexts can and cannot make available.

Rules and Structure
Before we move to consider some basic features of doctoring, it may be helpful to try and locate this essay in the general field of studies of doctor–patient interactions. Two main categories may be mentioned, the first of which concentrates on psychological aspects of the interaction between doctor and patient. Prominent in this category is the work on general practice of Balint and of the group following his work,[2] and also the school

[2] Balint (1957), *The Doctor, His Patient and the Illness.* See also such studies

of medical sociologists known as ethnomethodologists, conducting studies of verbal and behavioural exchanges in the consultation process.[3] The second category contains sociological studies of the doctor's prescribing habits, referral patterns and other countable and measurable aspects such as the distribution of doctors, the numbers of patients per diagnostic group, length of consultations turnover, patterns of complaints and so on.[4]

While each of these kinds of study may provide useful clarification of important characteristics of the doctor–patient relationship, each focusses almost exclusively on general practice, and therefore leaves open the question of how far statements about the doctor–patient relationship in other contexts can be derived from this one.

In short, neither group of studies makes sufficient allowance for the fact that the essence of the doctor–patient relationship lies in the nature of the 'contract' between doctor and patient, and that this 'contract', while it comes into being because of human need, and while it is naturally coloured by the personalities and states of mind of doctor and patient at any given time, as well as by the infinity of forces which bear on people generally, is quintessentially embodied in *the structure that creates and controls* the doctor–patient relationship.

'Structure' is used here to include a variety of rules: the rules governing the coming together and separation of doctor and patient; the rules governing the freedom of the doctor to take action in relation to the patient's state, such as what prescriptions he can lay down for diagnostic or therapeutic steps to be taken; the rules governing the responsibility of the doctor for the work he does with the patient. It is rules such as these which give meaning to doctor–patient exchanges. Conversely, discussion of the doctor–patient relationship without specifying the context of rules leaves the discussion unclear. It is like discussing travelling times without knowing what means of transport or other limiting conditions apply: does it take long to reach

---

as: Max Clyne (1961), *Night Calls*. Greco and Pittenger (1966), *One Man's Practice*.

[3] E.g. J. Jacobs (1971), 'Perplexity, Confusion and Suspicion'. J. R. Sorensen (1974/5),'Biomedical Innovation, Uncertainty, and Doctor–Patient Interaction'.

[4] E.g. J. R. Butler *et al.* (1973), *Family Doctor and Public Policy*.

Oxford from London? Four hours on horseback (and even then, what breed and condition of horse?), an hour by car, minutes by plane, etc. So also with the rights and responsibilities of doctors and patients: what kind of doctor, what kind of patient, what kind of rules determining their relationship? It is only when answers to these questions are specified that such further issues can be tackled as whether a doctor (or some other helper) is needed; or how responsibility for action is divided between doctor and patients; or what the position is when social or psychological factors arise; or what the doctor's role is when dealing with people who are not really ill, such as the healthy pregnant woman.

In summary, the discussion which follows will need to cover *both* what Hayek[5] calls 'spontaneous order' *and* what he terms 'organization'. In other words, we are dealing at one and the same time with orders of things which are beyond our complete knowledge or control (e.g. 'human nature') and with orders which can be constructed and explicitly stated, such as rules of professional conduct or regulations in respect of patients' rights, or the expectations and intentions structure of a given health service.

Hayek's distinction, which appears to be of great value in helping to clarify the limits of what men can consciously achieve, while respecting the 'spontaneous orders' which inhere in the world (including in men themselves) is itself a more explicit formulation of a distinction previously sensed by many. For example, the less-often remembered complement of Virgil's well-known 'Happy is the man who understands the cause of things, and treads under his feet all fear, relentless fate and the consuming roar of the greedy river of hell' (that is, who achieves rational understanding), runs thus: 'But happy too the man who knows the gods of the country, Pan and old Silvanus, and the Sister Nymphs'[6] (that is, who can feel at home with the inherent, spontaneous orders of nature over which he has no control but whose workings he needs to respect nonetheless). The 'spontaneous order' to be found in doctor–patient relationships will arise from, among other things, the nature of human

[5] F. A. Hayek (1973), *Law, Legislation and Liberty*. Vol. I: Rules and Order, pp. 35–54.
[6] Virgil, *Georgics*, 2, 490–494.

experience in illness and in confronting appeals for help. The 'organization' will be the particular rules adopted by social mechanisms such as the NHS as part of the means for getting doctoring work done. Examples of such organization are the mechanisms through which a 'personal doctor' is made available to each citizen.

The fact that so much discussion and criticism is heard from doctors, patients, and the general public alike about present arrangements in Britain suggests that our existing system does not altogether fill the various requirements expected: either because structures ignore natural order; or because the structures are inadequate; or perhaps both.[7]

In the context of doctor–patient relationships, Hayek's analysis suggests that certain features may be found to be constants; that in all such relationships spontaneous orders will be found which arise, for example, as a result of human make-up, whatever the organizational or political context in which the relationship functions. We therefore turn now to the question of natural orders in the doctor–patient relationship and indeed in all relationships of help and advice.

The Natural Order of Relationships of Help and Advice

Consideration of some basic features of such relationships will show that since individuals are in normal circumstances necessarily responsible for themselves, the structuring of relationships in which they receive help from others must requisitely preserve that responsibility, or at least do nothing to dilute or interfere with it. Particularly when confronted by difficult or frightening experiences, the individual may tend to seek comfort in the idea that someone else can 'take over' his life, including the unwanted problem. At the same time, such a move is felt to carry the drawback that the individual will lose the self-determination he values. What is required then is a structure that will allow the experiences of illness to be handled in such a way as to give the individual such help and relief as another person can realistically provide, while at the same time strengthening

[7] See, for example: Margot Jeffreys (1976), 'Measuring the Quality of GP Care'; Philip Rhodes (1976), *The Value of Medicine*; Ivan Illich (1973), *Medical Nemesis*.

so far as possible his sense of managing his own life. It is argued that this implies a 'personal doctor' for the patient.

An individual's life is his own. He has the power to determine his actions in whatever way he chooses (within limits of natural and artificial kinds such as his own capacities and resources, the reactions of his fellows, the law and other codes of rule) and can decide what steps to take or not about his health. He may even decide to end his life.

So far as relations with others are concerned, therefore, the adult individual decides what access and power to assign to them, so far as his own actions go.

This decision is an especially difficult one of course when the nature of the other's potential behaviour, contribution or effect on oneself is less clear, as is the case for example in courtship or in general social intercourse. In so far as work is concerned, the difficulty is exacerbated to the extent that the other's contribution is specialized and thus less easily assessable in any respect beforehand. What Rice[8] has noted in relation in the context of the group applies pretty well in the case of the individual:

> The introduction of a specialist can therefore be expected to give rise to a complex of feelings among the members of the community about both the specialist and his task, feelings which are likely to arouse attitudes towards the specialist and towards his task which may vary from open hostility to profound relief, but which, in most situations, can be expected to contain elements both of rejection and acceptance.
>
> Considerations about the introduction of any specialist into any community cannot therefore be concerned only with the kind of skill which the specialist brings, and which the community or parts of the community feel to be demanded by the needs of the situation, but must be concerned with the total social structure of the field he enters. That structure will be determined by a large number of social forces, and the arrival of a specialist will introduce into the field a new force which will affect to some extent all the other forces in the field, and consequently the social structure which they determine.

[8] A. K. Rice (1949), 'The Role of the Specialist in the Community', pp. 177–184.

In other words, the social structure is in part determined by the mixed feelings aroused by the introduction of the specialist.

The fact that people tolerate mixed feelings with difficulty is an important element of spontaneous order. The dilemma which arises when the help of another person is sought (and which indeed appears to some degree in all relationships) may be expressed as 'What will it cost me?' This is not a mean-minded, financial calculation but the expression of man's natural anxiety as a living being, aware of potential dangers even if the individual himself is a friendly and generous specimen. The individual seeking help therefore experiences simultaneously a wish for assistance *and* anxiety about the consequences of doing so.

Faced with this problem, two common responses may be noted, each set out in exaggerated form to point up the continuum as a whole. In the case of those better able to stand the painful mixture of feelings, the response is in effect: 'This is my problem. I wish to know what you can say or do about my problem which might help me to overcome it. I am asking you for your reaction or advice in the face of this problem, which I have described to you. When you have reacted, I hope I shall feel that your reaction is a helpful one. If I do, I shall somehow adopt it. If I do not, I shall use it very little, or perhaps not at all, and pursue some other course in the face of my problem.'

At the other end of the spectrum of reactions, the individual in effect says: 'I have a problem with which I cannot deal. You are an expert in these matters. Please solve this problem for me, on my behalf. Take it, make it your problem and let me have it back – solved. If you fail I shall blame you, or regard you as a false expert. If you succeed I shall extol your capacity for solving such problems and shall testify to your worth as a Great Expert.'

The concept of psychological ownership, introduced by Macdonald in Chapter 14 (see p. 260), is useful in formulating the reactions just described, which will be familiar in essence to anyone who has either practised in the role of expert (or doctor or management consultant or specialist adviser or parent) or who has found himself regarded in such a light, regardless of his own view of himself and his position.

The crucial point about an individual's relationship with a helper or adviser concerns the extent to which the individual feels or perceives himself to 'own' the problem. Taking the other end of the emotional spectrum, this can be expressed as the extent to which he disowns his problem and maintains that it belongs to the adviser. Not only do individuals differ in their capacity to own their problems; the same person's capacity may differ according to the nature of the difficulty. There may for example be strong ownership in matters of choice of material goods but very weak ownership (in other words, a strong tendency to seek some other owner) when it comes to complex choices about future aims, in such fields as for example education, life partnerships, or career.

The basic character of help and advice relationships invariably emerges clearly when action has to be taken. Helpers and advisers generally tend to find it a problem that while they are allowed to assess and to analyse the client's problem, the proposed solution is not necessarily acted on. In other words, where the question of action (decisions affecting the client's future) is involved, the 'handover' to the adviser of the client's problem can be seen to have a major proviso attached. Indeed, it is not in reality so much a question of handover as of referral for an opinion, following which the client will decide what to do. It is when action is contemplated that the adviser learns that no complete handover was ever made. In the same way, the patient is always free to reject or accept or modify the doctor's advice, which is in fact all he is offered.

For what else is the patient seeking when he consults a doctor? Is he not asking for advice and reserving the right to act as he pleases following the advice? In what real sense could he be 'putting himself into the doctor's hands', and presumably staying there until the doctor's hands no longer contain him and he finds himself back in his own?

From the specialist's (doctor's) point of view, it is often tempting to believe that the situation is of the second kind – 'this is *my* patient, I decide what is going to happen to him'. There is much behaviour by patients and relatives which can give apparent support to such a view of the situation: the eagerness with which the doctor's time and prescriptions for action are sought, suggesting that his opinion is valued; the deference with which he is treated when anxiety about the future runs high; the statutory rules which require a 'doctor's certificate' which determines what the accepted version of 'the facts' is to be: is he ill/isn't he? is it infectious or not? can he walk yet or not yet or never? All are momentous decisions for someone. Both parties are tempted to believe that the doctor decides *for* the patient, rather than simply giving an opinion for the patient to use.[9] The patient is apparently relieved of the responsibility for his own life: 'I had no choice, the doctor said . . .' The doctor not only receives the (to some) comforting idea of being able to know what is best for someone else; he is also relieved of the experience of an uncertain patient weighing up the decision, which may be in itself a relatively unpleasant experience and which may stir up corresponding doubts in the doctor. Uncertainty, like anxiety, has a way of spreading. There is therefore no shortage of people and procedures for eliminating it, whether it is justified or not. Against such a background, it can therefore come as something of a shock to both patients and doctors to realize that such a view, the more comforting in proportion as the anxiety involved rises, is not straightforward.

It is of course true that examples can be found where the doctor *in fact* takes over responsibility from the patient: following a trauma, when the patient is unconscious (say after an accident), and when the supposition is invoked that he wishes to retain life and function. The doctor and co-workers therefore act without waiting for permission from anyone. But outside such situations, the patient's life always remains his own. There is always more choice, even after a doctor's diagnosis and prescription, than some patients care to admit. Those who seek second and Nth opinions, or who ignore their physician's advice, are not hard to find. The literature on 'deviance' from doctor's instructions is in effect itself a vivid example of a particular notion at work: the notion that it is 'normal' *always* to take a doctor's advice – or more correctly the notion that a doctor's advice is or should be more binding than that of other advisers.[10] If this view is abandoned, then those who do not

[9] This view is essential to Parsons' classical analysis of the sick role. T. Parsons (1952), *The Social System*.

[10] See, e.g., G. Stimson (1974), 'Obeying Doctor's Orders: a view from the other side'.

take their pills cease to be 'deviants'; indeed they become independent individuals, and if independence of mind were to rise
in general social esteem, it might become necessary to question
the deviancy of those who always did what they were 'told' or,
in reality, *advised* to do.

What emerges from this review is that the 'natural order' of
things when a person falls ill, or suspects that he may be doing
so, is that he wishes to establish a relationship with another person whom he regards as a potential, or already trusted, helper.

It takes an individual to deal with an individual. In other
words, the fundamental tenet of the National Health Service,
that each person has the right to his or her own doctor, appears
to be grounded in a correct assessment of human experience
and requirements. It now remains to examine ways in which
the psychological realities discussed above can be translated
into social ones: in other words, to see precisely what follows
when we consider how to structure doctor–patient relationships
in the sense of describing limits to action so as to try and obtain
the kind of doctor–patient interaction which seems necessary.

'Organization' of the Doctor–Patient Relationship

We therefore now turn to consider the diversity of structures
within which doctors and patients interact.

First, account must be taken of the fact that whatever the
psychological realities, by no means all doctor–patient interactions which take place can take the individual patient's attitude into consideration. Such is the case for example under conditions of mass X-ray, or when an emergency arises and the
individual patient or doctor is simply 'the patient' and 'a
doctor': no questions are asked about choice, match, acceptance or intentions. It is simply not that kind of situation, either
because (as in the case of the mass X-ray) it is not intended
to deal with the individual *qua* individual but only as a pair
of lungs; or because (as in the case of an accident) the time-
scale of, say, loss of blood is understood to govern everyone's
actions as the most important factor until dealt with. Just as
the state of decoration of his house is less important to the starv-
ing man, so the nature of his link to the doctor is of less consequence to the man whose life is ebbing away than the need
for immediate technical intervention.

Similarly, if less dramatically, the organization of the doctor–patient relationship is different when a patient is admitted to hospital for a surgical procedure. His relationship with the surgeon may be so restricted that the two never meet when both are conscious, which must be reckoned a major constraint on the kind of interaction they can have.

Here, however, it becomes possible to see that the patient increasingly needs to establish his own relationship with the surgeon as the significance of the operation itself increases, or as the further developments are or become complex. At the one extreme would be, say, the straightforward removal of a corn or wisdom tooth: it is easier to tolerate procedures of this sort without establishing a personal relationship with the surgeon than it is in the case of experiences at the other extreme: say an operation of unknown dimensions, nature or consequences for cancer. In such a case, the idea of the operation being carried out by a stranger would no longer feel appropriate.

A comparable type of contact arises when a patient is referred to a specialist, say a neurologist or radiologist, so that the personal physician may have help in steering his relationship with the patient. In such contacts the parties are both conscious and interact verbally; most people would feel such doctor–patient relationships to differ markedly from that between a person and his 'own' doctor; yet the need arises to personalize the contact if matters are serious.

At this point it is necessary to recall the psychological analysis carried out earlier of the way in which doctor and patient between them deal with the patient's problem. The proposition pursued here is that the social consequences of a 'personal doctor' relationship must, as already mentioned, include nothing that interferes with the individual's attempts to own his own problems. For the sake of clarity, we need to bear in mind that in 'psychological ownership' we are dealing with a continuum, on which individuals inhabit preferred positions; we do not need to assume a fixed and unmoving anchorage. The type of structure implied by, or compatible with, the respective ends of the psychological ownership continuum may now be reviewed in turn.

Let us begin with the person who owns his problem to a high degree. Another way of expressing the same fact would be to say that he takes responsibility, feels concern, for his problem. His attitude to it is therefore something like that of a man who, appointed guardian of some valuable object, does not lightly allow it to be examined, advised upon or altered by anyone else. In the case of his own body (and perhaps even more so in the case of his own personality or state of mind) such a person will wish to establish with his doctor what is called a 'personal relationship'.

Just what does this term imply? It can hardly be called jargon; but nonetheless its meaning may bear a little thought.

The view argued here is that the term 'personal' here refers to an acknowledgement that *a person* is involved: rather than a discrete and disconnected lung, or hand, or piece of intestine, or mood. In other words, that in considering the symptomatically active part of the person, the rest is not to be forgotten. In some contexts the point is emphasized by use of the term 'a whole person', as though somehow the whole person is more than the person.

Because any human personality (person) is complex, it is a sizeable undertaking to try and establish a 'personal' relationship. We are not here concerned with *understanding* the person: merely the setting-up of a relationship which the individuals concerned would be likely to feel was personal to one of them.[11]

Such an imbalance is in fact appropriate: both doctor and patient seek to make their relationship one in which the patient as a person can be the object of the doctor's attention; but not *vice versa*.

What then are the external conditions or rules (organization) which such an aim requires? They would appear to include the following as necessary conditions.

First, there must be free choice on each side. The very existence of the idea of compatibility demonstrates that we discriminate clearly among those with whom we can or cannot easily

[11] One of the reasons for explicitly aimed-for lack of reciprocity in 'professional relationships' may be that it promotes the more efficient development of the professional's relationship with the client. If it were allowed to develop as ordinary social relationships do, something like double the amount of time and effort would presumably be required to build a 'both-ways personal relationship', as compared with the situation in which the patient has a 'personal doctor' while the latter does not have a 'personal patient' but rather 'many hundreds of patients whose personal doctor I am'.

associate. Not everyone is one's sort of person. This holds good for doctor and patient alike, since there is nothing to guarantee that A's fervent choice will stimulate the desired response in B. Each must be free to refuse the other. In view of the fact that people can change, even if it appears only that they change their outlooks, freedom to refuse must also be a *continuing* characteristic of the relationship.

Secondly, there must be reciprocity of number. One patient cannot have a 'personal' link in this sense with more than one doctor at a time. To be required to do so would entail the unrealistic requirement that the patient should be able to duplicate a relationship in all its detail and complexity.

Third, there must be adequate time in order for the one person to get to know the other, otherwise the latter will not be given 'personal' attention. Time is important in two respects: adequate time at each encounter; and an adequate expectation that the relationship will continue. The reasons for the second provision, which may appear less obvious than the first, are that the complexities of functioning and behaviour are known to be great and to change with such changes in state as maturation or ageing or disease; and that trust cannot develop unless there is a reasonable expectation that it is not being wasted or misplaced.[12]

But what of the requirements of the person at the other end of the continuum, who tends not to 'own' his problems? Just as the wish is *not* to take responsibility for his own experience, so such a person will tend to feel more comfortable if some way can be found for his problems to be attended to without their being forced on him. He is apparently eager to leave them to the experts.

It may be expected that those whose general position in life is of this kind will not press so strongly for relationships with their doctors of a 'personal' kind. Indeed they may explicitly reject and avoid such relationships.

[12] It may appear paradoxical that it seems as easy to trust the total stranger as the tried friend – but only if it appears certain that the stranger will remain so. The paradox is resolved if it is seen that safety is guaranteed in both cases, in contrast to the uncertain middle ground of associates who are neither sufficiently well-known to be trusted (or are sufficiently well-known not to be trusted), nor sufficiently not-associates (i.e. strangers) for confidences to be safe because they cannot be acted on.

It must be borne in mind here that where sickness is concerned we are dealing with matters which are by definition at the least alarming (however minor they may appear), and which, more commonly than is sometimes supposed, may be quite terrifying to the individual. Avoidance of a 'personal' doctor need not therefore imply that the individual is incapable of anything but distinct and fragmented relationships in all areas of his life: the pattern may be very much affected by the content of the experience in question.

All that has been said above from the point of view of the patient will of course also hold for the doctor. The practitioner who does not find it easy or congenial to deal with 'persons' will perhaps find it simpler to tackle 'parts of persons'. This may mean either specialization of a kind which creates contact with blood, or specimens, or particular parts of the body, or particular states of illness only; or of a kind which limits in time the contact with the patient – either time of interview, or time in the sense of the longer perspective as discussed above.[13]

The provisions of the National Health Service make it clear however that a personal doctor-patient relationship is what the Service provides, at least in the sense that that is the manifest statement of what is wanted. In other words, individuals (doctors and patients alike) who may feel that they wish to avoid one-to-one relationships are not supported in this aim by the provisions of the Health Service. On the contrary, the stated aim is to provide help by means of the one-to-one relationship. Naturally, those who feel less comfortable with such a structure will do their best to avoid it. A proportion of patients will continually change their doctor, not necessarily by formal means but through, for example, attending hospital Accident and Emergency departments rather than their GP. By such means they provide themselves with an agency service and avoid the personal relationship. But the requirements and intentions of the NHS remain clear.

---

[13] Again, it does not of course follow that anyone working in such a way necessarily functions in the manner of the psychological model under review. Only the opposite view is implied, namely that if the person prefers to work with the part-person, then certain work is more readily structured for him.

Trends and Prospects

Many complaints can be heard that thanks to such developments as large partnerships, group practices with *de facto*
'patients of the group', the housing of general practitioners in
health centres which themselves begin to include a number of
associated medical and support facilities and thus begin to
acquire the feel of a hospital, deputizing services, appointments
systems and perhaps above all the greatly diminished real
choice of practitioner,[14] the intentions of the NHS are gradually
being subverted. It is said the GP services all too often feel impersonal and agency-like.

The foregoing analysis suggests that if the intention remains
to provide personal doctoring in the sense discussed above, then
the organizational changes listed here must be closely examined, through the eyes both of patients and of doctors, in order
to establish at what point stated intentions and existing
structures become incompatible. The absence of genuine choice
of doctor is an obvious example. Doctors who feel that clinical
medicine can be practised only on a personal basis, with independent and personal status and with freedom of choice for both
parties to the relationship, and patients who instinctively
regard a relationship with a personal doctor as the best means
of obtaining medical care, both need to realize that changes
in organizational form, whatever their origins in financial or
professional forces, acquire importance because of their effects
on the behaviour of practitioners and patients alike.

[14] See for example the report of the Kensington and Chelsea and Westminster (South) CHC (1977), *The Family Doctor in Central London*, obtainable
from the CHC.

5

Professionals in Health and Social Services Organizations

Ralph Rowbottom

Introduction

Action-research[1] at BIOSS since the late 1960s in the health and social services field has provided a rich opportunity to study many basic questions about the way in which professionals may be organized. Work has been undertaken with a wide range of medical specialists, with general practitioners, nurses and midwives, remedial therapists, social workers, pharmacists, engineers and technicians, and a whole host of members of other paramedical and ancillary professions employed in the NHS or in local authority social services departments.

Some of the issues that have been encountered are to do with how far the external management or direction of professional work is appropriate or possible. Can doctors, nurses, social workers, engineers, and so on, be managed by their employers and, if so, in what sense of the word? Can they appropriately be put under the control of some senior lay administrator, some 'general manager'? How far can even the employing authorities themselves (the governing bodies that is, as distinct from their officers) properly guide or direct the work of their professional employees?

A second set of issues are to do generally with organizational relationships within particular professional groups. Put baldly, can even doctors appropriately manage other doctors, or nurses other nurses, or social workers other social workers, without improper interference with the exercise of professional judgment?

[1] For a full description of the specific method used, its subject field, scope, practice, and scientific status, see R. W. Rowbottom (1977), *Social Analysis.*

A third set are to do with relationships between professional or occupational groups as a whole. Some professions or occupations are (for whatever reason) manifestly of higher status than others. Does this higher status automatically confer authority in dealings with others of lower status? If doctors, for example, have authority over nurses or paramedical staff, how far does it extend, and what justifies it? Are doctors also justified in assuming authority over social workers or psychologists?

In general the question might be put: how much autonomy, how much independence is it appropriate for the members of any given profession to have where they are employed by public authorities or other bodies. Are there different answers for different types of profession or occupation, or for professions or occupations at different stages of development, or for different practice situations; and if so, from what do these differences spring?

In exploring these questions over the years[2] it has become clear that there is no one definite set of answers which applies equally to all the various occupational groups under consideration. It turns out that there are a number of different characteristics which basically distinguish the practice of one occupational group from another. Each of these characteristics where it arises carries its own particular and specific consequences for what is organizationally possible and appropriate. In brief, these four characteristics are:

1. *degree of professional development* – whether the occupational group possesses its own specific body of theory and practice which has moved beyond the stage where non-members can be expected to appreciate emerging possibilities for extension and further development;
2. *the practice assumption* – whether the assumptions, explicit or otherwise, of the nature of the practice in any given situation are consistent with what may be called 'agency service', or whether they demand what may be called 'independent practice' for the individual practitioner;
3. *existence of an 'encompassing' profession* – whether or not another

[2] An earlier version of the material to be presented was published jointly by the two Research Units in the form of a Working Paper, 'Professionals in Health and Social Services Organizations'.

occupation or profession exists which is regarded as having a deeper or more encompassing view of practice in the field concerned;

4. *primacy* – whether or not its members are recognized as automatically carrying prime responsibility where members of other occupational groups regularly work together with them on the same cases or projects.

The specific organizational consequences of these various characteristics are summarized in Table 5.1. As will be demonstrated, not all these characteristics are by any means inimical in principle to the development of straightforward hierarchical organization built upon extended lines of managerial relationships. It is only one of the characteristics here identified – the existence of practice-assumptions which demand 'independent practice', or the 'independent practitioner' – which is absolutely at odds with managerial relationships (in the precise definition of this term which we shall use). Thus, our general conclusion will be that it is not professionalism as such that is inimical to managerial organization, but only one and by no means universally occurring aspect of it.[3] However, all the characteristics described will be shown to have implications for organization, more or less radical, even where managerial structure is in general possible.

The four characteristics listed and their various organizational implications are discussed one by one in the sections that follow. First, some consideration will be given to the idea of 'profession' – a word which (naturally enough) figures prominently in discussions.

[3] Care must be taken here to avoid any too ready equation of 'managerial organization' with 'bureaucracy'. From the time of Weber onwards, the conception of bureaucracy has carried ambivalent, if not outright pejorative, overtones. If 'bureaucracy' is taken to imply rulebound organization, the removal of all discretion and freedom, a machine-like impersonality, rigidity of structure, identification with narrow cost-scraping aims, etc., it will be little surprise if professionals (amongst others) find bureaucratic environments highly uncongenial!

Again, within any given organization, bureaucratic or other, the particular *ethos* that has developed may or may not be in conflict with the prevailing ethos of any given professional group at any time. (An accountant, a doctor, and a physicist, for example, may find himself feeling very differently about employment in a highly profit-conscious commercial company as opposed

TABLE 5.1: Various characteristics of occupational groups and their organizational consequences

Occupational characteristic	*Organizational consequence*
1. Existence of an advanced degree of professional development.	*Management* by non-members of the occupational group becomes increasingly inappropriate.
2. Practice assumptions adopted in any situation:	
(a) are compatible with *agency service*	Possibility of *managerial* organization.
(b) demand *independent practice (independent practitioners)*.	Impossibility of *managerial* organization (trainees apart) even within the same occupational group, but possibility of *monitoring* and *co-ordinating* roles.
3. Existence of a profession with a deeper or more encompassing knowledge-base in the field.	Possibility of members in the encompassing profession carrying *prescribing* authority.
4. Existence of primacy, i.e. members of the occupational group or sub-group automatically take prime responsibility in work with other groups or sub-groups in the same field.	Leads to *co-ordinating* roles for those carrying primacy.

Attempts to Define 'Profession'

When particular occupational groups in health or social services are pressing for greater independence, or defending existing situations of independence, it is common for them to place much weight on their claimed 'professional status' in arguing their case. Even before the validity of such arguments can be assessed

to a public service or voluntary organization.) It should be stressed that what is being considered in this paper are any implicit conflicts in authority structures – whether any one may properly have *authority* to direct certain kinds of professionals, assess their work, reallocate it, etc., whatever the particular objects of the organization in question, its prevailing ethos, or the rigidity or flexibility of its structure.

there is of course a prior problem of pinning an exact meaning to this phrase, and of finding a definition which will provide an unambiguous and generally acceptable means of deciding whether the claim of professional status is in fact justified in any particular instance.

The considerable sociological literature on professions is filled with attempts to find an adequate definition. Things such as possession of a body of particular and specialized knowledge, adoption of a service ethic, existence of a professional association, control of training and testing of competence, public registration, length of training, and many other factors have been given due weight by various commentators.[4] Others again claim that the whole attempt to find a rational definition is misguided: that professions are simply those occupational groups who have been lucky or clever enough to negotiate themselves into a situation of high status and power.[5]

It is our own belief that there is some significant and useful definition of 'profession' to be discovered. Clearly, the word has everyday currency, and as it is used conveys something over and beyond the more general term 'occupation'. A theory developed from this same research programme on the subject of the stratification of organized work offers one lead. In brief, this theory distinguishes a number of distinguishable bands or strata of work in all organizations. In the first stratum the outputs desired can be specifically prescribed before work commences and demands can be taken as they stand. The second and higher strata have in common the requirement to exercise judgment in assessing the precise needs in various situations, and hence judgment in constructing the exact responses which they call for.[6] It seems likely that one element lurking in everyday usage of profession is the idea of ability to work somewhere within these higher strata: of ability, that is, to penetrate from demands-as-given to underlying needs. (Of course, this alone does not define professional work, just as there are many who might not

[4] See H. L. Wilensky (1964), 'The Professionalisation of Everyone?'; W. J. Goode (1969), 'The Theoretical Limits of Professionalisation'; and D. J. Hickson and M. W. Thomas (1969), 'Professionalisation in Britain, a Preliminary Measurement'.

[5] T. J. Johnson (1972), *Professions and Power*.

[6] See Chapter 7, 'The Stratification of Work and Organizational Design'.

qualify on other counts as 'professionals' who nevertheless show ability to do work at such levels.)

There is surely also in everyday usage an implication that being a 'professional' means bringing specific theoretical knowledge and insight to bear which non-professionals do not have, or have in lower degree, in this process of assessing real needs and appropriate responses. Further still, there is an implicit expectation that the true professional practitioner will exercise his own judgment in particular cases as impartially and objectively as possible. In other words, there is an implication of some particular kind of accompanying *ethic*.

Throughout the remainder of this chapter where the word 'professional' is used, it will be used then in this broad sense: of a person capable of applying special theoretical knowledge or insight in cases where objective and impartial judgment of both needs and appropriate responses is called for.[7] Now, this still does not amount to an exact definition, or at least one that could act as a precise criterion in situations of contention. However, it may be noted that none of the propositions or arguments which follow depend on the existence of an exact definition of 'profession' for their validity, so that a broad definition will serve well enough for the present discussion.

Degree of Professional Development

As has already been noted, a question which regularly arises in health and welfare organizations is, how far it is possible or appropriate for so-called 'senior administrators' or 'general managers' to control doctors, nurses, paramedics, engineers, social workers, or members of various other professions or occupational groups.

The issue here is not whether such 'generalists' could actually do with equal proficiency all the work of those of various specific professions or crafts of whom they were in charge. Nor is it whether they could give detailed 'technical' instructions to such; for where even a moderate level of special knowledge or competence is called for this is readily conceded to be difficult if not impossible for non-members. The real issue is whether

[7] Compare Goode's two 'central generating qualities' of profession as (1) a basic body of abstract knowledge and (2) the ideal of service. W. J. Goode (1969), op. cit.

they could be expected to understand enough about the work and the specific needs which it has to meet, to *manage* the performers of that work.

Here of course, we are obliged to clarify what is meant by 'manage'. The word is, in fact, commonly employed in a whole range of somewhat different circumstances. We ourselves start from the specific notion of a manager as one who is accountable for his subordinates' work in all its aspects; who is able to assess the quality and effectiveness of his subordinates' work as it is done, and who has the authority to make any further prescriptions or re-assignments of work which he may judge to be necessary (see Appendix). Beyond this there is an implication that an effective manager, at any rate one who is capable of working at Stratum-3 or higher,[8] is able to lead his subordinates in new developments in approach and practice. There is also the implication that he must understand the needs and characteristics of developing practice thoroughly enough to be able to represent their ideas and views adequately in external discussion and negotiation.

Clearly, the more developed an occupational or professional group becomes, the more difficult it is for a non-member, however generally capable, to perform these managerial functions adequately. Where a so-called manager cannot really help his subordinates with technical problems encountered, where he cannot really judge the all-round competence of his subordinates in any precise degree, and where he lacks any feel for emerging possibilities of general developments in practice, it is necessary to question in exactly what sense the word 'manager' is being used.

The following situation may illuminate these points further. In our earlier project work in health services we frequently came across senior hospital 'lay' administrators who were willing to assert (privately, if not publicly) their collective competence to 'manage' doctors or members of any other professions deployed in hospitals, however specialized or advanced the nature of their work. However, further exploration would invariably demonstrate that these same administrators did not mean by this that they would feel able, for example, to assign particular clinical cases to doctors, or to make effective

[8] See Chapter 7, 'The Stratification of Work and Organizational Design'.

assessments of their clinical as well as general abilities. Nor would they feel able to carry full accountability for all aspects of the work of doctors, or indeed of many other professionals, in the same way that they would quite naturally do for the work of their own immediate assistants. Nor would they feel competent to guide doctors in important developments in medical practice.

However, these same senior administrators were clearly carrying some relationship of control or guidance, even if not managerial, in respect of doctors and other professionals employed in the hospital. Two further distinct kinds of relationship were identified and described by the terms 'monitoring' and 'co-ordinating', respectively. Brief definitions of these two relationships are given in Appendix B. What neither relationship includes is either the right to issue final or binding prescriptions in the face of strongly conflicting views, or the right to make or act upon fine assessments of performance of personal competence, as is expected in the managerial relationship. Thus, hospital administrators might take action where one of the doctors had gone sharply off the rails; but they had no rights to instruct him in such matters of judgment as exact choice of treatment methods, or where expensive drugs were to be used and where not, or at what rate to clear beds by discharging patients from hospital, for example.[9]

Generalizing, it can be seen that as any profession develops an increasing body of specific knowledge, ideas, and practice of its own, it will be natural for a number of things to follow. First, it will be natural for members to seek to interact with one another through specifically-formed professional associations in order to forward the development of their common practice and knowledge. (This is over and above any desire to associate in order to protect their collective interests, a desire which they may share with less well-developed occupational groups.) Second, it will be natural for them to begin to take an increasing interest in training and the setting of qualification for practice. Thirdly, they will tend to want control of their own practice development in specific organizations where they are employed in large numbers, and they will look to the establishment of management posts to be filled by their own

[9] See R. W. Rowbottom *et al.* (1973), *Hospital Organization*, Chapter 9.

members, and the direct access of such members to policy forming bodies. (This leaves aside for the moment the special case
to be discussed below where managerial relationships are prohi-
bited even within the profession.)

Of course, there are many cases where there is no suggestion
that the specialized knowledge and practice of an occupational
group has got to a stage where management by a non-member
is impossible in principle. To extend the example considered
above, it appears to be accepted that health service administrators may readily manage personnel and supplies specialists, or
catering and cleaning staff, notwithstanding any special skills
and expertise which the latter might be expected to possess. It
has not, however, been generally accepted that the same administrators may manage engineering and building staff, or
nurses, or members of the paramedical occupations. In a different field the gathering together in recent years of all social
workers in separate social services departments, headed by
Directors who are increasingly chosen from the ranks of qualified social workers themselves, suggests recognition that social
workers too have reached a stage of professional development
which prohibits effective management by non-members.

Binding Standards
As an occupational group or profession evolves it develops not
only an underlying body of knowledge but also certain very
specific standards and norms of behaviour. Certain things are
invariably (and therefore 'properly') done this way; other
things should always be avoided. What is of particular interest
from the organizational point of view are any standards or conditions which are regarded at any time as absolute and binding;
standards which are not to be abandoned in deference to the
judgment of some superior, however highly placed, capable or
better qualified. Thus, engineers will not be expected to install
plant which is unsafe, however badly needed; pharmacists will
not be expected to supply certain dangerous combinations of
drugs; accountants will not be expected to cook the books in
order to help cover overspending or to prove a case for more
investment; nurses will not be expected to undertake certain
clinical procedures which are reckoned to be beyond nursing
competence.

Where (as in all the cases quoted) professional associations already exist, they will serve as a source of potential external support should excessive pressures be applied to change or ignore such standards. Where, as in the case of many professions in the health field, there is public registration as well, then the threat of being struck off the register for 'unprofessional conduct' will act as a further reinforcement.

The organizational effect of such binding standards where they occur is thus to impose certain *limits* on possible direction by superior officers or bodies. They can be added to other more general limits which exist for all employees, professional or not, such as not being required to carry out illegal actions or acts which go beyond the bounds of what is considered to be decent and acceptable human behaviour. It may be noted that the existence of any such binding professional standards do not in themselves prohibit in principle the establishment of managerial or any other directive relationships, either by other members of the same profession or by non-members. However, it will usually be the case that the emergence of various constraints which are universal and binding reflects a general degree of professional development that already makes effective management by non-members difficult if not impossible (as discussed above).

Agency Service and Independent Practice

In terms of possibilities for managerial organization the occupational characteristics described so far have significant but not radical implications. They condition, but they do not prohibit, managerial forms. Either the occupational group or profession concerned can be incorporated into pre-existing managerial hierarchies (Figure 5.1a), or they may need the creation of an independent managerial hierarchy of their own under the employing authority (Figure 5.1b). 'Bureaucratic' organization (using the term neutrally) is thus still, in a general sense, possible.

The next characteristic to be discussed raises more profound issues. It is best expressed in terms of the distinction between two kinds of practice assumptions: those compatible with what may be called 'agency service' and those demanding 'independent practice'. The distinction may be illustrated sharply in

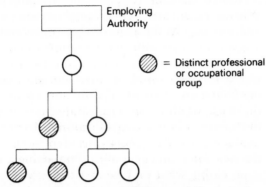

(a) Distinct profession or occupational group integrated into pre-existing managerial hierarchy

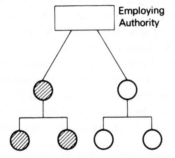

(b) Distinct profession or occupational group as separate managerial hierarchy

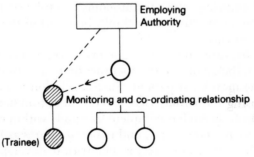

(c) Distinct professional in independent practice

FIGURE 5.1

relation to the different position of hospital doctors and nurses. When a patient arrives in hospital he expects both medical care and nursing. As far as nursing is concerned, although he sees and no doubt identifies with a number of individual nurses, he is nevertheless in the hands of the local nursing service as a whole. It is up to the chief nurse and, ultimately, to the employing body to see that he gets the nursing that he needs around the clock, whatever the immediate changes in nursing staff due to absence, shift-working, or transfers. In this situation any particular nurse is acting not as an independent professional practitioner but as an agent of the employing authority. He or she is providing what may be called *agency service*.

On the other hand, the patient arriving in hospital finds his medical care in the hands of particular and identified consultant – Dr X. The referral to Dr X as an identified person may well have been advised after careful thought by the general medical practitioner who first dealt with the patient. He is now described as 'Dr X's patient'; he is in 'Dr X's beds'; dealt with by 'Dr X's house officer', or 'Dr X's registrar'. Moreover, he hopes and expects to be examined or attended to at some point (in anything but the most trivial cases) by Dr X in person. The exact choice and quality of medical service which he gets will (within the limits of what is available) be entirely determined by Dr X, or his assistants who are understood to be acting on Dr X's behalf. Dr X will not think of himself as employed to execute the specific policies and programmes of the employing authority. He will think of himself as an independent practitioner, enjoying 'clinical autonomy', employed to pursue his professional practice as he thinks best within the broad terms of his contract.

In most situations where doctors work, a very high value is set upon the quality of the therapeutic relationship established with the individual patient. Such a relationship obviously revolves upon individual trust, and the more confident the patient that his physician has complete freedom (within certain broad limits) to diagnose, treat, and make prognosis as he personally judges best, the more likely is such trust to develop. Thus, independent practice is linked in this particular case to the requirement to establish a strong therapeutic relationship. This in turn implies the possibility of choice; the ability of the patient to choose or change his doctor, and indeed, the ability of the doctor to transfer his patient where a minimal necessary level of trust and co-operation cannot be established.

What then is the justification for establishing doctors in independent practice where there is no effective choice – where as often happens, one psychiatrist or one geriatrician automatically deals with all cases arising in one predetermined geographical 'sector'? What is the justification for establishing, say, pathologists, radiologists, or anaesthetists in independent practice, who rarely if ever have patients of their own, and where patient-choice is again usually non-existent? Are biochemists, physicists, and other clinical scientists to be thought of as in independent practice? So far, we have found no general answers to these questions. We have been able to establish only the one firm ground for independent practice. This is acceptance of a pre-eminent need to establish a voluntarily maintained relationship of trust and co-operation between a specifically identified professional practitioner and a specifically identified 'patient' or 'client'.[10] However, it may be that there are other good grounds for establishing situations of independent practice. Perhaps, for example, the requirement of the academic to have 'academic freedom' to teach and think what he wills is another and quite different ground in certain situations. Perhaps the freedom of the judge to pursue justice in individual cases before him irrespective of governmental policy or intervention is another again.[11]

---

[10] It is for this reason that what we are now calling 'independent practice' was in earlier work described by us as 'personalized service' – implying both the personal identification of the service-giver in the eyes of the client, and client-choice. It now seems better, however, to regard 'personalized service' (see the definition in Chapter 9, 'Physiotherapy and Occupational Therapy') as one only of a possible range of situations which may demand 'independent practice'.

[11] The supposition that it is the 'service ethic' of professionals which makes it impossible to assimilate them fully into bureaucracies, a position sometimes adopted in the sociological literature, seems far too sweeping. To state the obvious point again, the 'service ethic' of the professional need not necessarily conflict with either the avowed aims, or the actual and existing ethos, of the employing organization. Far more specific reasons are required to explain, or justify, the granting of what we are specifically defining here as *independent practitioner* status.

The Implications of Independent Practice

Where independent practice arises, whatever the justification for it, the organizational implications are, as we have said, profound. Not only is one talking about the inapplicability of management by non-members of the profession concerned, but also by other members too. For should a manager be appointed, either from within the professional group or from outside, the reality of independent practice could no longer be sustained. No longer could the user or the hirer of the service see only a professional acting in his own name and entirely at the dictates of his own skill and conscience; but behind him a figure, or whole line of figures, each with power to direct, adjust, or override. Where many professionals work together in independent practice then, however unequal their individual capabilities or personal reputation, in the organizational sense all must be equal colleagues; none subordinate to another. Here, and in this particular circumstance only is the true peer-group, true collegiate organization.[12]

Two important provisos must be made, however. The first is that there are naturally limits to freedom even in independent practice. 'Limitless freedom' is a meaningless conception. In fact, the limits and the sanctions which may be brought to bear if they are infringed, for example in medicine, can be quite readily and explicitly drawn out. They include the constraints of common and criminal law; the limits of acceptable professional practice; and, in the case of those employed, the limits explicit or implicit within particular employment contracts.

The second proviso is that although established practitioners will be allowed a wide scope for free and unreviewed action in this situation, those on the way up – the trainees, accolytes and apprentices – will be very much subject to the review and prescription of their masters. (Hierarchic authority will be present in this particular respect then, which may broadly be

[12] We must of course avoid the error – see for example P. M. Blau and W. R. Scott (1963), *Formal Organizations*, Chapter 3 – of confusing *professional associations*, that is associations formed to protect and forward the interests of members themselves, with the various organizations in which professionals are actually *employed*. The former, like all prime associations, are non-hierarchic in form. The real issue is under what circumstances the *employment* organization of professionals needs to be non-hierarchic.

described as 'managerial' even though it partakes something of the flavour of an older 'master-apprentice' quality.) Furthermore, where practitioners are in crucial positions to affect the future life and happiness of their clientele – as is clearly the case in medicine – there will be predictable social pressures for there to be a prolonged period of learning and test for apprentices, and for the proof of accredited qualifications at the end of it.

Indeed, if the work-stratum theory is considered, a further proposition about the requisite level of work for independent practice may be posed. If the practitioner is to be given complete freedom to work on his own it seems reasonable to require not only that he is able to cope with work at the 'situational response' level (i.e. Stratum-2), but also with work at the 'systematic service provision' level (Stratum-3). In other words, it seems reasonable to require that such practitioners would have the ability to be developing continually for themselves (and in conjunction with their colleagues) better general methods, procedures, and frameworks, for the application of their skills in particular cases. If this point is valid it implies, for example, that both medical consultants and general medical practitioners should be capable of Stratum-3 work at minimum. It has the same implications for those social workers, psychologists, and psychotherapists who aspire to independent practice in fields such as child guidance, or for physiotherapists and occupational therapists with the same aspirations in other settings.[13]

Various Arrangements for Independent Practice

With the exception of the case of trainees then, managerial relationships as we have defined them, or indeed other prescriptive relationships, are inconsistent with independent practice. What comes in as it were to fill the vacuum where independent practitioners work together, or with others, are two different kinds of relationships which have already been identified – the *monitoring* relationship and the *co-ordinating* relationship (see Figure 5.1c). For, in the first place, although fully fledged practitioners cannot in these circumstances be managed, there is nevertheless

[13] See Chapter 10, 'The Future of Child Guidance', and Chapter 9, 'Physiotherapy and Occupational Therapy'.

the possibility of – and arguably from a broader social view, the necessity for – monitoring their adherence to the kinds of limits described above. And again, though their work cannot be managed, there is nevertheless the need to see that it is co-ordinated and integrated with other contingent work and developments.

One ready way of achieving independent practice is by setting up in private practice. Frequently in this situation mutual support and protection without loss of autonomy can be secured through the device of the partnership-in-law. Such is found, for example, in medical practice, or in law, or in accountancy. Where 'senior' partners emerge this title implies not a *managerial* role but rather a *monitoring* and co-ordinating one (as each of these terms have been here defined) carrying a limited authority within, and only within, the general terms of any policies or practices adopted by the partnership as a whole.

Even for professionals intent on staying in independent practice, however, there are many obvious advantages to working in a larger organization. There are a number of ways of arranging this. Some will take the legal form of 'contract *for* services'. Others will be situations of straightforward salaried employment, i.e. 'contract *of* service'. In this latter case the professional finds himself working alongside other fellow-professionals, some of whom may be more senior or eminent; but again, if independent practice is truly required, this is inimical to the establishment of managerial relationships. Even the employing body itself will have no right to impose particular rules or policies, or to demand that specific tasks be accomplished, or that specific methods be followed, unless each or any of these have been the subject of specific contract negotiation. If there is any system of discretionary pay awards, it is likely to be applied in effect by the profession itself rather than the employing authority.

Thus, general medical practitioners, dentists, or ophthalmic opticians, all of whom have contracts-for-services within the NHS, recognize no right on the part of their sponsoring bodies, the Family Practitioner Committees, to tell them how to diagnose or treat, or what priorities to give to patients, or how to organize their work. And although medical consultants are actually in the salaried employment of Health Authorities who provide their premises, supporting staff, equipment, and materials, they too recognize no contraints on work that are not the subject of specific agreement. Any change in work arises by a kind of continuous negotiation and re-negotiation of the employment contract.[14] (However, the point must be noted that the employing bodies in this and the previous case obviously have ultimate rights to set policies – unilaterally if necessary – on the availability and use of resources.) Merit payments for medical consultants in the NHS are determined by a National Distinction Awards Committee appointed by the Secretary of State but composed of doctors, i.e. fellow-professionals.

Sometimes the professional practitioner in such situations will be grouped with his fellows in 'divisions', 'departments', and 'firms', or the like, and it will be usual for one of the most senior chosen by the group itself to act both as spokesman to the external world and as a co-ordinator within the group; acting always within the framework of agreed policies and practices. However, the role of such elected representatives has its limits, and in no way can they be held accountable by the employing authority. In addition then, there will need to be certain designated senior staff, not necessarily of the same professional group, who act unequivocally as agents or 'officers' of the employing authority, with the job of carrying out such additional and broader-focussed co-ordination as is necessary, as well as monitoring adherence to contract conditions.

Where a number of distinct specialties exist, that is a number of sub-groups within the main profession, questions will arise about how many of them have their own separate representatives to speak and negotiate on their behalf. For example, in medicine there are questions of how many specialties are banded together in each 'Cogwheel' division, and which specialties are directly represented in negotiations with Health Authorities and their officers.[15] The basic problem here is one

[14] The exact legal situation of employing and contracting authorities as far as their responsibility for the work of doctors is concerned is complex, and indeed in some respects debatable. Nothing, however, in the present legal situation contradicts the propositions just advanced, as far as we are aware.

[15] See Department of Health and Social Security (1967 and 1972), First and Second Reports of the Joint Working Party on the *Organization of Medical Work in Hospitals* ('Cogwheel').

already touched on above. It is the difficulty of non-members of any distinct professional group (or in this case sub-profession) being able to command adequate understanding of the specific needs and emerging possibilities for new developments in order to act as effective spokesmen.

Where Independent Practice is Appropriate

It should be noted that it is not the existence of a medical qualification, but the need for the establishment of strong one-to-one therapeutic relationships which argues for independent practice in medicine. In situations where doctors are employed outside clinical work with individuals (as in epidemiological work or medical administration), or in clinical work where the same emphasis does not fall on the establishment of individual therapeutic links (as in large-scale screening or immunization programmes), the same arguments do not apply, whatever others may be brought to bear.

Moreover, the case for independent practice is not specific to medicine, even in the health field. Considerable work with child psychotherapists has revealed their explicit preference for this mode. Educational psychologists and social workers employed in child guidance work, school psychological services or child psychiatric clinics, lean towards it as well.[16]

By contrast, there is continuing confirmation over the years that the bulk of social workers employed in local authority social services departments see themselves in fact as working in agency service.[17] This, of course, does not rule out any possibility of seeing social workers as true professionals, certainly not in the meaning of the term established earlier.[18] The main prob-

[16] See Chapter 10, 'The Future of Child Guidance'.

[17] See BIOSS, Social Services Organization Research Unit (1974), *Social Services Departments*.

[18] The dangers can be noted here of making the choice of organizational forms turn upon some attempted distinction of 'professionals' from 'semi-professionals' and 'non-professionals'. See A. Etzioni (1964), *Modern Organization*, and A. Etzioni (ed.) (1969), *The Semi-Professions*. The main thesis of this chapter is that much more specific determinants than these can be found; and whilst those who on virtually any grounds would be judged true 'professionals' may well be fitted with perfect adequacy into managerial hierarchies in some situation, others, whose claim to general 'professional' status is far more arguable, may nevertheless clearly require to be acknowledged as independent practitioners.

lem for the moment appears to be how much delegated discretion social workers at various stages of career development should carry.[19] However, tendencies towards independent practice can be observed strongly in those parts of social work that approach psychotherapy. They can also be observed in 'community work' and it may be that the model of the free-floating, independent 'change-agent' who helps community groups to look after themselves and fight for themselves, is absolutely inconsistent with the idea of 'agency service'-type employment, given the strong fiduciary bond with the client that is implicit in such work.

Existence of Encompassing Professions
We turn now to the third characteristic identified at the start of the chapter – the idea of 'encompassing' professions. It is a commonplace observation that members of certain occupations carry more status, influence or power than others, but it is rarely enquired what legitimate *authority* might exist between them. Once attention is turned to this feature, the striking point emerges that certain professions or occupations do in fact carry quite clear-cut authority in relation to others, certainly as regards decisions about what work or action should be undertaken in particular cases or circumstances. Our own research has revealed for example, as a clear social fact acted upon universally, the right of doctors to prescribe specific medical treatment to be carried out by nurses, or by remedial therapists.[20] (The personal attitudes and styles adopted in interaction is of course another matter again. Having authority does not necessarily mean behaving in an authoritarian way. Encouraging participation in decision-making does not necessarily mean relinquishing authority.)

On the other hand, our own research has shown that no prescriptive rights exist between doctor and doctor, other than

[19] See Chapter 7, 'The Stratification of Work and Organizational Design'.
[20] This statement applies at any rate to the administration of drugs and other physical treatments or procedures, where clear and explicit prescriptions can readily be given. In other matters, our own research has revealed that the authority of doctors in relation to nurses may be much more problematic – for example in respect of the general regime in psychiatric hospitals. See R. W. Rowbottom *et al.*, op. cit., Chapters 5 and 7. See also A. Strauss *et al.* (1963), 'The Hospital and its Negotiated Order'.

where the second doctor is in training or specifically employed as an assistant.[21] This applies even where prescription might at first sight have been expected, for example between surgeons and anaesthetists, or physicians and pathologists. It has also observed, for example, the strong move for social work to establish itself as a profession independent of medicine, even where the two professions work closely together as they do in the hospital setting. And it has observed a state of some tension in fields such as psychotherapy, psychology, and other clinical sciences where many practitioners would also wish to establish a clear independence of doctors, but are not sure whether they have it at the moment.

Where any state of authority exists or is claimed to exist between any two professional groups, what then legitimates the claim? It is suggested that any justifications must turn, and can only turn again on questions of knowledge or competence. For it seems reasonable to suggest that one occupational or professional group should have prescriptive rights over the work of another if, and only if, the first is generally accepted as having a better or broader competence to assess the 'real' needs or problems in the field concerned. Thus, the right of doctors to prescribe to nurses can be rationally supported only if it can be shown that medical education gives better grounds for diagnosing disease and physical malfunction, and deciding what is best done about it, than a nursing education.

Clearly, where any contrast arises between those we might think of as craftsmen or technicians on the one hand, and those we might readily think of as higher professionals in the same field on the other, there is always likely, according to this argument, to be an authoritative relationship between the two. For whereas 'craft' or 'technical skill' implies no more than special competence in the execution of certain kinds of tasks, 'profession' here implies a deeper understanding of the nature of the field, and an accepted competence in exploring complex problems and penetrating to fundamental needs. Thus, to stick to the health field, the laboratory technician will always be subordinate in technical matters to the qualified pathologist or biochemist; the orthoptist will be subordinate to the qualified ophthalmologist; the audiometrician to the audiologist; the

[21] R. W. Rowbottom *et al.*, op. cit.

radiographer to the radiologist – and so it turns out in practice.[22]

But beyond this there are cases where a group, which is itself
naturally thought of as a profession in its own right rather than
a craft, is nevertheless subject to at least a certain level of prescription from members of another professional group. Physiotherapy provides a good case in point. Trained physiotherapists
with whom discussions have been held laid claims not only to
competence in executing certain therapeutic procedures but
also to competence in making, in some degree at least,
judgments about their patients' physical condition, problems,
and capabilities, in deciding which particular set of therapeutic
procedures to apply. By this criterion, as has been suggested,
they justify a 'professional' rather than a 'craft' label. Nevertheless, it appears in this situation not only that prime responsibility (a concept which will be explored later) for the patient
usually rests with a doctor rather than with the physiotherapist,
it also appears that the doctor carries an accepted right to determine what treatment objectives and boundaries should be set
in any case, even though he may on many occasions do no more
than invite, either directly or by implication, standard therapeutic treatment for the condition concerned.[23]

We may recognize, then, that there are certain crafts or professions which may in principle be subject to prescriptions from
some other profession with a deeper or more embracing knowledge in the same field of endeavour. The words 'in principle'
have to be added to cover the point just made. There is no need
to assume that members of the first group of crafts or professions
operate only upon receipt of prescriptions. Much of the nurses'
work, like seeing to the comfort, general care, and cleanliness
of patients, for example, arises at their own initiative, though
always within the assumption that what is done would not run
counter to any obvious medical prescription likely to be issued.

Where such encompassing professions exist then, there is
always an underlying authority-base which would allow the
prescription of certain specific actions required – what has been
identified in our own research as a *prescribing* relationship (see
Appendix B). Indeed certain (though not necessarily all) of the

[22] R. W. Rowbottom *et al.*, op. cit., Chapter 6.
[23] See Chapter 9, 'Physiotherapy and Occupational Therapy'.

pre-conditions discussed above for establishing full *managerial* relationships, are already met by definition. In general, a number of more or less complex organizational arrangements may follow. For example:

(a) members of the profession or craft in question can be organized in a separate managerial hierarchy, subject to specific prescriptions in its lower reaches from members of the encompassing profession – as for example in hospital nursing;

(b) members of the profession or craft in question, though themselves hierarchically organized if employed in sufficient numbers, can be organized directly under the managerial control of a member of the encompassing profession, as where medical pathologists directly manage a group of laboratory technicians, or manage a chief technician who himself manages a group of such technicians;

(c) specific members of the profession or craft in question can be *attached* to specific members or groups of the encompassing profession to work permanently under their direction, but whilst still retaining a superior manager in their own profession. This sometimes arises in physiotherapy for example.[24] (For a precise definition of attachment see Appendix B.)

In general, it may be taken that models of the second kind (b), that is those where members of an encompassing profession carry a full managerial role, will be appropriate only where the prime profession or occupation concerned is at a relatively low level of professional development. In other cases all the arguments already explored will apply. Although members of the profession concerned will be willing to accept prescriptions on specific pieces of work referred to them, they will be looking to the establishment of managerial posts at Stratum-3 or higher in their own profession to give the lead in the general development of professional practice. Moreover, they will be wanting such senior managers to have direct access to resource-allocating groups and, indeed in the ultimate, to the employing authority itself.

[24] See Chapter 9, 'Physiotherapy and Occupational Therapy'.

Prime Responsibility

Finally we come to the fourth feature identified at the start of the paper – the idea of 'primacy', and (what it springs from) that of 'prime responsibility'. One of the noteworthy and oft-noted features of social and health services in advanced societies is the increasing variety of professionals who may be called upon to contribute to some personal or social problem posed by an individual. The illness which was formerly dealt with by the all-purpose doctor may now involve, besides the general practitioner, the work of half a dozen or more different kinds of medical specialists, clinical scientists, ancillary therapists and technicians. The social distress once dealt with by a charitable visitor might now involve several different social workers, a 'home help', a volunteer delivering 'meals on wheels', and perhaps an occupational therapist as well. In situations such as those to be found for example in child guidance clinics, psychiatric hospitals, or special schools, even more complex combinations of professionals are called for, drawn not just from one but from several separate fields of work – health, education, and social welfare.

In our experience such situations are invariably seen as more or less problematic by those within them. Immediate expressions of anxiety are often accompanied by strong statements of the need for greater 'team spirit', but further exploration nearly always reveals structural problems. For a start there is frequently doubt as to the state of relative authority or independence of the particular professional groups involved. In the mental health field, for example, there is often doubt as to whether the psychotherapist, or the psychologist, or the social worker, or the psychiatric nurse, is really independent of the psychiatrist's prescription.[25]

Even where there is clear understanding that no prescriptive authority exists between one professional group and another, there is frequently an uncertainty about who is 'in charge of the case'. Who is meant to be seeing that as many different specialists are involved in any case as are required, that their work is co-ordinated, and that necessary actions or decisions are taken in situations of ambiguity or uncertainty? Who is meant to be seeing that the underlying needs of the case or

[25] See Chapter 10, 'The Future of Child Guidance'.

person in question do not pass undealt with through any holes or gaps in the system?

What is at issue here can be described more precisely as *prime responsibility*. When fully spelt out this appears to involve the person who carries it in the following duties:

(a) making a personal assessment of the general needs of the case at the time of assumption of prime responsibility;

(b) undertaking personally any action needed in consequence, or initiating such action through subordinate or ancillary staff;

(c) referring as necessary to colleagues and other independent agencies for collaboration in further assesssment or action, or for action in parallel;

(d) keeping continuous awareness of the progress of the case, and taking further initiative as necessary;

(e) deciding when to relinquish extended collaboration with colleagues, or when to terminate all further action on the case. (This perhaps applies only when the person concerned is in *independent practice*.)

The exercise of the first four functions above implies what has already been defined as *co-ordinative* authority. Again, it may be noted that such authority does not include either the right to issue final or binding prescriptions in the face of strongly conflicting views, or the right to make assessments of overall performance or personal competence of other workers involved, as arises in the managerial relationship. It does not therefore cut at the roots of the independent professional practice of any other members of the team concerned.

In addition, however, where *independent practice* is concerned, there appears to be a right implied in the fifth function, (e) above, to withdraw the request for continued help from colleagues when, in the judgment of the independent practitioner concerned, such further help is not called for. For example the surgeon may judge when to call on the services of the radiologists, and judge also when further radiological exploration appears (to him) to be unnecessary. In agency service, the situation may be somewhat different. By definition some higher authority exists with rights to adjudicate where the judgments of collaborating professionals may disagree. Thus, even if a field social worker carries clear prime responsibility for the case of a child in residential care, it is doubtful whether this should encompass the right to withdraw that child from residential care unilaterally, as it were, and irrespective of the judgment of the professional residential social worker involved. If the two disagree, there will always be some more senior officer, ultimately the Director of Social Services, to act as an arbiter.

Primacy
The desirability of having prime responsibility clearly identified and clearly assigned to some one particular professional practitioner in each particular case can easily be argued. The deeper issues which arise, however, are not just to do with individual cases, but whether there are any valid generalizations about the particular professional groups or sub-groups who most appropriately carry prime responsibility where several work together; and if so, about the boundaries of the kinds of work to which the claim is valid.

It seems, for example in the health field, that there are certain sorts of doctors who regularly carry prime responsibility as defined above, and others who do not. The first includes all those who are in a position to talk about 'their' patients – general practitioners, surgeons, physicians, psychiatrists, and so on. On the other hand, anaesthetists and radiologists (in contrast to radiotherapists) are not likely in the nature of things to carry prime responsibility. Neither are clinical scientists like biologists or physicists, who are not medically qualified, even though they may act independently of medical prescription. Nor do nurses or members of paramedical professions carry primacy. By and large, there appears to be a very well-developed 'etiquette' in medicine itself as to who carries prime responsibility in any case, and at what point it transfers. However, even in this highly developed professional field there are still significant pockets of doubt, for example as our own researches have shown in transactions between consultants and general practitioners in relation to patients in 'cottage' hospitals.[26]

In the social services field, project work has frequently revealed confusion over the location of prime responsibility in particular cases, and whether any automatic primacy exists.

[26] See R. W. Rowbottom *et al.*, op. cit., Chapter 5.

There is often confusion, for example, where residential staff and field social workers are continuously concerned with the same child in care, or where home help organizers, specialist workers with the handicapped, and field social workers are concerned with the same handicapped person who is living at home.

On the second issue, the extent and limit of the area within which prime responsibility is carried, it now seems likely in the kinds of situation we have been examining that important boundaries are to be discerned between the health field and the field of social welfare (and perhaps between both of these and field of education). It appears, for example, that though hospital doctors of certain kinds may carry prime responsibility for the health care of their 'patients', to the extent that these same people are seen as 'clients' for social aid, responsibility for co-ordinating arrangements for their welfare has to be understood as resting with the hospital social workers. Conversely, where 'clients' of social services are in residential care, once a doctor has been called in to deal with clear symptoms of 'illness' of some kind, prime responsibility for medical treatment thereafter (in contrast to social welfare) will rest with him. In both situations doctors may find themselves co-ordinating members of other groups of health professionals, whilst social workers simultaneously co-ordinate the work of various ancillary welfare workers.

Thus, if it is desired to establish the existence of what may be called primacy, that is the automatic allocation of prime responsibility (as we have just defined it) to one particular occupational group or sub-group where several work together, it is apparent that such a concept must always be limited to some particular field of work. One may properly and usefully talk about carrying prime responsibility for the health care of a person, or his social well-being, or his educational well-being; but not about prime responsibility for all aspects of a person's life or activity. (Again, special problems may be noted in a field of psychiatry, where it is often debatable whether it is 'illness' that is at issue, 'social rehabilitation', or 'personal re-education'. Issues of the limits of prime responsibility are correspondingly debatable as well.)

Summary and Conclusion

We started with a statement of some of the problems encountered over the years in health and social services as regards the situation of professionals who work there. In its most general form the issue be said to be that of how much independence professionals should have when they are employed in organizations.

In effect, we have seen that there is no general answer to this question. There are a number of different characteristics of professional or occupational groups, which bear on the issue of appropriate organizational accommodation. And each of these characteristics poses definite and specific organizational requirements. We have seen:

(a) that where the work assumptions of the occupational group in certain situations demand independent practice (such as in many branches of medicine, or in psychotherapy, for example), that this is absolutely inconsistent with managerial hierarchy or technical direction; and that the appropriate organizational form will be collegial, strengthened and interwoven with co-ordinating and monitoring relationships at various points;

(b) that where the specific body of knowledge, ideas, and practice of an occupational group has developed beyond a certain stage (as is the case in nursing, social work, clinical science, and physiotherapy, for example) there will be strong arguments for management by members of the profession only (assuming that the practice assumptions allow any extended managerial structure) with the direct access of the senior manager to policy-making bodies and to the employing authority;

(c) that over and above this, certain intrinsic relationships may exist between various professional or occupational groups – the intrinsic 'prescribing' authority of one to the other as far as specific action is concerned, or the 'primacy' of one of two or more professions who regularly work together in the same field – and that these will have particular organizational consequences which can be built into a variety of organizational forms, either basically hierarchical or basically collegial.

These specific propositions, it may be suggested, provide the key to many organizational issues in the health and social services field. They offer some answer, for example, to the question of why such complex organization arises in health services, given its wide range of developed professions and its mixture of independent practice and agency service. They provide clues to some of the tensions emerging in social services departments, given social workers who are pulled by the contradictory practice assumptions of counselling, psychotherapeutic, or community work, approaches on the one hand, and agency service needs on the other. They provide insights into some of the increasing problems of multi-disciplinary teamwork in and across various public agencies, given the complex mixture of developed and developing professions often to be discovered there. Over and above this, they offer definite statements about the conditions under which any professional may be assimilated into bureaucratic organization, and the specific circumstances in which radically different organizational arrangements become necessary – an area in which it is all too easy to be borne aloft in contemplation of the broad generalities of ideological conflict and 'ideal types', without ever descending to concrete propositions which can be put to the test in practice.

6

Work Levels and Grading

Elliott Jaques

One of the most general problems in the organization of the NHS, as indeed of employment work systems in general, is the failure to distinguish between two different systems of levels or stratification. First is the system of levels needed for organizing the work to be done: we shall refer to them as *work-strata*. These work-strata are needed for setting the different levels at which, for example, various types of professional roles should be established, and for arranging managerial levels.

Second is the system of levels or bands needed for grading roles for purposes of arranging for status, differential rewards, and for career progression. We shall refer to these bands by the common term of *grades*.

Work-strata and grades need to be separated from each other, because experience shows that about three times as many grading bands are required as work-strata. If the two systems are not separated from each other, the grading system tends to be used as the basis for establishing work-organization, the result being the setting up of far too many work-levels; showing, for example, in unnecessarily long, unwieldy, and unrealistic lines of command.

In this chapter we shall present evidence for the existence of one uniform underlying system of work-strata – the same for all types of work; and shall describe the manner in which those work-strata can be subdivided into grades, giving the possibility of one common grading structure for all occupational groups and professions in the NHS, and in other institutions as well.

Confusion Between Work and Grading Strata
The lack of a systematic basis for grading systems can be seen in the enormously wide variations in practice in different work

systems. There is no detectable common framework of any kind. In the British Civil Service there are some 8,500 different grades with different titles: something like 1,400 occupational groups (classes), each class in turn divided into anywhere between three and fifteen separate grades. In the National Health Service there are some forty or fifty different grading schemes, one for each service – for example, ten nursing grades, fifteen clerical and administrative grades, twelve physiotherapy grades – and some grades are further divided into 'steps'. Most large employment systems have such grading schemes, and rarely only one set of grades – there are usually different schemes of grading for hourly rated operators, for clerical and office staff, for senior staff, and there are usually the so-called management grades as well.

The one thing common to these grading schemes is that they are all used for conferring differential status, and they all have pay brackets associated with them, each grade having a related pay range. Even for these purposes, however, they tend to be incomplete. It is possible to identify which roles are of higher and which of lower status *within* the same occupational group; but it is not always easy to compare the relative status of roles in different occupational groups; for example, nurses as compared with administrators or physiotherapists. And with respect to pay brackets, sometimes the brackets are distinct – that is, each higher bracket begins above the top of the next lower bracket – and sometimes they overlap.

The main difficulty is that in the absence of any equally explicit systems of work-strata or levels, an explicit grading system tends to take over the function of a system of work organization as well. The net effect is to proliferate far too many management levels – a sociological disease which is pandemic in all industrial nations.

The mechanism works as follows. A manager in Grade M (say) has subordinates in Grade K. These subordinates experience a missing promotion opportunity in Grade L, and proceed to negotiate to have a role established there. If eventually they succeed, then one of them may get promoted. In the normal course of events, that person will be treated as an interposed manager, perhaps called deputy department head or some such title, and the new structure will appear as shown in Figure 6.1,

Grade

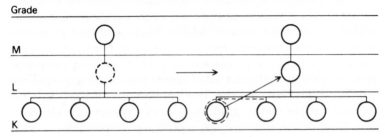

FIGURE 6.1

with one additional managerial level built in. In this way, it not uncommonly occurs that the roles at all levels in the grading system get filled, giving excessively long lines of command – a recipe for the creation of red tape.

An associated effect of this mixing of grading and work-strata is the introduction of an inflexibility in both organization and career progression. It may be noted from the foregoing illustration that for one of the subordinates to be upgraded from K to L required a reorganization of the managerial structure. Such a requirement makes upgrading a much more complex and difficult exercise. An example of a related difficulty is shown here. In order for subordinate R to be upgraded he must be promoted either to become a direct subordinate of P, his manager-once-removed, and hence to become a colleague of his former manager, or to become a subordinate of some other manager at the same level as his manager-once-removed. Some of these complexities are unnecessary if provision is made for several grades within each work-stratum. One of the minor tragedies of work organization is that employees often believe that

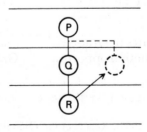

FIGURE 6.2

they can automatically enhance their career prospects by negotiating larger numbers of grading levels which then tend to
double up as management levels. What so often happens,
however, is that the new levels simply push the existing level
lower in status, in responsibility, and eventually in pay, thus
worsening the situation for all. This commonly occurring effect
can be illustrated by the implementation of the Salmon
Scheme[1] into nursing organization in the National Health Service. Intended to improve the career opportunities for nurses,
it substituted a new grading structure for the then existing

Previous Grades	Salmon Gradings	
	CNO	10
Matron	PNO	9
Asst. Matron	SNO	7
	NO	8
Ward Sister	Ward sister	6
	Staff Nurse	5

FIGURE 6.3

structure. The net effect was that matrons sought to become
Chief Nursing Officers though some remained as Principal
Nursing Officers. Assistant Matrons strove to become Principal
Nursing Officers or at least Senior Nursing Officers. And the
good experienced ward sisters sought upgrading to Grade 7
Nursing Officer in charge of two or three wards.

The result was that the best ward sisters tended to be creamed
off the wards to be upgraded to become Nursing Officers
(Grade 7). Because Grade 7 was considered to be managerially
in charge of Grade 6, the Grade 7 Nursing Officers had too
little to do and the ward sister roles tended to be submerged
under the sheer mass of the four-level superstructure under
which they now struggled. Within a few years the level of work

[1] Ministry of Health (1966), Report of the Committee on Senior Nursing
Staff Structure.

of ward sisters was generally held to have decreased. Many experienced ward sisters were no longer on the wards; they had achieved promotion into what in many cases proved to be administrative dead-end posts, with little increase in reward and with decrease in career satisfaction and prospects.

Consequences of 'Too Many' Levels of Organization

It is an almost universal disease of work systems that they have too many levels of organization. This disease manifests itself in a number of commonly known symptoms. Among these familiar symptoms are: the occurrence of much by-passing because of excessively long lines of command; uncertainty as to whether a person's manager is really the next one up on the organization chart, or the one above him, or even the one above him; uncertainty as to whether a manager's subordinates are really just the ones immediately below him on the organization chart, or perhaps the ones below them as well; too much passing of paper up and down too many levels – the red tape phenomenon; a feeling on the part of subordinates of being too close to their managers as shown on the chart; a feeling of organizational clutter, of managers 'breathing down their subordinates' necks' of too many levels involved in any problem, of too many cooks, of too much interference, of not being allowed to get on with the work in hand.

True Managers, Quasi-managers, and Bureaucratic Levels

Consideration of these symptoms raises the question of just how many levels there ought to be in a work hierarchy. This problem of how many working levels there ought to be can be illustrated by reference to a number of different types of hierarchy. Here, for example, are descriptions of three lines of command (examination will show them to be based upon gradings) as set out in the manifest organization charts in a factory, in a scientific laboratory department, and in a hospital nursing organization. Let us examine each in turn in terms of one factor: namely, who is experienced as manager of whom.

In the factory, if you ask the operator who is manager, he will probably ask if what you mean by his manager is his 'boss'. He will then want to know whether you mean his 'boss' or his 'real boss'. The distinction here is between what the operator would call 'my real boss' – the one from whom he feels he stands a chance of getting a decision about himself – and the 'middle-men' or 'straw bosses' who are pushed in between him and his real boss, and through whom he must go if he wants to see his boss. The operator would then probably pick the assistant foreman or foreman as his real boss, with the charge hand and

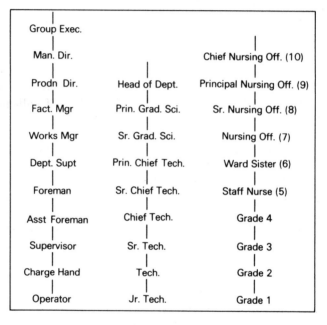

FIGURE 6.4

supervisor (and possibly the assistant foreman) as middlemen or straw bosses.

The same phenomenon occurs in the laboratory as well. For example, the chief technician might well refer to the senior chief technician as his manager for 'administrative purposes', but the principal chief technician as his direct manager where 'real technical work' is concerned; and the principal chief technician would certainly see the head of department as his real manager, and not the intervening graduate scientists. Nowhere in the line of command is it possible to predict whether or not a subordinate will experience the next up on the organization chart (the manifest situation) as his real manager (the extant situation).

From the manager's point of view a mirror image is obtained. He may wish to appear well organized, and emphasize that his immediate subordinates are those shown immediately below him on the chart. But he too will admit that it does not necessarily always work quite that way, and that he must often make direct contact with subordinates two and three levels down 'in order to get work done'. This by-passing is seen as necessary even though it might not make good management theory!

In a nursing organization, a Chief Nursing Officer (CNO) of a hospital group describes her relationship with her manifestly subordinate Principal Nursing Officers (PNOs) as one in which 'I am really the co-ordinator of a group of colleagues and not really their manager. You can't work in nursing with these strong managerial relationships. You all have to work together in the interests of the patients.' The extant situation is that the CNO is a co-ordinative colleague, in contrast to the manifest manager–subordinate relationship.

The conclusion from these and other experiences is that it is never possible to tell from an organization chart just who is manager of whom; in effect, it is a wise manager (or subordinate) who knows his own subordinate (or manager).

Just how confusing it can all become can readily be seen the moment the concepts of deputy and assistant are introduced. Is a deputy administrator, or deputy secretary, or deputy manager, or deputy catering officer, or deputy engineer, or deputy scientist, or deputy accountant, and so on ('assistant' for 'deputy' can be substituted in each case) a genuine managerial level, or is he merely someone who acts for the manager when he is away? It is usually difficult to know just what is the extant situation – the occupants of the roles being confused. Organizational confusion of this kind is tailor-made for buck-passing, everyone willing to be manager in accord with the manifest organization chart when everything is going well, but retreating to the extant situation when things are going badly.

Time-span Boundaries and Managerial Strata

The manifest picture of organization is a confusing one. There appears to be no rhyme or reason for the structures that are developed, in number of levels, in titling, or even in the mean-

ing to be attached to the $\begin{array}{c} \bigcirc \text{Mgr} \\ | \\ \bigcirc \text{Sub} \end{array}$ linkage. That there may be

more reason than meets the eye, however, in the underlying
or depth-structure of work hierarchies become apparent from
an accidental series of observations, hit upon quite separately
and independently in Holland and in England during 1957
and 1958. The findings were accidental in the sense that they
were discovered in the course of studies being carried out for
other purposes. The same findings have since been obtained
in many other countries and in all types of work system including civil service, industry and commerce, local government,
social services, and education.

The findings are based upon the use of a measuring instrument called the time-span of discretion.[2] This measure is based
on discovering those tasks or task sequences in a role which have
the longest time targets, from the start to the point where the
person has been targeted to complete the task. It is the maximum period during which the individual is required actively
to plan and carry out particular tasks. Examples would be: a
ward sister organizing the training process for a student nurse
assigned for three months on a ward; or a sector administrator
monitoring and co-ordinating and pushing forward a particular building upgrading programme to be completed in eighteen
months; or a speech therapist carrying out a prescribed six
months' treatment programme with a patient, before a case
conference review.

The findings may perhaps best be described as follows. Figure
6.5 on p. 105 shows a series of lines of command in which time-
spans have been measured for each role. The diagram is sche-
matized to show the time-span bands within which each role
falls. It will be noted that as one moves higher up the hierarchy
there is a fanning out of the time-spans, a phenomenon which
occurs universally. The arrows from each role denote the occu-

---

[2] This method of measurement is described in detail in Jaques (1961), *Equitable Payment*, and (1964) *Time-Span Handbook*.

pant's feeling of where his real manager is situated as against his manifest manager.

What might at first sight appear to be a rather messy diagram reveals on closer examination the following interesting regularities: everyone in a role below 3-month time-span feels the occupant of the first role above 3-month time-span to be his real manager; between 3-month and 1-year time-span the occupant of the first role above 1-year time-span is felt to be the real manager; between 1- and 2-year time-span, the occupant of the first role above the 2-year time-span is felt to be the real

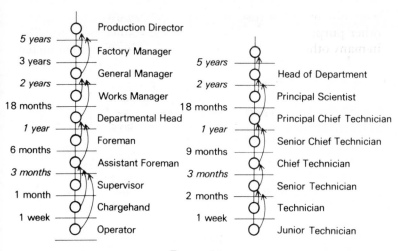

FIGURE 6.5

manager; between 2- and 5-year time-span, the occupant of the first role above the 5-year time-span is felt to be the real manager; between 5- and 10-year time-span, the occupant of the first role above the 10-year time-span is felt to be the real manager. Sufficient data have not been obtained to show where the cut-off points are above 10-year time-span, but preliminary findings suggest a boundary at the 20-year year.

This regularity – and it has so far appeared constantly in over 100 studies – points to the existence of a structure underlying bureaucratic organization, a sub-structure or a structure in depth, composed of managerial strata with consistent boundaries measured in time-span as illustrated. The data extend to over 15-year time-span, and there has been the suggestion of a boundary at 20-year time-span in some very large employment systems, although this finding has not been confirmed by measurement.

The data suggest that this apparently general depth-structure of stratification is universally applicable, and that it gives a formula for the design of work organization. The formula is easily applied. Measure the level of work in time-span of any role, managerial or not, and that time-span will give the stratum in which that role should be placed. For example,

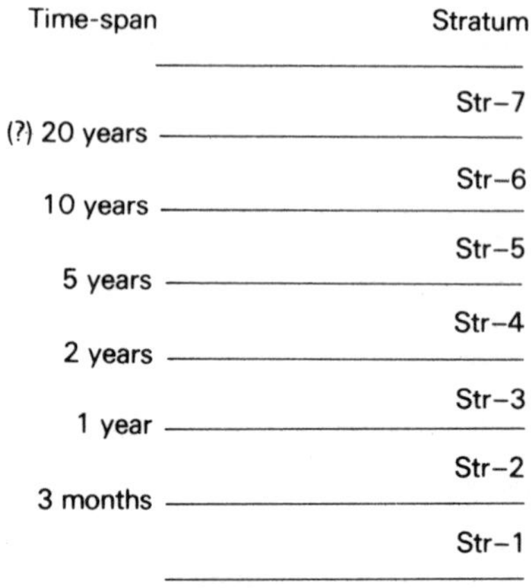

Time-span	Stratum
	Str–7
(?) 20 years	
	Str–6
10 years	
	Str–5
5 years	
	Str–4
2 years	
	Str–3
1 year	
	Str–2
3 months	
	Str–1

FIGURE 6.6

if the time-span is 18 months, that makes it a Stratum-3 role; or 9 months, a Stratum-2 role.

If the role is a managerial role, not only can the stratum of the role be ascertained, but also how many strata of organization there should requisitely be, including shop- or office-floor Stratum-1 roles if any. Measure the level of work in time-span of the top role of the hierarchy – say, departmental head of a department – and that time-span will give the stratum in which that role will fall, and therefore the number of organizational strata required below that role. For example, if the role time-spans at 3 years, it makes the hierarchy a Stratum-4 institution, and calls for four levels of work organization including the top role and the shop- or office-floor if the work roles go down to that level. If the bottom work role, however, is above the 3-month time-span – say, for example, 6 months, as may be the case in some types of professional institution – then the institution will require only three levels of work organization, namely, Stratum-4, an intermediate Stratum-3, and the bottom professional Stratum-2.

Pilot Project in the NHS
The structure was recently confirmed in a systematic study in South District of the Kensington and Chelsea and Westminster AHA.

Fourteen departments and fifty-four individuals were involved in the study, including: X-ray diagnosis, physiotherapy, pharmacy, catering, building, medical records, administration, midwifery, nursing education, nursing administration, medical nursing, surgical nursing, children's nursing, and community nursing.

The procedure used was to obtain time-span measurements for a head of department and each of the subordinates in the line of command within that department to and including the bottom level. Each individual's sense of his position in the managerial structure was discussed, and his feeling of fair pay for the work he was currently being given to do.

It was possible to measure time-span in all cases. The results ranged from 5 years to 1 hour.

The roles in the 2- to 5-year time-span were all senior roles, and consistent with Stratum-4 managerial status. Those in the 1- to 2-year band were middle managerial level. Those in the 3-month to 1-year band were either full professional roles without subordinates, or else first line managerial roles. No full professional or actual managerial roles were found below 3 months time-span (whatever the titles may have suggested).

In addition it appeared possible to use the time-span results to differentiate about 3 separate grades within each of the work-strata.

Participants in the project were also asked in confidence about their felt fair pay: that is, their perception of the payment consonant with the work they were doing, regardless of NHS or national constraints. These results were not to be made public but it can be noted that individuals' perceptions of their felt fair pay showed consistency with time-span findings, and when plotted on a graph showed a curve characteristic of findings in many other studies.

The pilot project suggested that time-span measurement gave an evaluation of level-of-work of any type of NHS role, and allowed cross comparisons between all disciplines on a uniform basis.

The results suggested that the measurements might be useful for:

(a) constructing systematic managerial organization structures;

(b) separating grading levels from managerial levels;

(c) establishing appropriate levels for professional roles which are non-managerial;

(d) providing (in the long term) a possible basis for establishing differential pay structures.

Summary of Work-strata

In summary, then, what is postulated is the existence of a universal bureaucratic depth-structure, composed of organizational strata with boundaries at levels of work represented by time-spans of 3 months, 1 year, 2 years, 5 years, 10 years, and possibly 20 years and higher. These strata are real strata in the geological sense, with observable boundaries and discontinuity. They are not mere shadings and gradations. Requisite organization must be designed in such a way that manager–subordinate role relationships will be established at one-stratum distance.

A description of the content of these work-strata is given in the succeeding chapter by Rowbottom and Billis. The concepts will be found applied in detail in the organization analyses pursued Chapters 9 and 10 on PT and OT and child guidance, and in Chapter 17, on collaboration between health and social services.

A General Grading Scheme

The bands established for work-strata have, however, consistently been experienced as too wide for grading purposes: that is to say for career progression, for recognition of differences in ability and responsibility within the same work-strata, and for fixing payment brackets. The Salmon Report, for example, recognized the need for a distinction in its subdividing each of its management levels into two grades, and the bottom non-managerial level into four grades.

Extensive experience has suggested that each work-stratum needs to be subdivided into about three grading subdivisions; the lowest level requiring about four. Such a subdividing of the work-strata seems to give a psychologically comfortable fit: it gives opportunity for upgrading within a given managerial stratum or professional work-stratum – that is to say, upgrading

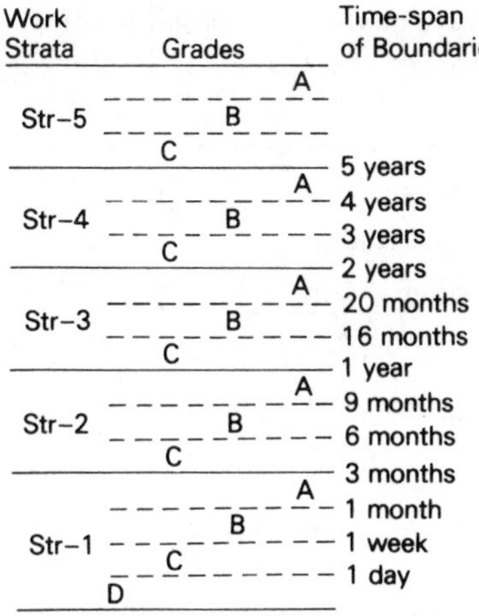

FIGURE 6.7. Grading schema

recognition for carrying out the same general level of work but at a recognized higher level of competence. And it provides what are felt to be reasonably wide payment brackets for each grade. This type of recognition is illustrated in detail in Chapter 9 on PTs and OTs.

This type of subdivision of work-strata into grades is illustrated in Figure 6.7.

This general grading schema is applicable to any and all hierarchical work systems and to any and all departments or occupational groups within such systems. What would be optimum organizationally would be for each work system to be organized in the first place into the work-strata which have here been set out as requisite. But the condition is not absolute. It is possible to apply the generalized grading schema by using the time-span definition of the grade boundaries, without necessarily implementing the system of requisite work-strata.

The combined use of requisite work-strata and the generalized grading schema, however, will give the firmest grip upon work organizational structure. Excess levels of work organization cannot proliferate, precisely because the work system is separated from the grading system. New work-strata need to be added only with significant stages in organization growth.

The fact that about three times as many grades as work levels are provided for, means that it is possible for a manager to have subordinates in any of the three (or in the case of Stratum-1,

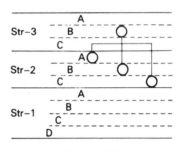

FIGURE 6.8

the four) grades in the next lower work-stratum. Thus Figure 6.8 shows a manager in a Stratum-3B role with immediate subordinates in Stratum-2A, B, and C roles. In these circumstances the subordinate in the Stratum-2C role can be progressed not only within his grade, he can also be upgraded from 2C to 2B and to 2A if his personal capacity and work opportunity combine to make this possible, while still remaining subordinate to the same manager and without its being necessary to recognize the work structure.

Only when a subordinate reaches the top of the highest grade in a stratum do the more complex problems arise. That is the point at which promotion to the next higher stratum must be considered. If the subordinate is promoted he must at that stage move from the command of his immediate manager to that of a manager in a higher stratum. It is for this reason that it has proved so useful to have the upper boundary of the highest grade and the bottom boundary of the lowest grade in any given work-stratum coincide with the boundaries of the stratum itself. Promotion across the boundary from one stratum to the next can take place simultaneously with upgrading.

By providing for several grades in each work-stratum the generalized grading schema makes it possible, where necessary, for people to obtain recognized progression in work and status without necessarily having to take on managerial duties. In the case of the nursing organization described earlier, for example, it becomes possible to provide for ward sister roles to be established at three different grades – reflecting differences in level of work which may be caused by such factors as size of ward and technical difficulties in the work. Thus, as a ward sister became more proficient she could be upgraded without having to take over the unsatisfactory pseudo-managerial responsibilities of a nursing officer. She could remain on the ward, doing nursing work, but with adequate status and pay. If she became ready for promotion to a genuine managerial role in the next higher stratum, the schema would accommodate such a change – but it would be a realistic and serious move.

This solution to the nursing problem is relevant to innumerable situations in which professional staff are employed. It makes it possible for the individual to receive adequate advancement in terms of level of professional work and professional competence alone, without having to accept unsought administrative work so as to be able to collect the increasing number of subordinates needed to gain higher status. Too often 'head counting' becomes the major criterion for progression.

Merit Progression, Upgrading and Promotion, and the Use of Timespan in Job Evaluation
It may be noted that we have distinguished from one another three types of progression of individuals.

The first is that of increases in payment and level of work within a grade. These increases may be automatic annual increments, as can be provided by grant-income institutions. Or they may be based on merit review, as must obtain in earned-income institutions. Such increases may be termed *merit progression*.

The second is the movement of an individual from one grade

to a higher grade but within the same work-stratum. Reorganization is not necessarily involved. The individual is simply brought up to the next higher grade and continues to have the same manager, subordinates (if any), and colleagues. Such progress may be termed *upgrading*.

The third is the movement of an individual from one work-stratum to a higher one (and inevitably a higher grade). Such a move involves reorganization. The individual must have a new manager. If he had subordinates, they will have to be assigned to a new manager. Colleague relationships will change, with even the possibility, if the person is moved up to replace his own manager, that he will become the manager of his former colleagues. Such a change may be termed *promotion*.

Of the three changes defined, only promotion calls for evidence of emerging capacity in the individual at a new level of abstraction.

Use of these concepts requires that the role a person occupies must be capable of being evaluated for grading purposes. It is in this situation that time-span measurement comes into its own as a method of job evaluation. By means of time-span measurement any role can be allocated to a grade in the generalized grading schema presented. That allocation establishes the pay bracket for the role. The actual pay received by a person occupying the role would be determined by the merit progression through the grade.[3]

---

[3] A systematic progression and payment procedure using these concepts will be found in my (1961) *Equitable Payment*, Chapters 14 and 15. The supporting procedures are described in (1964) *Time-span Handbook* and (1968) *Progression Handbook*.

7

The Stratification of Work and Organizational Design[1]

Ralph Rowbottom and David Billis

To try to deepen an understanding of what hierarchies of management levels are about, a descriptive theory is offered of the existence of a natural stratification of the work to be done in organizations. It is based on action-research over a number of years in social services departments in England and Wales. It appears that the first five successive organizational levels are concerned with what may briefly be categorized as: prescribed output *work*, situational response *work*, systematic service provision *work*, comprehensive service provision *work, and* comprehensive field coverage *work. Examples are quoted of how this conceptual framework has been used in practice* (a) *to clarify and simplify existing managerial structures, and* (b) *to help design total organization according to the quality of response to the environment which is required.*

What is the hierarchy of management levels in organizations *about*? In keeping with the spirit of their age, the earliest writers on management, the so-called 'classical' school – the Fayols, Taylors, and Urwicks – simply took them for granted. These people were not so much concerned with why management levels were there, as how to strengthen them and improve their efficiency. In a different way the subsequent Human Relations writers also took them for granted, in their case by largely ignoring the 'formal' system in the pursuit of supportive, participatory processes. It was not until the advent of the later, more sociology-minded and systems-minded researchers, that managerial systems as such came under stern and critical review. Generalizing very broadly, two models were identified. The first was a conventional or traditional model variously described as 'hierarchical', 'bureaucratic', 'mechanistic', and 'authoritarian'. The second was a new, emerging model, by im-

[1] Reprinted from *Human Relations*, Vol. 30, No. 1, 1977.

plication more suited to the turbulent social environment of the twentieth century, and variously described as 'nonhierarchical', 'anti-bureaucratic', 'organic', 'responsive', and 'democratic'. [We might take as key works here those of McGregor (1960), Burns and Stalker (1961), and Emery and Trist (1965).] But a whole host of other names could be added to the founders of, and subscribers to, this now-dominant ideology – Argyris, Bennis, Blake and Mouton, Katz and Kahn, Lawrence and Lorsch, etc.

However, in spite of the general enthusiastic espousal of the second vision, not only by the academics and commentators but by many of the more lively and forward-looking of managers themselves, strong elements of hierarchical structure still manifestly and stubbornly abound in most real-life organizations, public as well as private. The men at the top (or more modishly, the 'centre') still seem to carry significant extra increments of power and authority, not to speak of pay and status.

In this chapter we shall be examining a detailed thesis which serves to explain this persistence of hierarchical structure on the general grounds that there are different kinds of work to be carried out in organizations which can quite reasonably be described as 'higher' and 'lower'. Although we shall not be concerned with how these different kinds of work might justify differences in pay or status, we shall be very much concerned with what they imply in terms of authority. We shall also be concerned with the question of how the existence of work at a variety of levels is related to differing capacities amongst organization members and, more especially, to the way in which the capacity of any one individual member may develop through time. Here we may note the considerable influence on the ideas expressed in this chapter of the theories and findings of Elliott Jaques on these same subjects.[2] We may also note, without

---

[2] See Jaques, 1965a, 1965b, 1967, 1976. His own inititial conception of the stratification of work was based on empirical observations of a natural spacing of managerial tiers in terms of 'time-span' measures of levels of work (Jaques, 1965a). If the two approaches, his and the one described here, are consistent (as it is assumed they are) then his critical time-span boundaries between strata – 3 months, 1 year, 2 years, 5 years, and 10 years – will correspond to the boundaries between successive strata of work identified in the qualitative terms used below. In the various descriptions of work-strata offered below the links may also be noted with the idea of the 'perceptual–concrete' nature

further pursuing, the links at this point with more general issues of 'social stratification'.[3]

Origin of the Work-stratum Model
The ideas to be described arose from an action–research programme which has been in progress since 1969 in the new social services departments (SSDs) in local authorities (Social Services Organization Research Unit, 1974). In the course of work with a number of these departments one of the recurrent problems noted was that of the precise role within the hierarchy of certain particular groups of senior staff. Time and again in field or seminar discussions members of departments would spontaneously refer to the difficult organizational position of social work 'team leaders' or 'seniors', in relation to the members of their teams; or of 'homes advisers' in relation to the heads of the various residential homes for children that they were expected to supervise; or of 'specialist advisers', 'principal officers', and the like at headquarters in relation to teams of social workers at Area Offices; or of 'deputy directors' in relation to 'assistant directors'.

Although each of these groups of staff were shown 'higher' on the charts than their counterparts, and were often indeed in more highly-graded posts, analysis often revealed considerable uncertainties or disagreements about the extent of their managerial authority. There would be doubt as to how far they had the right to set policies or general authoritative guides for work which were binding on their counterparts, or to make authoritative appraisals of their performance, their suitability for promotion, etc. There would be doubt as to how far it would

---

of the lowest stratum of human capacity; the 'imaginal–concrete' nature of the second stratum, and the 'conceptual–concrete' nature of the third stratum (Jaques, 1965b).

[3] For the general terms of the social-stratification discussion see the Davis and Moore versus Tumin debate (Bendix and Lipset, 1953) and also Dahrendorf (1968). Specifically, the issue may be noted of how far, in general, differences in power, status, and wealth in society may be explained or justified either in terms of the need to have a variety of different social functions carried out (which bears an obvious relation to the present discussion of 'work-strata'), or in terms of the existence of a given 'natural' distribution of human abilities (which bears an obvious relation to Jaques' notion of 'capacity').

be right to describe them as accountable for the work of their counterparts.

By contrast, none of these same doubts would usually exist to any significant extent for certain other posts in the hierarchy – 'area officers' in relation to 'team leaders'; 'heads of homes' in relation to the staff of the home; 'assistant directors' in relation to 'principal officers'; or indeed directors of departments in relation to any or all other staff.

The attempt to probe further into why these distinctions should arise (and the answer was obviously more general than that of the personal strength or weaknesses of particular individuals) led to a general consideration of the *kinds* of work carried out in these various positions, and whether any significant stratification in the work itself might be observable. Clearly these 'kinds' of work would be perceived as not just different, but themselves as 'higher' or 'lower' in responsibility. However, there would be no need to deny as well the presence of some continuing scale of responsibility within each discrete kind or category. Hence, what we should be seeking to identify would be a series of discrete, qualitatively different *strata* of work, superimposed on a continuous scale of work of increasing responsibility from bottom to top of the organization.

In the attempt to identify these various work-strata some immediate observations appeared relevant. Ignoring the manifest hierarchy of authority and grades it was noteworthy:

(a) that certain social workers talked of 'their' caseload, and apparently carried a full measure of responsibility for each case within it;

(b) that others – students, trainees, and assistants, for example – did not talk in quite the same way and apparently did not carry full case responsibility, but carried out work under the close supervision and direction of some of the first group of staff; and

(c) that there were others again – more senior social workers, area officers, and specialist advisers, for example – who often spoke with regret about being unable at this stage of their careers to carry a personal caseload, and who seemed to be more concerned with general systems of provision and general procedures for work, training, administration, etc., than getting involved in particular cases.

Gradually from these beginnings a general thesis grew; and as it grew it seemed that it might be applicable not only to social services departments but to a much wider range of organizations. In essence the thesis was this:

1. that the work to be done in organizations falls into a hierarchy of discrete strata in which the range of the ends or objectives to be achieved and the range of environmental circumstances to be taken into account both broadens and changes in quality at successive steps;
2. that the work at successively higher strata is judged to be more responsible, but that significant differences of responsibility are also felt to arise *within* strata; i.e., that these qualitative strata form stages within a continuous scale of increasing levels of work or responsibility;
3. that at least five such possible strata can be precisely identified in qualitative terms; in successive order and starting from the lowest: *prescribed output, situational response, systematic service provision, comprehensive service provision,* and *comprehensive field coverage;*
4. that these strata form a natural chain for delegating work and hence provide the basis for constructing an effective chain of successive managerial levels within the organization; and
5. that the understanding of these strata can also provide a practical guide to designing new organizations (or part-organizations) according to the kind and level of organizational response required in relation to the social and physical environment in which the organization is to operate.

One important proviso needs to be added to the fourth point just made. It is assumed there (and for the rest of this chapter) that managerial relationships are not for any reason inappropriate in principle. It should be noted that there are some situations in which the development of full managerial relationships (in the precise sense in which 'managerial' is defined later in the chapter) appears for good reasons to be specifically excluded – as, for example, in the organization of medical consultants (Rowbottom, 1973b). However, even in these situations the questions of the various levels or kinds of work to be done still remains, as well as the question of who is expected to carry them out.

This descriptive model of the natural hierarchy of work in organizations outlined above has been tested and developed over the year or so since its first formulation in a series of seminar discussions with groups of senior staff from social services throughout the country.[4] More specifically it has been employed in a series of exploratory projects during this period (some of which are described below) undertaken within specific social services departments, and has already been absorbed into executive action in several of these projects.

The main features of each stratum of work in the model are summarized in Table 7.1 and elaborated one by one below. Illustrative examples are taken from the project work described in social services, but since the thesis is in such general terms, tentative illustrations have been offered as well drawing upon recent work in the field of health services (Rowbottom *et al.*, 1973) and certain other material from the authors' combined experience. In addition precise definitions of the boundary between strata are given in clear-cut terms of the kinds of decisions which the worker at any level is or is not expected to make in the course of his work. (These boundary definitions provide the ultimate test in practice in classifying the kind of work required in specific given jobs.)

Stratum-1 – Prescribed Output

At the lowest stratum of work the output required of the worker is completely prescribed or prescribable, as are the specific circumstances in which this or that task should be pursued. If he is in doubt as to which task to pursue, it is prescribed that he take the matter up with his immediate superior. Work consists of such things as rendering given services, collecting given information, making prescribed checks or tests, producing predetermined products. What is to be done, in terms of the kind or

[4] The Social Services Organization Research Unit at Brunel has been running a continuing series of research conferences and seminars now in its sixth year, specifically with the purposes of disseminating and simultaneously testing organizational theories emerging from its field project work.

TABLE 7.1 Summary of work-strata

Stratum	Description of work	Upper boundary
1	*Prescribed output* – working toward objectives which can be completely specified (as far as is significant) beforehand, according to defined circumstances which may present themselves.	Not expected to make any significant judgments on what output to aim for or under what circumstances to aim for it.
2	*Situational response* – carrying out work where the precise objectives to be pursued have to be judged according to the needs of each specific concrete situation which presents itself.	Not expected to make any decisions, i.e., commitments on how future possible situations are to be dealt with.
3	*Systematic service provision* – making systematic provision of services of some given kinds shaped to the needs of a continuous sequence of concrete situations which present themselves.	Not expected to make any decisions on the reallocation of resources to meet as yet unmanifested needs (for the given kinds of services) within some given territorial or organizational society.
4	*Comprehensive service provision* – making comprehensive provision of services of some given kinds according to the total and continuing needs for them throughout some given territorial or organizational society.	Not expected to make any decisions on the reallocation of resources to meet needs for services of different or new kinds.
5	*Comprehensive field coverage* – making comprehensive provision of services within some general field of need throughout some given territorial or organizational society.	Not expected to make any decisions on the reallocation of resources to provide services outside the given field of need.

form of results to be achieved, does not have to be decided. This will (either) have been specifically prescribed for the occasion or (frequently) have been communicated during the process of induction to the job as the sorts of response required when certain stimuli are experienced. If there is any doubt about the result required it can be dispelled by further description or demonstration to the point where more detailed discrimination becomes irrelevant to the quality of result required. What does need to be decided – and this may not necessarily be at all straightforward – is just how to produce the results required, that is, by what method and also with what priority. Thus, greater or lesser exercise of discretion is necessary – the work is far from being prescribed in totality.

The personal qualities called for within this stratum include possession of knowledge of the range of demands to be expected in daily work, knowledge of the proper responses called for, skills in carrying out these various responses and, not least, appropriate attitudes to the work in question and the people to be dealt with.

And so within this stratum we have the typical work of those in social services departments described as social work assistants, care assistants, cleaners, cooks, drivers, and clerks. More generally, it may be assumed that most artisans and craftsmen work within this stratum, and also those professional trainees and apprentices destined for work at higher levels who are as yet in some early and preparatory stages of their career.

Stratum-2 – Situational Response

Within the second stratum the ends to be pursued are again in the form of results required in specific situations, but here the output required can be partially, and only partially, specified beforehand. The appropriate results or output must now depend to a significant degree on assessments of the social or physical nature of the situation which presents itself and in which the task is to be carried out. The work is such that it is impossible in principle to demonstrate fully beforehand just what the final outcome should look like – this could only be established by actually going through the task concerned. However, by way of limit, no decisions, that is no commitments to future action, are called for in respect to possible future situations which may arise. The work is still concerned with the concrete and the particular.

Rather than collecting given information, or making prescribed tests or checks as in Stratum-1, the task would now be redefined in Stratum-2 in the more general form of producing an appraisal or making an assessment. Rather than rendering a prescribed service or making a prescribed product, the task would now be redefined as producing a service or product of a certain kind but shaped according to the judged needs of the particular situation. The 'judged needs' might, for example, be those of a person in distress (social services), or a child at school (education), or a customer (commerce). Within this stratum 'demands' can never be taken at their face value : there is always an implicit requirement to explore and assess what the 'real' needs of the situation are.

Thus in addition to the technical skills of the Stratum-1 worker, the worker in Stratum-2 must have the ability to penetrate to the underlying nature of the specific situations with which he finds himself in contact. Indeed it is this latter ability, based on some body of explicit theoretical knowledge, which perhaps distinguishes the true 'professional' in his particular field from the 'craftsman' or 'technician' who is only equipped to work within the first stratum described above.[5] However, this is not to imply that only members of the acknowledged professions may work at this stratum or higher ones. The ability itself is the thing in question, not any body of explicit theory.

Within this stratum the sort of managerial roles can be expected to emerge which carry full accountability for the work of Stratum-1 workers and duties of assessing their needs and capabilities in allocating work and promoting their personal development. (In contrast, what might be called 'supervisory'

[5] The introduction of ideas of discrete work-strata into theories of occupation and profession presents intriguing prospects. Apart from the possible distinction of 'craftsmen' and 'technicians' from 'professionals', just described, it also draws attention to the likely presence of many different strata or levels within any one occupational group – or, putting it another way, of finding social workers, teachers, doctors, etc., within any one of Strata-2, 3, 4, etc. This stratification *within* occupational groups is usually obscured by a sociological habit of treating each group as if its members had one unique status or prestige level – treating the house-surgeon as identical with the President of the Royal College of Surgeons, for example.

roles may exist in the upper reaches of Stratum-1, but those in them will not be expected to make rounded appraisals of the ability and need of subordinate staff, but rather to carry out such prescribed tasks as instructing staff in their work, allocating specific jobs and dealing with specific queries.) However, it is not at all necessary to assume that all roles within this stratum have a managerial content, and indeed the kind of definitions proposed here and below surmount the problem of being forced to describe higher-than-basic strata of work in a way which automatically links them to the carrying of managerial or supervisory responsibility. The example of the experienced social worker who takes full responsibility for cases but works without subordinates has already been cited.

Stratum 3 – Systematic Service Provision
At Stratum-3 it is required to go beyond responding to specific situations case by case, however adequately. It is required to envisage the needs of a continuing sequence of situations, some as yet in the future and unmaterialized, in terms of the patterns of response which may be established. Relationships of one situation to another and the characteristics of the sequence as a whole are crucial. In order to design appropriate responses some general specifications of the kinds of services which are required must be available.

Thus, in social services departments an example of Stratum-3 work would be the development of intake and assessment procedures for all those clients who apply to, or are referred to, a particular Area Office; or the development of standard assessment procedures for the range of children being referred by existing field-work services for residential care. In health services an example might be the development of systematic accident and emergency services in a particular hospital. In education, it might be the development of a general curriculum for all the infants who present themselves at a particular school for primary education. In manufacturing, it might be developing a system for handling orders for a particular kind of product.

Within this stratum, however, work is confined to dealing with some particular flow or sequence of situations which naturally arises from the given organizational provision. The work does not extend to considering and dealing with various situations of need that do not, without further investments of resource, yet manifest themselves in any particular organizational or territorial society – for example, needs for social work that might be manifested were additional local offices to be opened in new districts. Although staff working within Stratum-3 may draw attention to the possibilities of such new investments, they will not be expected to make any *decisions* about them.

Stratum-3 work is essentially concerned with developing systems and procedures which prescribe the way future situational-response work is to be carried out. There is seemingly similar work in Stratum-2 which consists of laying down general rules, methods or standards. However, this, if it is indeed within Stratum-2, will be pitched in terms of the totally prescribed responses required in completely specifiable circumstances. Thus at Stratum-3 the first genuine policy-making type work emerges: that is, the laying down of general prescriptions which guide, without precisely specifying. In using the word 'system' here we are referring to prescriptions of this general type. Characteristically, the work involves initial discussions and negotiations with a number of fellow workers and co-ordinating with them the introduction of new schemes. Necessarily, it involves some use of conceptualization, both of types of situations likely to be faced and of appropriate kinds of response.

Within SSDs it has become clear that many 'specialist advisers' and 'development officers' work at this level; and also the 'area officers' in charge of large local offices containing several teams of social workers and ancillary staff.

Stratum-4 – Comprehensive Service Provision

At Stratum-4 the definition of the aims of work and the environmental situation to be encompassed takes a decisive jump again. No longer is it sufficient to stay passively within the bounds of the succession of situations with which contact arises in the normal course of things. Now further initiative is required. It is required to take account systematically of the need for service as it exists and wherever it exists in some given society, territorially or organizationally defined. However, within this stratum the identification of the need to be met is still limited by a particular conception of the kinds of service which the organization is understood to be legitimately providing. Let us elaborate this last point.

At Stratum-2 the identification of need which can be met is limited both by the existence of certain systems and procedures and the existence (or non-existence) of substantive organizational resources with which to carry out work at a given point in the broader society concerned. At Stratum-3 the former constraint disappears but the latter remains. But at Stratum-4 both these constraints disappear. The only constraint on developing new services or proposals for new services is the constraint of given policy, explicit or understood, on the particular kind of services which will be regarded as well-established, sanctioned, and legitimated.

The starting question at Stratum-4 is: what is the extent of the need for services of these kinds throughout the given territorial or organizational society? New information about the various ranges of past situations encountered is not enough. More information must be fed in, of the kind that can often be discovered only by systematic survey or deliberate 'intelligence' work.

Thus, in social services the starting point may be all those in a given county or borough, known or unknown, needing advice or material aid or other specific services because of their physical disabilities; or all those who could benefit, for one reason or another from, say, 'meals on wheels' or 'home help' services. In commerce, it might be all those in some given regional, national, or international territory who would be potential customers for certain established ranges of product or service. Within any given organizational society, it might be the internal needs for facilities to carry out various kinds of personnel, administrative or financial work.

At Stratum-4 then, the essence of the work is concerned with developing comprehensive provision of services or products of a specified kind throughout some defined society. Financial investment in plant and buildings and, in general, recruitment and training programmes are a natural concomitant. Since new capital investment of any significant size is always a sensitive matter, the final sanction for it may often rest at higher organization levels, or indeed within governing bodies of various kinds. Organization members within Stratum-4 may not themselves have authority to make the final decision on investment therefore, but at least they will need some degree of authority to reallocate existing resources so as to cope with emerging or as yet untapped areas of need within the society concerned.

Within this Stratum are to be found in SSDs various 'assistant directors' and 'divisional directors'. In health services it is presumed that most of the new community physicians, the chief nurses, and the administrators at Area and District level are also working within this stratum. It appears unlikely that any people within this fourth stratum can carry out their work without assistance; all appear to need access to subordinate or ancillary staff.

Stratum-5 – Comprehensive Field Coverage

At Stratum-5 need has to be considered again in its complete incidence throughout some given territorial or organizational society, but the scope is broadened by moving from a framework of accepted, specified, and sanctioned kinds of service on offer to a framework which simply defines some general field of need. The work consists essentially of developing whatever comprehensive provision may be required within this given general field. Thus, in social services departments, in moving from Stratum-4 to Stratum-5, the focus changes from things like needs for homes for the elderly, case work with problem families, provision of home help, to the general question 'how can social distress in this district, in all its forms, best be prevented or alleviated?' In health services the question changes from 'what sorts of hospital, general practice, and public health services are needed throughout this district?' (with the meanings that these terms already attract) to 'what are the basic health needs of this district, group by group, and how they may best be met in any combination of old or new services?' Other general fields of need in the public sector whose nature would imply potential Stratum-5 work would include education, leisure, housing, physical environment, transportation, etc., where similar questions might be posed. In industry, needs in Stratum-4 terms for things like 'overcoats', 'telephones', or 'calculators' would presumably become redefined as needs for 'clothing', 'communication systems', and 'data processing', respectively, in Stratum-5 terms.

Thus there is an important distinction to be observed here between what we have called *particular kinds of service* and *general fields of need*. As we are using it, the phrase 'particular kinds of service' is one which at a given point of cultural development would conjure up a precise picture of what the services comprised and what kinds of physical facilities and staff were needed to provide them. On the other hand, a field-of-need description would convey no such precise image. (Presumably, in the normal course of social development many terms, which initially imply little more than fields of possible need, later acquire much more concrete connotations. Think, for example, of the now-specific connotations of such phrases as 'general medical practice' or 'social casework' or 'television services' or 'life insurance' compared with their imprecise significance at earlier points of social history.)

Work within this stratum involves much interaction with directing and sponsoring bodies of various kinds – boards of directors or other governing bodies, financial bodies, trusts, public authorities, and the like. Inevitably, staff within this stratum spend much time 'outside' the immediate operational zone of the organization.

Within this stratum then, we should expect to find the chief officers of at least the major departments in local authorities, some senior executive posts (as yet not altogether clear) in the new Health Authorities, and the chief executives of many large commercial operating organizations, freestanding or part of larger financial groupings.

Possible Higher Strata
So far we have described five discrete strata of work but there seems no necessary reason to stop here. Jaques (1965a), for example, has assumed on the basis of his own observations of viable managerial structures in a number of varied organizational settings that at least seven distinct levels can be identified. There is evidently further work above the fifth stratum concerned with the interaction of many fields of need at local, regional, national, or even international levels. There is the need within local authorities to produce plans which intermesh

the whole range of public services – education, social services, planning, leisure, etc. – provided at local level. The same inter-meshing of various broad fields of public service, together with nationalized industries, arises at national level. In the private sector there is the increasing growth of national or multi-national conglomerates bringing together operating divisions or subsidiaries in many broad fields. For the moment the exist-ence of such higher level work is noted, but no definite classifica-tion can be advanced.

'Zooming' and 'Transitional Phases'
Before passing on, however, two important elaborations of the thesis which have been developed in discussions of its applic-ability to social services departments must be mentioned. The first is the idea of 'zooming'; the second what might be called the 'transitional phase'.

It is evident that staff at Stratum-3 and upward are not able to spend, and do not spend, all their time simply considering extended ranges of work and needs, as it were, in abstraction. Stratum-5 staff will frequently get involved in discussions of the comprehensive provision of existing kinds of services, the estab-lishment of specific systems, or the correct handling of the spe-cific and perhaps quite crucial cases; Stratum-4 staff will quite frequently get involved with particular systems or they too with particular cases; and so on. Such phenomena may be described as 'zooming' (Evans, 1970). There may be a variety of causes: direct externally given requirements, such as insistence by the governing body that the head or director of a public agency looks into a particular case; or the need to help some subordi-nate in difficulty; or a laudable aim to get the 'feel' of lower level and more concrete realities, from time to time; or even perhaps the occasional attempted flight from higher demands!

Does this mean that more senior people commonly act at several different levels of work, concurrently or in rapid succes-sion? To assume this would in fact be to assume that they experienced rapid expansion and contraction of personal capacity, one moment only capable of seeing aims and situa-tions in a narrow context, and the next far more broadly – which seem implausible. On the contrary, it is readily observ-able that when people capable of operating at higher levels get involved in work which is at *apparently* lower levels, that they tackle them in crucially different ways, ways which constantly exhibit the characteristics of the higher level approach. Where people with Stratum-3 capacity become involved in concrete situations needing their attention, these specific situations are rapidly seized on as illustrative instances of a general problem demanding a more systematic response. Where Stratum-4 people become involved with particular ailing systems or procedures their interventions inevitably lead to considerations of how the benefits might be extended comprehensively throughout the organization concerned.

An actual illustration of this process which has come to our notice is that of the industrial chief executive who asked his secretary to prepare and to maintain in an up-to-date state an organization chart of his company for the wall of his office. Given the written, highly explicit accounts of jobs and organization which were current in this particular company, this task would appear to have been straightforward enough, but nevertheless the chief executive found himself dissatisfied in this instance with the results of his secretary's work. As anyone knows who has tried to draw charts of the detailed and complex relationships, however well-established, in large organizations, the sheer job of charting itself is not so simple as it might seem. The chief executive grappled with it for several hours – indeed all evening. What he began to devise was not simply an answer to his immediate problem (Stratum-2) but the outlines of a general system of organizational charting (Stratum-3). Moreover, having devised such a system he proceeded to think about, and later to act upon, the possibility of its useful employment throughout the company (Stratum-4). (Whether he proceeded to any further action which indicated a Stratum-5 or higher outlook is not known; however, the point is made.)

What this suggests then is that 'zooming' is a normal or proper part of executive work, and must be thought of as not simply a 'zoom down' into a lower stratum of work (leaving apart, that is, the case where the person concerned is not in fact capable of operating at the higher stratum) but also properly a subsequent 'zoom up', or return, the total sweep in fact providing valuable concrete experience for the more abstract work to be carried out.

The second phenomenon which must be taken into account is that of the *transitional phase*, which is to do with the observable development in people's abilities as they approach the points in their careers where they are ready to take on work at the next higher stratum. Now it is possible, as described above, to define a completely sharp boundary between strata in terms of certain kinds of decisions which may or may not be made, but it is not easy to believe that human capacity develops in the same completely discontinuous way. One does not go to bed one night unable to think beyond the case in hand and wake up next morning unable to do other than see cases as illustrative of whole ranges of work to be tackled accordingly.

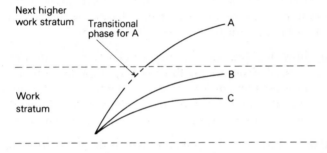

FIGURE 7.1. Differing patterns of development of personal capacity

There is evidence that personal capacity to do work at various levels develops in a continuous pattern over time though at different rates for different people – as A, B, and C in Figure 7.1 (Jaques, 1967). Moreover, for those like A who are on their way to achieving not merely a higher ability within a given stratum, but ability of a different and higher kind (and only for those people), observation now suggests that they begin to show evidences of this higher ability in a nascent form well before it has reached its fully realized state. The 1- or 2-year practical postqualification experience in 'responsible positions' required by many professional bodies, before full-professional registration is awarded, is no doubt a particular recognition of this phenomenon at the Stratum 1–2 boundary.

The organizational consequences of this phenomenon are as follows. Whereas the manager within the next higher stratum, say, for example, the *systematic service provision* stratum, Stratum-3, may involve A, B, and C, who are all at this moment of their careers in Stratum-2, in discussion about new policies (say, the introduction of new systems or procedures) he is likely, it seems, to get contributions of a different quality from A than from B or C. Such discussion may help to train A for his forthcoming leap. Indeed, he may be asked to do such things as chairing working parties to produce ideas for new policies, though at this stage of his career he will not be judged quite ready to take full responsibility for the final formulation of such policies or responsibility for their implementation following approval.

Applications of the Model
Having now laid out the model, at least in its present stage of development, the remainder of the chapter is devoted to the uses to which it can be put. We shall consider:

   (a) how the ideas can be used to clarify roles and organizational structure within existing organization; and
   (b) how the ideas may help to design new organizations considered as total systems from which a particular quality of response is required in relation to their environment.

Illustrations of both applications will be given from actual developmental project work that has been carried out in particular social services departments.

The Clarification of Existing Organizational Roles and Structure
As has been noted, the theory under discussion grew out of observations of the equivocal position of certain apparently managerial posts in many SSDs. Such posts seemed regularly to attract conflicts about their status and authority in a way not true of other posts within the hierarchy. Earlier studies in manufacturing and nursing organizations had revealed similar phenomena (Brown, 1960; Rowbottom *et al.*, 1973). Generalizing, it seems that if a hierarchy is set up in any organization on the basis of all the various different grades of post which may exist or be required in the given organization, then not all of them will turn out in practice to carry the same relationship to those beneath them. Moreover, to the extent that this phenomenon is denied officially, or by those in the particular

posts concerned, certain inevitable and quite painful stresses and conflicts will result.

Let us start with a definition. Let us describe the strongest, most secure, most authoritative posts in the hierarchy as 'fully managerial' or simply 'managerial'. We shall associate these with unquestioned rights to set or sanction general aims and guides for subordinates, and with rights to appraise their performance and capacity in practice and to assign or reassign work to them accordingly. Then we may pose a simple proposition: that no more than one of these managerial posts can be sustained in any one stratum of work (as here defined) within the hierarchy. Thus, knowing the range of strata of work to be carried out within any organization, we can readily compute the maximum number of viable managerial posts in the hierarchy. In the case of social services departments for example, assuming the desire to carry out work at all five of the strata identified above, there would only be room for four such managerial posts in any strand of the hierarchy.

However, as it happens, there are something of the order of ten or twelve main *grades* of post in SSDs, and indeed it seems quite usual for organizations to generate many more steps in their grading hierarchies than can be justified in terms of the basic managerial hierarchy required. What is the position of the people in all these other posts? Judging from project work in various fields that has been quoted, the answer, it appears, is that they will in reality tend to carry roles which are less than, and crucially different from, full managerial roles as they have just been described. At least four possible alternative roles have been identified in these various fields of project work – 'co-ordinating roles', 'monitoring roles', 'staff-officer roles', and 'supervisory roles' (Brown, 1960; Rowbottom *et al.*, 1973; Social Services Organisation Research Unit, 1974). Each has its distinct qualities, but in general none of these types of role carries authority to set general aims and guides for those in posts of lower grade, or to appraise their performance and capacity, or to assign or reassign work accordingly.

In other words, these other people will not naturally and readily be identified as the 'boss'. It will be more natural and satisfactory to have a 'boss' who is (and is capable of) working at the next higher stratum of work, and one who is therefore able to make a radical adjustment to the whole *setting* within which work is carried out when major problems loom. What is unsatisfactory and a constant source of tension is a supposed boss who goes through some motions of appraising performance and setting general aims and guides, even though in reality he is only carrying out work of essentially the same kind himself, and therefore needs to refer any major difficulties requiring radical readjustments in work or circumstance to some further point still in the hierarchy. This is indeed 'bureaucracy' with a vengeance!

Some Examples from Social Services

Let us briefly illustrate how this idea of linking managerial roles with different strata of work has been applied in actual projects in SSDs.

One project (still in hand) is concerned with the managerial structure of an Area Social Work Office and in particular with the role of the Team Leader, which has been left in this department as elsewhere to raise considerable problems. There are four teams in this particular office and each Team Leader is 'in charge' of a team of up to a dozen or so people. Manifestly, the hierarchy is as shown in Figure 7.2a. On the surface it appears that all members of the team are managed, directly or indirectly, by the Team Leader. Collaborative analyses, using these ideas of discrete strata of work and managerial and other roles, have revealed a very different situation, one much closer to the model of Figure 7.2b, which, now it has been made explicit, seems to command considerable approval. In reality it appears that Team Leaders, Senior Social Workers, and certain of the more experienced Basic Grade workers are all working within the same 'situational response' stratum – they are all carrying full 'professional' responsibility for their cases, drawing only on voluntary consultation with colleagues as and when they require it. Moreover, when large issues appear on the scene, they all tend to look directly to the Area Officer for guidance rather than the Team Leader. In respect of the other workers at this second stratum then, the Team Leader has essentially a *co-ordinative* role – co-ordinating the daily flow of work, co-ordinating duty arrangements, chairing team meetings, etc. – though in addition he provides advice to his col-

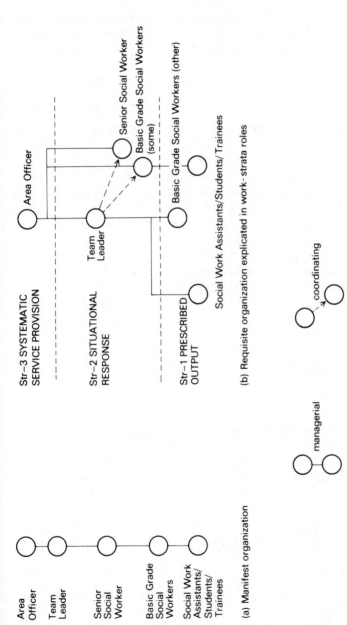

FIGURE 7.2 Organization of an area social work team

leagues, when asked. In contrast, the social work assistants, the trainees and students, and other of the Basic Grade social workers, both unqualified and newly qualified, are still working in Stratum-1, although many of them, particularly the students and newly qualified social workers, may be expected to be within the 'transitional phase' leading to Stratum-2. This latter group clearly requires a special treatment. However, since none of these people has actually realized a Stratum-2 capability, they can all be expected to find it acceptable to see the Team Leader (or perhaps one of the other Stratum-2 workers to whom they may be attached for training purposes in the case of students) in a managerial role – in conventional social work terminology as a realistic and accepted 'supervisor'.[6] Thus, what could easily be seen and interpreted (or misinterpreted) as a long, complex hierarchy within the Area Office can now be seen in a much clearer, simpler, and more functional form, with only one intermediate management level, and that not applying to all staff within the office.

Another project has been concerned with helping the top management group of an SSD to redefine and clarify their own roles and relationships. One issue concerned the role of the Deputy Director. His position was publicly portrayed as in Figure 7.3a. His role was generally described in terms like 'doubling for the Director' and 'dealing with day-to-day matters', but carried some specific areas of responsibility as well. Although on examination the roles of the Assistant Directors revealed clear Stratum-4 work, examination of the Deputy's role failed to reveal the same. The new organization (Figure 7.3b) which was introduced made specific use of the idea of work-strata, and failing to find room for any intermediate managerial level between the work of the Director (Stratum-5) and his Assistant Directors (Stratum-4), the Deputy was assigned a senior Stratum-4 post, with responsibility in this case for the comprehensive provision of all 'field-work' services.

---

[6] It may be noted that the term 'supervisor' as used in social work practice implies in fact a range of authority and accountabillty commensurate with a 'managerial' role as defined above. However, the term 'supervisor' in the Glacier Project (Brown, 1960) and later work was used, in keeping with industrial and certain other practice, to define a role with precisely *less* than full managerial characteristics.

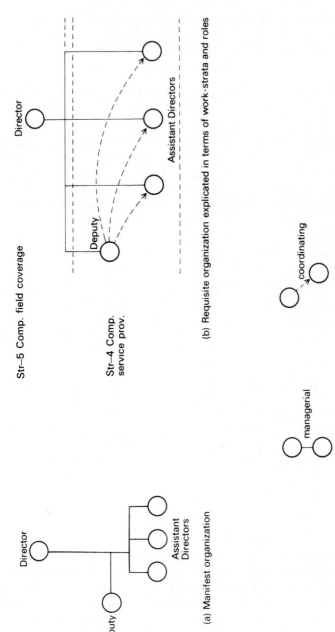

FIGURE 7.3. Top management structure of a social services department

Although a significant co-ordinative role was also recognized in relation to his other Stratum-4 colleagues, it was clearly established that all these people were to regard the Director and not the Deputy as their immediate manager.

A third project (supported by seminar work of the kind described above) has been concerned with the nationally important question of the future role and organization of the Education Welfare Service, at present usually attached to education departments but with strong links to SSDs. The distinction between Stratum-1 and Stratum-2 definition of the role of the Education Welfare Officer turns out to be of central significance. In a Stratum-1 conception, his work is describable in terms like enforcing school attendance, providing specific information to parents, and providing or arranging specific material aids. In a Stratum-2 conception his work becomes redefinable in terms such as dealing in a flexible, responsive way with problems of non-attendance and their social causes, with a view to promoting a situation in which the child can best benefit from the educational facilities available. The indications are that the strong preference will be for the second definition of the role – a decision with profound implications for the training and deployment of staff – with perhaps recognition of the need for the provision of ancillary staff at Stratum-1 as well.

Other projects have applied similar analyses to the kind of work required of heads of homes in residential social work – whether it should be at Stratum-1 or 2 (Billis, 1975); to the kind of work required of so-called 'training officers' – whether it should be at Stratum-2 or 3; and to the kind of work required of those developing new types of social work with disturbed adolescents known as 'intermediate treatment' – again, whether at Stratum-2 or 3.

Designing New Organizational Structure
The examples quoted so far have all been of situations where staff and organization already exist and the problem is to clarify the levels of work to be done, and the consequent managerial and other role structure called for. In a more fundamental application, the theory can also be applied to the design and establishment of new organizations by posing the question:

what strata of work is the organization as a whole required to encompass?

A current example from our own project work is that of the setting up, or rather re-establishment, of hospital social work organization following the recent transfer of hospital social workers en bloc from Health Authorities to social services departments. We have become involved in helping in this task of integration in three departments. Nationally, the difficulties of integration have been much exacerbated by uncertainties about relative gradings. Although the same sort of grade-titles have traditionally been used in both hospital social work and local authority services – 'principal', 'senior', and 'basic' grade – the actual associated salary scales have been lower for workers in hospitals. There has been considerable argument as to whether this in fact betokens less responsibility, grade-title for grade-title; or whether it simply reflects the continuous history of comparative underpayment of hospital workers.

Here, the Work-Stratum theory has provided a useful cutting edge in project work. Separating and leaving aside for the moment any questions of grade and pay, it has been possible to expose the basic issue: what kind of work is required to be carried out in hospital settings of various types? The answer from the field has been unanimous on the need in all hospital settings for work of at least Stratum-2 the total 'situational response' of the fully responsible case-worker. The remaining issue is then seen to be whether to provide on site, in any hospital or group of hospitals, an organization capable of carrying out systematic provision of social work services (that is, Stratum-3 work), or to leave the on-site organization as one merely capable of co-ordinated Stratum-2 work, the necessary higher level work being done by others not specifically associated with the particular hospitals concerned.

Given this analysis, the three project departments concerned are now in processes of making explicit choices, and seem in fact to be opting for full Stratum-3 organizations in the larger hospitals or hospital groups, and Stratum-2 individual posts or teams in the smaller hospitals. Questions of appropriate grading can properly follow, starting with the question of whether there could be any justification for lower grades for the same stratum of work in one setting or the other.

Thus, the Work-Stratum theory appears to offer a new way, not only of deciding the design of extensions to existing organizations, but of designing organizations from new. It is a way which starts from the question of the *kind* of impact which is required on some given social and physical environment. At the same time it is a way which does not seek to deny the fundamental reality of the stratification of authority in many situations. Such stratification is justified in defensible terms of higher and lower kinds of work to be performed, rather than in such crude arguments as the inevitability of having those who direct and those who obey.

It may be stressed that the quality of organizational impact on, or response to, its environment can be a matter of *choice*. As Silverman (1970) and Child (1972) separately observe, organizations are the creation of conscious decision-taking actors, not simply a product of a 'causal' environment. Much has been written about the correlations between various kinds of organizational structure and organizational environment, but not a lot has been said about the precise mechanisms by which managers might create so-called 'organic' or 'mechanistic' organizations. Apart from some of the Tavistock work on detailed systems design, using ideas of 'primary tasks' and 'sentient groups' (see, for example, Miller and Rice, 1967), the literature is content for the most part to rest at broad descriptive or ideological levels; or to observe empirical correlation in certain organizational and environmental characteristics. But the levers of change are rarely revealed.

The Work-Stratum model, as described here, offers one very concrete way in which organizations may be designed to react in various ways, or various degrees of depth, to their environment. Thus, a Stratum-3 system will respond in quite a different and perhaps more 'organic' way than a Stratum-2 system. Conversely, the model also offers a precise way of categorizing the various possible stages of evolution of any given organization from the Stratum-1 'solitary-jobber' type of organization, capable only of a prescribed response to its environment, right through to the fully mature Stratum-5 type of organization. (This may be compared with other published descriptions of organizational evolution such as those of Chandler, 1963, Jaques, 1965a, Greiner, 1972.)

From this viewpoint the Stratum-5 organization with its fully realized capability for self-development emerges as the system of special interest. It appears to offer one concrete answer to the general problem posed by Schon (1971) of how society is to produce organizations, both public and private, capable of coping with the demands of an increasingly unstable world. The increasing establishment of Stratum-5 organizations at the 'periphery' (in Schon's term) seems to offer a means of getting away from a society dominated by the exclusive development of new ideas at the 'centre', and their diffusion on a 'centre periphery' model, with all the attendant problems he so ably identifies. It offers a means of retaining coherent organizational structure. At the same time it does not exclude the possibility of basic political and legal control from the centre. Thus, to stick to the examples quoted extensively in this chapter, the current establishment in Britain of new organizations at local level in the fields of both social services and health services, capable of working to the most general, i.e., Stratum-5 terms of reference, while still subject to the overall legal–political control of central government, seems a development to be welcomed.

At this point the thesis leaves us with some large questions: Are there other public services which could benefit from establishment in Stratum-5 organizations, either by extension or reduction of their present structure? What is the justification for the many large national public services which presumably require more than four-level executive structures, but with a brief which suggests only a Stratum-4 definition of need, such as providing comprehensive national rail services or a national supply of coal? What is the social justification for the existence of larger-than-Stratum-5 industrial and commercial organizations? How far might we see the proliferation of these as symptomatic of a society over-obsessed with advantages of the economy of size and scale, and neglectful of the needs for more convivial institutions in which men can live and work?

References
R. BENDIX and S. M. LIPSET (Eds.), *Class, Status and Power*, London: Routledge, 1953.
D. BILLIS, 'Managing to care', *Social Work Today*, 1975, *6*, 2, 38–43.

W. BROWN, *Exploration in Management*, London: Heinemann, 1960.

T. BURNS and G. M. STALKER, *The Management of Innovation*, London: Tavistock, 1961.

A. D. CHANDLER, *Strategy and Structure*, Cambridge, Mass.: M.I.T. Press, 1963.

J. CHILD, 'Organisational structure, environment and performance: The role of strategic choice', *Sociology*, 1972, *6*, 1, 2–22.

R. DAHRENDORF, On the origin of inequality among men, *Essays in the Theory of Society*, London: Routledge, 1968.

F. E. EMERY and E. L. TRIST, 'The causal texture of organisational environments', *Human Relations*, 1965, *18*, 21–32.

J. S. EVANS, 'Managerial accountability – chief officers, consultants and boards', unpublished paper, Brunel University, 1970.

E. L. Greiner, 'Evolution and revolution as organisations grow', *Harvard Business Review*, 1972, *50*, 4, 37–46.

E. JAQUES, 'Preliminary sketch of a general structure of executive strata', in W. Brown and E. Jaques, *Glacier Project Papers*, London: Heinemann, 1965a.

E. JAQUES, 'Speculations concerning level of capacity', in W. Brown and E. Jaques, *Glacier Project Papers*, London: Heinemann, 1965b.

E. JAQUES, *Equitable Payment* (2nd ed.), Harmondsworth: Penguin, 1967.

E. JAQUES, *A General Theory of Bureaucracy*, London: Heinemann, 1976.

D. McGREGOR, *The Human Side of Enterprise*, New York: McGraw-Hill, 1960.

E. J. MILLER and A. K. RICE, *Systems of Organisation*, London: Tavistock, 1967.

R. W. ROWBOTTOM, 'Organizing social services, hierarchy or . . . ?', *Public Administration*, 1973b, *51*, 291–301.

R. W. ROWBOTTOM, J. BALLE, S. CANG, M. DIXON, E. JAQUES, T. PACKWOOD and H. TOLLIDAY, *Hospital Organisation*, London: Heinemann, 1973.

D. A. SCHON, *Beyond the Stable State*, London: Temple Smith, 1971.

D. SILVERMAN, *The Theory of Organisations*, London: Heinemann, 1970.

SOCIAL SERVICES ORGANISATION RESEARCH UNIT, Brunel Institute of Organisation and Social Studies, *Social Services Departments: Developing Patterns of Work and Organisation*, London: Heinemann, 1974.

8

Teams and Leadership

Elliott Jaques

One of the most difficult issues in health services organization is that of the development of an adequate managerial structure. The common desire in most industrial countries is to establish a unified managerial structure, neatly and tidily organized under a single 'chief executive officer' at the top. As those involved in hospital and health services organization are well aware, no such solution is realistically available.

This problem was faced in the discussion leading up to the reorganization of the NHS in 1974. We shall in this chapter consider the problems as they were faced in the organization of health Districts, immediately subordinate to Area Health Authorities. In order to present certain principles as sharply as possible, we shall confine our attention to the case of a single district Area – referring to it as the District.

The object of the chapter will be to show how complex team structures can be established and made to work, so long as their structure, and the functions and duties of their members are sufficiently carefully and clearly enunciated.

Various Organization Possibilities
One of the first possibilities to be considered by the Management Steering Committee which was charged with the responsibility for proposing a possible structure for the reorganization, was to have an Area Chief Executive Officer, 'in charge of everything'. This proposal was rejected on the grounds that consultants and GPs cannot have managers. It is not organizationally possible to place a chief executive officer in a position of managerial accountability in relation to consultants and GPs and to retain clinical autonomy as the foundation of personalized services for patients. It is not possible to do so even if the

chief executive were himself to be a doctor. (This argument is pursued in detail in Chapter 5.)

The second possibility which was then considered was to separate the doctors from the rest of the services. A role might then be established which could carry co-ordinative authority only in relation to the doctors, but managerial authority with respect to all the other services.

This concept, however, also proved unacceptable, since it was found to run counter to the professional independence required in the wide range of medical services provided, including, for example, nursing, community medicine and medical administration, many of the paramedical services, and the administrative services. All these services are provided in their own right directly to patients and the community and cannot be subordinated one to the other, for reasons which are argued in detail in the essay on professionals in health and social services.

The District Management Team

At this stage it was recognized that each of the major services ancillary to medicine – such as physiotherapy, nursing, pathology, radiology, psychotherapy, and the other thirty or more therapeutic and scientific and technical services – required to be established as independent hierarchically organized services, separate from the consultants and GPs. A further feature was then recognized: namely, that only a few of these services were concerned with the totality of services in the District, whereas the others were concerned only with specialized services.

Those concerned with the planning and development of the totality of service included: the consultants and GPs; the District Community Physician (DCP) (concerned with epidemiology); the District Administrator (DA); the District Nursing Officer (DNO); and the District Finance Officer (DFO). The consultants and GPs were organized in a committee structure at the top of which was the District Medical Committee which could elect a District Consultant Representative and a District GP Representative. The other four, however, the DCP, DA, DNO and DFO, were all appointed officers, each head of a managerial hierarchy (although the role of the DCP as a manager is less clearly established). Who could be 'head' of such a group? Or could it perhaps successfully function as a team? The latter course was chosen, in the light of previous experience of similar teams in the pre-reorganization hospital service.

The function of such a team would not be to 'manage' the District. It would be accountable for keeping District services under review, proposing annual plans and budgets to the AHA, and monitoring and co-ordinating the implementation of AHA policies by all services within the District. The question then was whether it was possible for such a group to function effectively as a team, and if so, how?

Development of the Various Team Roles

The team to be considered, then, was composed of six members: two elected members – the consultant and GP representatives; and four appointed members – the DCP, DA, DNO, and DFO. It was recognized that the various services would have to be bound together by co-ordinative mechanisms. One possibility, therefore, was to establish a separate free-standing co-ordinative role, the occupant of which would be called *district co-ordinator*. This co-ordinator might be from any discipline. He would not be head of any department, but would be full-time engaged in co-ordinating the activities of the team as a whole, and might be of higher status and pay.

Consideration of the possible co-ordinator role highlighted the fact that it was essential that all members of the District team should be ordinary members of the team in the sense of being there because they were in charge of a department, or because they were elected representatives of clinicians. There was no room for a free-standing co-ordinator who might come to be perceived as 'over' the other members. Moreover, each of the members had co-ordinative duties in connection with his or her own work, and if this co-ordinative work were done properly there would be no need for an extra co-ordinator.

This last finding led to the conception of each member of the team carrying out *functional co-ordination*, that is to say co-ordination in connection with each one's own field of work, while the *general co-ordination* required to pull the total programme together might be carried out by a member of the team appointed to do that work. This member might be from any discipline, could act as *chairman* of the team, and might receive extra remuneration for these special duties.

Consideration of the proposed chairman and general co-ordinator role led to further clarification. In fact, what was referred to as general co-ordination was nothing more than the normal role of the administrator engaged in knitting together and consolidation of the various parts of a programme, and ensuring the successful co-ordination of its progress according to schedule and planned expenditure. If the administrator carried out this function, and other members of the team carried out their own co-ordinative functions, as for example, the District Community Physician co-ordinating medical service projects, then the work of the team could be effectively co-ordinated. There might additionally be a need for a chairman role, but that was a matter to be considered in the light of the leadership requirement.

Leadership in a Team Situation

These developments are briefly reviewed in order to show that there exists a problem in formulating how leadership shall be exercised in district teams. Because the NHS is a complex organization it is unlikely that any attempt to define who is 'the' leader of a team will be successful, because leadership is not concentrated exclusively in one single role. It is essential rather to define the various types of leadership role which will be required, and to prescribe how these various roles should be set up and how they should work together so as to achieve harmonious and efficient functioning of the team.

The following roles would appear to carry leadership functions in connection with district, area, and regional teams:

AHA chairman;
possible team chairman role;
team members as functional co-ordinators,
including the administrator engaged in general co-ordinative work;
the elected clinician representatives, with a leadership role in relation to their constituents.

The qualities required in each of these leadership roles are briefly indicated in the following paragraphs. Once these qualities are defined it may then be possible to consider the particular leadership requirements for the team as a whole.

AHA Chairmanship: These roles are co-ordinative chairmen roles. They call for a chairman who can ensure that his committee works effectively and that the agendas are well constructed in relation to the work to be done. He must have an experienced judgment of health service needs and priorities, and be able to judge the effectiveness of performance of appointed officers singly and as a team. He must be able to give leadership to the DMT members in the sense of influencing them on behalf of the AHA to use their best endeavours, in instructing them where necessary and appropriate, and in helping them to co-ordinate their efforts by resolving any differences which might arise or by referring intractable problems to the Authority.

Team Chairmanship: Team chairmen would not only be group relations chairmen but also co-ordinative chairmen. They would take the chair at meetings, in order to help the team to work together effectively in arriving at consensus decisions. They would be assisted in this function by the co-ordinating member for each agenda item who would take the role of leader of the debate. In between meetings the chairman would be kept informed by the administrator about general progress, and would use his influence to overcome obstacles due to inadequate working relationships among the team members. He would have to have the personal confidence of all the team members in order to carry out his functions, a factor which is the main reason why he should be an elected chairman.

Co-ordinative Leadership: Each of the team members must give leadership with respect to the functions which he is accountable for co-ordinating. This leadership calls for the capacity to gain co-operation by influence and persuasion, and by being able to co-operate with the others in working towards the common objectives. The co-ordinator must be able to show why given actions are necessary, and must be flexible enough for give and take in getting the best result when difficulties arise and adjustments to programme have to be made. The co-ordinator must be able to report on progress in his own field, and to act as point of contact for these activities.

The administrators carry the heaviest co-ordinative role, in that they must knit together and consolidate the total programme, and see to its progress as well as co-ordinate administrative developments; they must in addition provide administrative services to other members of the team to assist their own activities including their co-ordinative work; they must also act as a general point of contact for all members of the team, ensuring that communications are routed to the correct role.

The District Community Physicians carry the major co-ordinative role for the planning and progress of medical service projects, including the planning of proposals for capital projects, and the planning of modifications to services or the introduction of new services.

District Nursing Officers carry co-ordinative leadership for the modification of nursing services and their organization.

District Treasurers, in addition to their interpretation and monitoring of trends of expenditure against budget, are accountable for co-ordinating the preparation of budget proposals.

Medical Committee Chairmanship: These roles are co-ordinative chairmen roles. The chairman is in a representative rather than a delegate role, and must thus exercise a leadership function in agreeing policies. He must not only see that his committee works effectively but must use his influence to see that individual constituents – consultants or GPs – co-operate in accepting the policies and programmes agreed on their behalf by their representatives on the DMT. He must be the kind of person who can take initiative in seeing non-co-operative members and attempting to persuade them to change, and if unsuccessful, to see that the matter is referred higher. He must be able to gain and retain the confidence of his constituents and to lead in such a way as to gain their active co-operation in putting forward their views on service development needs, and in helping to formulate proposals.

Consensus Decision-Making and Veto Voting

Given these definitions of various roles, the remaining question was that of how DMT decisions could be made. Majority voting can readily be seen to be unworkable. If any single one of the team members has strong reason to be opposed, say, to a team plan to be proposed to the AHA, then it is not a workable plan. For in effect, the consultant or GP representative would be saying that he could not get sufficient support from his constituent colleagues; and each of the four officers would be saying that it was unworkable for his particular department.

What was required was a working-through of problems and difficulties by the team, to the point where all the members could agree that a particular proposal, if not perfect, was at least not only the best under the circumstances but also workable and implementable. That is to say, the team would work through to the point of unanimous acceptance of the team decisions.

This notion of unanimous functioning proved of great practical importance. Thus, for example, the consultants and GPs would have been unlikely to allow themselves to become involved in a planning team where they could be committed to unacceptable policies by being out-voted in a majority voting procedure. With unanimous consensus, however, they could readily take part in the team and its planning functions, knowing that decisions would have to be worked through to the point where all team members were at least minimally satisfied.

Should it on occasion become impossible to arrive at unanimous agreement in the team, the AHA Chairman has an important role. Such an intractable situation may arise from a variety of causes – from serious differences of opinion on the content of an issue to perhaps personality clashes or inadequacy of one or other member. It is for the Chairman to help to sort out these difficulties, consulting with his Authority colleagues – perhaps bringing an unresolved issue for debate within the Authority, or helping to resolve interpersonal stresses among team members, and finally acting as a first screen in assessing the competence of individual appointed officers.

In this latter regard, the AHA Chairman cannot, of course, assess the competence of the consultant and GP representatives since they have been elected by their colleagues. But the AHA and its Chairman can make direct approaches to all consultants or all GPs, if they feel that the doctors are pressing for unreasonable or unrealistic policies in the DMT.

Managerial Leadership contrasted with Team Membership
If the above organization of duties seems untidy, there is considerable experience from former Regional Hospital Boards

and from teaching hospitals that it can work quite effectively. It is an organizational pattern called forth by the complexity of co-ordinating the health services so that they work as an efficient whole. Clear formulation of each person's role in the collective effort can facilitate the operation of the conjoint teams.

It is important, however, to note that the above organization is for the limited object of drawing together and co-ordinating the various services – mainly for planning, for assessment of progress and performance, and for modifying and adjusting plans and objectives. The day-to-day work of actually carrying out the plans is carried by the specialists and GPs in their clinical roles, and by the nurses, administrators, services, and paramedical and technical staffs, in their managerial organizations.

The effective functioning of the service thus depends upon the individual sense of responsibility of clinicians, and upon the quality of managerial leadership in the rest of the service. It is for that reason that the roles of the 25,000 or more managers in the service should be made clear.

Good managerial leadership requires that the managerial roles should be specified, so that constructive managerial behaviour can be supported and reinforced. It is first of all essential that managers be held accountable by their own superiors not only for the quality of their own work but also for the quality of the work of their subordinates. This accountability is the keystone of effective management.

Second, it is essential that the authority of managers be made absolutely clear. This authority is very different from the persuasive authority of the monitoring and co-ordinative role or of the various chairman roles. Comparison between managerial and co-ordinative authority may make the matter clear.

Managerial authority must make it possible in the final analysis for the manager to instruct his subordinate what to do, whereas co-ordination, for example, allows the co-ordinator only to persuade, and in the final analysis where there is disagreement, not to instruct but to refer the matter higher.

In the case of new appointments, a manager must take part in selection and would not ordinarily have a strongly unacceptable candidate forced upon him as a subordinate. A co-ordinator need not be involved in selection at all. Equally, a manager must have the authority to decide the assessment of the quality of performance of his subordinates, and in the final analysis to initiate transfer of a subordinate who has been shown to be unable, even with training, to meet the standards of performance set. A co-ordinator does not decide the assessment of the quality of performance of the colleagues with whom he works.

The establishment of strong managerial accountability and authority can be enhanced by proper individual appeals mechanisms and by institutions which give members employed in managerial hierarchies the opportunity to participate through elected representatives in influencing the chief officer of the hierarchy with respect to policy.

Given these safeguards, a manager can be enabled to exercise effective managerial leadership if he has the ability to do so. He must be able to maintain due consultation with his subordinates, to take account of subordinates' views, and to be decisive with respect to setting out the work to be done. Although he may not himself be able to do the subordinate's work, he must be competent to judge what to expect of a subordinate and to determine how well that subordinate is doing. He must further be able to translate policies and agreed team decisions into work programmes, to delegate various aspects of the programmes to subordinates, and to progress work so as to ensure that it is done.

Good managerial leadership is needed to make the whole system work effectively. The various co-ordinative functions must also be well carried out. The success of the integration of the services thus calls for sound interaction between co-ordinative, chairmanship, professional, and managerial activities, and that in turn demands clear definition of differences in role and type of leadership for each function.

Multi-Disciplinary Clinical Teams

A final observation on the nature of teams may be added with respect to the widespread growth of so-called multi-disciplinary teams in clinical work. The functioning of such teams in the child guidance field is considered in Chapter 10. Some more general comments may, however, be useful.

Multi-disciplinary clinical teams are small groups, always including a doctor, plus a few other professionals engaged in patient care – say two or three from among perhaps a nurse, a social worker, a psychotherapist, a clinical psychologist, a physiotherapist, an occupational therapist. These teams can be identified by the fact that the particular individuals concerned work together for relatively long periods of time; their existence as a working group is explicitly recognized. They meet regularly to discuss the cases under their care.

The activities of these multi-disciplinary teams include: reception and diagnostic procedures for new cases; discussion as a group, and decisions upon disposal of cases; determination of treatment; follow-up discussion of treatment; and decisions eventually upon termination of treatment and disposal.

Such teams are to be found frequently in out-patient clinics; in primary health care services in connection with general practice; in the less clearly organized services such as geriatrics; or in the services which do not fit so readily under the bio-medical model, such as the services for the mentally ill and the mentally handicapped.

The general point would seem to be that multi-disciplinary clinical teams come into existence where no particular professional group has clearly acceptable primacy; that is to say, where the clinical leadership and control of the medical profession is not accepted as inevitable or necessarily essential. Under such circumstances, if in addition there are individual members of other professional groups who have achieved *de facto* independent practitioner status, these individuals will tend to seek to become colleagues of the doctors with whom they work. Many speech therapists, for example, have been in such a position for many years.

In the absence of explicit recognition of the possibility of any professional group other than doctors having primacy in the NHS, and in the absence of provision for such primacy, the pressures by some members of other professions towards a sharing of primacy with doctors would not be surprising, and indeed, are to be expected. It is these pressures which are leading to a gradual spread of the multi-disciplinary clinical teams in which this sharing can occur.

It is suggested, then, that the multi-disciplinary clinical team is one in which there is an undermining of primacy of the medical profession. Prime responsibility is substituted for primacy, the team deciding which of its individual members will take prime responsibility for any particular patient. In the absence of a clear and explicit formulation of this state of affairs, however, much confusion inevitably arises, and many different working arrangements are arrived at, depending upon the 'personalities' of the members of any particular team.

The central questions which arise almost universally are: first, who should be the 'leader' of the team? and second, who, 'in the final analysis' should be responsible – that is to say, who should be responsible if anything goes seriously wrong with diagnosis and treatment, and who should be responsible for prognosis? It is these questions which reflect the lack of provision for *explicit* allocation of primacy or prime responsibility to professions other than medicine. For if primacy or prime responsibility could be explicitly allocated to one or other member of a team, then the uncertainty with respect to leadership and final responsibility would not arise.

A major point to be noted is that these problems cannot be simply resolved by saying that the team shall decide. Team decisions imply responsibility of the whole group for the care of an individual patient: such an arrangement vitiates the right of the patient to a personal confidential relationship with one person in connection with his health care, and undermines the ultimate sense of responsibility of individual professionals for patient care. When things go wrong, individual accountability is all too readily lost or hidden in the group. Or else, the problems are referred back to the medical member of the team. Where the latter solution is the underlying mechanism, the doctor inevitably remains the truly accountable member, and the notion of the team is in actuality a myth.

It is unlikely that the unclarity about leadership and responsibility in multi-disciplinary clinical teams can be finally clarified until some of the problems of the role of the senior members of the emerging professional groups in the NHS are resolved. As the status of physicists, speech therapists, clinical psychologists, specialist nurses, and so on, is resolved, so the question of the nature of the working relationship between these members and the doctors will be able to be answered.

Moreover, to answer some of these questions may require that some of more general questions raised in other chapters will have to be answered: questions to do with the nature of the health services themselves, and the conditions under which parts of such services as rehabilitation and re-education; or provision for the mentally handicapped and the chronic mentally ill or for the elderly, should be under the health service umbrella or the responsibility of some other service in which doctors do not have a prime role.

Given answers to these major questions about the organization of services and the status of professions, many of the problems of multi-disciplinary clinical teams would disappear. It might be, moreover, that the need for such teams would diminish, to be replaced by the ordinary collateral working relationships between colleagues, which can exist where true colleague status has been established.

The one area in which multi-disciplinary clinical teams might conceivably be required would be where professionals from related services have to work together on an equal footing; for example, where health services have to combine with housing, social services, education, or employment, to provide a composite service for, say, the mentally handicapped or the mentally ill. Even with this kind of inter-service collaboration, however, it is likely that network organization rather than multi-disciplinary teams would work most effectively, as described, for example, in Chapter 10, on Child Guidance services.

Part Two

Specific Services

9

Physiotherapy and Occupational Therapy

Heather Tolliday and Elliott Jaques

Introduction

The organization of professional services – both established professions and newly emerging ones – creates a widespread problem in health, education, and social and welfare services. This problem occurs not only in the UK: it is widespread in most countries with developed professional services. The central feature of the problem is that of the degree of independence or autonomy of the professional in making judgments and in determining action – the model which is most commonly aspired towards being that of the clinical doctor who is seen as having achieved the maximum of clinical freedom.

There are two general reasons for these growing stresses. First, with the increase in educational facilities and the raising of entry requirements, many fields of work are recruiting an increasing proportion of individuals with levels of ability consistent with recognition for professional independence. Second, in many of these fields the work has been undertaken predominantly by women; the increasing independence of women in society has been a considerable force in the direction of such groups seeking to manage their own work with full recognition of their abilities regardless of sex.

The problem of professional organization is at its most acute, however, in health services, for a number of reasons in addition to the two just mentioned. First, there is the clinical autonomy of doctors which is immediately present, as a reminder of what might be achieved. This effect of the clinical autonomy of doctors is reinforced by their central role as responsible for diagnosis, treatment, and prognosis for individual patients, setting limits within which the work of all the other professional groups is constrained.

Second, there is the existence of a very wide range of different services which are becoming increasingly professionalized. Many of these services have hitherto been managed by doctors. As they develop in professional status, under medical management, there eventually emerges the desire for managerial autonomy, of which the achieved autonomy in this respect of the nurses is often taken as the model.[1]

Third, there is the fact that the basic model for the relationship between doctors and other professional groups was established in that field of activity concerned with the treatment of physical illness by physical (as against psychological) methods of treatment, where the doctor carries primary responsibility. There is a changing relationship, however, between doctors and other groups in such fields as psychotherapy, and in educational methods of assisting individuals better to use their physiological and psychological resources, where with new developments the need for primacy of the doctor with medical degree is no longer so self-evident.[2]

Some of the difficulties have been present in the NHS from its beginning – a continuation of difficulties which existed long before the NHS was born. The trouble has been exacerbated, however, within the NHS; first, because of the scale of each of the services brought together within one national service; and second, because of the considerable increase in the number of newly emerging professions, and the rapid growth of all professional services, which have been the consequence of recent scientific and technical advances in health services.

It is the object of this chapter to examine some of these difficulties in professional organization, but with particular reference to the remedial professions of physiotherapy and occupational therapy. The material comes from work carried out during the past ten years by members of HSORU in fieldwork projects and in research conferences. Some hundreds of

---

[1] The recommendation of *The Report of the Committee on Senior Nursing Staff Structure* (London: HMSO, 1966) established chief nurses in the NHS managerially independent of either doctors or administrators.

[2] For a discussion of the position of doctors in health services, see Chapter 11.

individuals have been seen, many of them on repeated occasions over many years, as new organizational patterns were tested.

Professional Levels in Physiotherapy (PT) and Occupational Therapy (OT)

The starting point for any clarification of organization is to determine the work that has to be done, and the level of responsibility in that work. In the case of PT and OT, the main work is that of the clinical practitioner professional giving treatment to patients. It is the content of that clinical work which determines the basic level of professional work for PT and OT, upon which the organization of these services will depend.

The results of the research work of the HSORU to date indicate that there is no single or simple answer to the question of what levels of professional work in PT and OT are currently being called for in the NHS. There would appear to be a number of different levels depending upon the type of work and the circumstances. In particular, we shall outline our findings to the present time for PT and OT roles in three main fields of clinical work: physical treatment; psychological treatment; education for environmental adaptation; as well as in work concerned with the growth and development of therapy services.

ORGANIZATION FOR CLINICAL SERVICE OR FOR CAREER? Although what ought to be done may seem self-evident, it is not always clear in practice whether NHS organization has been designed primarily to provide career structures for staff, or deploy staff in order to treat patients. There is a widespread tendency – in many other public services as well as in the NHS – to assume that the provision of a good career structure will automatically ensure efficient functioning.

This view of the importance of career structure has proved to be misguided, as seen for example, in experience of the way in which the Salmon Report[3] proposals were implemented in many parts of the country.[4] Despite the nurses' experience and the stated wish of PTs and OTs to avoid 'Salmonization', the automatic equation of management with grading structures led

[3] Report of the Committee on Senior Nursing Staff Structure (1966).
[4] See Chapter 6, p. 100.

to the paragraphs on management structure in the McMillan Report[5] being headed Career Structure.

The danger in starting with careers in establishing organization is that without initial agreement on the work required, and the grounding of organization firmly upon this work, structures are created which frequently fail to facilitate the doing of effective work, fail to establish true higher levels of work for promoted staff, and fail to establish grades which reflect actual allocation of responsibility. Thus, for example, one of the reasons for therapists' concern about setting up District Therapists' roles as new and additional roles was that if it turned out that there was not full-time work of the right kind for such roles, these would not in fact prove to be attractive career posts.

In discussions of these issues with PTs and OTs, it became clear that in looking at the nature of PT and OT work, PTs and OTs distinguished differences both in the kind of work and in the level of work in different roles. Even where roles carried the same grading and titles, there could nevertheless be important differences in the kind and weight of work carried; these differences could be obscured because of there being no satisfactory work criteria by means of which grades could be assigned on a common and agreed basis throughout the country.

A number of criteria had been tried out for assessing the various degrees of responsibility in work, but with not much success. For example, descriptions of the knowledge being used in work by members of the same profession in different settings, or by members of different professions, might help to some extent to give a rough sense of differences in level of work, but did not discriminate finely enough to give a practical assessment of the full differences that people experienced. Nor did consideration of the sorts of problems to which this knowledge is applied get at the differences; for instance an aide might undertake a task which, ten years before might have been undertaken only by a qualified PT – but few would argue that this meant that the work of the aide was now strictly comparable to that of the PT ten years ago.

EMERGENCE OF DIFFERENT LEVELS OF WORK OR WORK-STRATA.
Despite these failures to specify in any exact and practically

[5] McMillan Report, paras. 36–51.

useful way the level of work in various types of OT and PT role, there was a considerable consistency in the intuitive judgments which PTs and OTs made about the relative levels of their roles as compared with each other and with other professions as well. Work with them on formulating the criteria that they were intuitively using led to the emergence of statements of four main kinds of work which were best expressed as levels in a hierarchy.

The starting point for the discussions was the level of basic professional work, that is to say the level of work expected of all fully established members of the OT and PT professions. This was the sort of work carried by the therapist who had had sufficient experience to undertake the full range of normal clinical work unsupervised. This base coincided in the judgment of therapists with what an experienced ward sister or a local authority employed social worker with his own case load did. Therapists at this level were expected to be able to use their own judgment in assessing patient needs, within the framework set by the patient's doctor.

Below this level there were the therapist aides who were not expected to exercise discretion in determining what treatment was necessary.

A third level, one above the basic professional level, was perceived in the role of the full-scale superintendent or department head. The reference here was to the superintendent who was truly the manager of a department of professional therapists, one who directed their work and was able to be held accountable for the quality of the work done by the therapists. A managerial district therapist role might also be at this level. This superintendent role was contrasted with another role which might carry the same title, but which was really at the same level as the other therapists; namely, the role of a therapist with her own case load who additionally was responsible for co-ordinating the work of the department but was not the accountable manager.

In some few fields of work (for example, where a therapist was independently engaged in psychotherapy) the professional and clinical content of work in the role was itself thought by some to warrant recognition at the same level as a full-scale department head; that is to say, at the third level.

There were thus thought to be at least three distinct levels and probably now a fourth. The work that some principals of NHS PT schools and the district therapists were undertaking, not just responding to demand but identifying gaps in provision and creating ways of filling the gaps, was felt by some to be of a different order from that done by most superintendents, and this was assumed to constitute a fourth level.

GRADING OF ROLES WITHIN LEVELS. In addition to these broad band organization levels or work-strata, there was also thought to be a need for grading subdivisions within each one. These grading subdivisions were held to be necessary to allow a person to progress within his work role, as he became increasingly experienced and competent and able to exercise greater independence over a wider range of activities.

In the case of therapists, for example, such grading subdivisions would make it possible for a fully qualified therapist to have a full career, if she so wished, as a clinical therapist, gaining advancement in grading as she became more clinically competent, without necessarily having to take on an administrative post in order to advance.

The most commonly expressed view was that several grades should be allowed for within each organization level. A person could thus gain progress within a grade, or upgrading from one grade to another, without necessarily having to move to an entirely different professional level, or to take on unwanted administrative and managerial duties.

LEVEL OF PT AND OT CLINICAL ROLES. These views of the PTs and OTs corresponded closely with the general structure of work-strata and grading described above in Chapters 6 and 7. With these concepts of work-strata, grading, and manager–subordinate relationships, it became possible to consider in more detail the question of the level of various types of PT and OT clinical practitioner and managerial roles.

Although many OTs and PTs do work without the help of subordinates there is general agreement among them that their entry training and qualification standards are not appropriate to work at level or Stratum-1. The lowest level (the basic professional level) at which all fully recognized members of the PT and OT professions expect to work is Stratum-2. They feel over-qualified for what they do if clinicians treat them as if they were capable only of working in a Stratum-1 way by detailing precisely the treatment to be given. And this is what many therapists complain of. They feel that they are competent to work at Stratum-2, and if they are not allowed to decide for themselves what PT or OT can achieve for a particular patient, their work is depressed to a Stratum-1 level and they feel they are working below their competence.

Moreover work with administrators, doctors, and others confirms the view of PTs and OTs that the expectation in the NHS is that PTs and OTs should, at a minimum, be aiming at competence in, or be competent in, work at Stratum-2. This conclusion is based on the fact that the full-fledged therapist must be capable of interpreting the specific treatment needs for each referral, and cannot have their work completely specified. It is only so specified where students or newly qualified therapists working under supervision until competence at Stratum-2 is demonstrated.

However, in some fields of NHS activity in which PTs and OTs may be found – that in which the prime aim is to change states of mind, or to change behaviour, or to carry out special long-term treatment – in addition to Stratum-2 clinical practitioners' work there may also be opportunities for PTs and OTs to do full-time Stratum-3 clinical practitioner work. These situations may occur, for example, in some PT work with the cerebral palsied and with some OT work in psycho-dynamically oriented day centres.

The reasons for these possible differences in the levels in full-time clinical practitioner PT and OT in the different fields are not yet clear. One reason may be a difference between the knowledge and skill assumed to be acquired by each of the professions in each field and the knowledge and skills applied in actual work. In the field of changing physical states, medicine is the encompassing profession. Doctors' training is based on the assumption that they are required to know more about the human physical organism than do members of other professions working in the same field. Thus doctors take the lead in determining what can be done for patients and how it is to be achieved. However, where it is a matter of changing not physical states but of changing states of mind and changing behaviour, some doctors and therapists hold the view that doctors are not necessarily always best qualified to take the lead. And, in practice, it is not inevitably the case that a doctor takes the prime responsibility *vis-à-vis* clients/patients in these fields.

LEVEL OF PT AND OT MANAGERIAL ROLES. In those Health Districts which offer work opportunities to PTs and OTs limited to clinically based Stratum-2 practitioner roles, one of the clinical PTs and one of the clinical OTs usually carries an additional responsibility. This responsibility is for bringing together her colleagues where issues concerning their work arise and for seeing whether they can formulate a common view. This additional responsibility is usually recognized by means of a higher grading.

The higher grading in such situations should not be assumed automatically to confer managerial authority over the other clinical therapists. Research findings support the proposition that managerial relationships can be established only between people who are at least at one stratum distance in work and capacity. If the more highly graded clinical therapist is in the same work-stratum as the other clinical therapists, then she is a colleague and not a manager, but a colleague who has a *monitoring and co-ordinating* role in relation to the others when general issues affecting them all need to be tackled. In exercising that co-ordinating authority she has the authority to call her colleagues together to discuss an issue, but if they fail to come to agreement she cannot impose a solution on them – something she could do if she were their manager. A co-ordinating relationship is one in which the co-ordinator is expected to take the lead in suggesting specific actions or programmes, and in reviewing actual progress; but does not have *managerial* rights to appraise personal performance or to take action in consequence, nor to issue binding rulings or instructions in situations of sustained disagreement. In a monitoring relationship the monitor is expected to keep himself aware of certain specifically defined areas or aspects of activity, to discuss deviations from acceptable standards in these areas and to report continued or serious deviations to higher authority. In carrying out this function the monitor has neither *managerial* nor *prescribing* authority, but only authority to explore, warn, discuss, and (ultimately) report.

There are other districts in which there are PTs and OTs in charge of departments, who are working at Stratum-3, and doing both clinical and administrative work. PTs and OTs undertaking this type of Stratum-3 work often have the title superintendent or head. It is important to distinguish them from the Stratum-2 co-ordinators described in the previous paragraph who may, in many cases, carry similar titles.

Where there is provision for Stratum-3 PT or OT roles in Districts it is usually appropriate for them to be established as the *managers* of the Stratum-2 clinical practitioner therapists. This is only so, however, where the Stratum-3 and Stratum-2 therapists are members of the same profession *and* work in the same field of activity.[6] The Stratum-3 managerial therapists undertake clinical work mainly to keep themselves in touch with the problems that their subordinate therapists encounter. This enables them to take these factors into account in devising systems, and to remain proficient in specialized clinical techniques for teaching purposes. It is interesting to note that where Stratum-2 clinical OTs are working with psycho-dynamic techniques to change states of mind, they tend not to be managed by a Stratum-3 OT unless she too is fully engaged in the same field. The same applies to PTs working in the behaviour changing field.

DISTRICT ROLES. Following the reorganization and the amalgamation into Districts of groups of hospitals formerly managed by the Hospital Management Committees, some Districts had more than one post which would appear to be a Stratum-3 OT or PT post. Under such circumstances, what tended to happen was that one of them assumed a co-ordinative role among her Stratum-3 colleagues to establish a District-wide PT or OT view. Where the Stratum-3 therapists are working in the same field several Stratum-3 managerial posts can be justified if the District is large. These Stratum-3 posts would be managed in turn by a Stratum-4 District Therapist. But where the Stratum-4 posts are concerned with PT or OT work in different fields, it is possible that more than one Stratum-4 managerial post can

[6] This theme is elaborated in Chapter 4.

be justified because of the difficulties of managing therapists who are in other fields. In that case, the only way of providing for a single PT or OT focus in that District would be for one of the PTs or OTs to assume a co-ordinative District-wide duty when the need for it arose.

In summary, it can be said that opportunities for PTs and OTs are currently to be found both in clinical practice which is definable as Stratum-2 work (with a few opportunities for additional District-wide co-ordinative duty where there is no provision for PT or OT managerial work), and in managerial roles and some clinical roles which, in the language of this paper, are at Stratum-3 or at Stratum-4. Experience of the ultimate nature of District Therapist work among the professions suggests that it is in line with what is here described as Stratum-4 work: but it is important to note that such roles could be either that of a District manager, or of a District co-ordinator of other Stratum-3 department heads.

LEVEL OF PT AND OT DEVELOPMENT ROLES. There are some PTs and OTs who argue that there is a need for high-level work of a developmental kind, of the type associated with comprehensive service provision at Stratum-4. With the rapid changes in the NHS they believe that to get the best out of PT and OT there should be an on-going comparison of actual with potential service provision, and the devising of ways of filling gaps in provision. It is not certain, however, that it is only members of the professions concerned who can undertake this sort of work in the development of services. Neither the NHS nor the professions could afford to make PTs and OTs available full-time to each district for such work. Many therapists would nonetheless like to see such developmental posts established at least within each region if not also within each area.

Whatever decisions are taken about the range of opportunities for PTs and OTs in the reorganized NHS – whether or not the range is to be standardized throughout all districts and new levels of PT and OT work to be established throughout the country – it will have to take into account the relationship between clinical and teaching PT staff in particular. Research findings suggest that there are at least some principals in PT training schools doing work which fits the description of

Stratum-4 work. If it were decided to set up PT development roles, questions would have to be asked about the way in which those roles would link with principal roles in schools.

The Relationships Between Clinicians and PTs and OTs

If the analysis thus far is accepted, what then is the appropriate relationship between doctors and PTs and OTs? In exploring this question, GPs and consultants will be considered separately from community physicians. The reason for this is that, although all are members of the medical profession, the involvement of PTs and OTs with GPs and consultants requires a different form of control from that required by community physicians. GPs and consultants carry personal responsibility to their patients for the services they draw on for them, whereas community physicians have no personal responsibility for individual patients – their responsibility is to ensure that services within communities meet the general needs of those communities.

SHOULD THERAPISTS BE MANAGED BY DOCTORS? The central question, which is continually encountered in discussions with PTs and OTs, is whether these remedial services should be managed by doctors – whether by consultant, or GP, or by community physicians. For many years PTs and OTs have been seeking to gain the right to manage their own affairs. They have argued that they should not be organized under anyone other than members of their own professions, as this alone can ensure that their professional voice is heard by employing authorities. Despite this view, the inclination of the NHS has always been to organize them within multi-professional service hierarchies headed by doctors or administrators. This arrangement was made largely on the grounds that employing authorities' management structures would otherwise be unduly fragmented, or, where doctors were put at the top of PT, OT and other hierarchies, that doctors needed to have some control over the resources available to their patients.

Of recent years, however, management of PTs and OTs by doctors has been subject to increasing strain, not only because of PT and OT professional opposition but also because if one clinician, say a consultant in rheumatology and rehabilitation, manages PTs and OTs this deprives other consultants with special requirements of the control they need.

A major influence in the situation was produced with the passing of the Professions Supplementary to Medicine Act in 1960, when PTs and OTs achieved the right and accepted the obligation, through majority membership on their Boards, to negotiate the scope of PT and OT directly with the state. In doing so, they determine the future of their professions and must, therefore, be able to ensure that the local conditions in which their members are employed permit them to fulfil the commitments they establish nationally. They need therefore to be able to negotiate directly with employing authorities rather than through the intermediary of a member of a separate profession. In effect, the demands of PTs and OTs for self-management has become a logical consequence of their having become state registered.

PROFESSIONAL INDEPENDENCE. The increasing organizational independence of therapists requires careful definition of the range of working relationships between therapists and doctors. First, it is necessary to define the binding professional standards which set the limits for what professionals can do, and to which all those who use their services must adhere. Then there is the question of the degree of independence which therapists have in relation to patients. This question of independence is connected with the question of who in any particular case carries prime responsibility for the care of the patient, bringing others in as necessary. And, finally, there are the organizational issues of the direct working relationships between therapists and heads of therapy departments, and the doctors with whom they work.

The definition of what constitutes a profession and a professional is far more than a merely verbal exercise. It is of the highest importance to some hundreds of thousands of members of the NHS – administrators, technicians, therapists of various kinds – who are seeking the status and authority that can accompany professional recognition. In the analysis to follow, the following concepts, described in Chapter 5 above, will be used: binding professional standards; agency service; personalized service; independent practice; primacy and prime responsibility.

PRESCRIBING AND REFERRAL. The practitioner carrying prime responsibility for the care of a patient will have the authority to draw upon other services. He will be able to prescribe, for example, what treatment shall be given, or what diagnostic procedures shall be carried out, or will be able to refer cases to colleagues for second opinion or for treatment. The Research Unit has not yet succeeded in defining clearly the differences between prescribing and referral. It is recognized that to use the term 'prescribing' for all referrals for treatment from a doctor to a PT or OT has too narrow a feel. The definition of prescribing relationship currently used by the Unit is shown in Appendix B, but we shall also use the term 'referral' in what follows.

The relationship between GPs, consultants, and OTs and PTs can be established only if the conditions in which it arises are clear. Where medicine is concerned with changing the physical state of patients, for example, those patients get access to non-medical and dental services only because their named personal doctor or dentist believes it would be useful in fulfilling the objective of the diagnostic or treatment programme established by him. The GP, or, more usually, the consultant, has to know enough of the range of NHS services to know which might usefully contribute to the management of his patient and to have some idea of the point at which another's contribution should be sought.

Where it is the GP or consultant's duty to establish the overall objective of NHS treatment for individual patients, and the stratum at which PT or OT is expected to carry out work with patients is Stratum-2, a relationship has to be devised which accommodates both factors. In the case here where the professions concerned – OT and PT – are professions encompassed by the medical profession, a relation arises in which the PT or OT contributes to patient care within the context established by the doctor. Such a context will include a statement of the diagnosis and any complications.

This relationship assures the patient's doctor the right to frame the PT's or OT's contribution in terms of his overall objectives for the patient, while leaving space to the PT or OT to decide just how to reach a PT or OT objective given her judgment of the individual patient's needs and responses. This situation is to be contrasted with that in which the medical profession does not encompass that of the person to be involved in the case. There a referral implies that the doctor is asking another to collaborate as a colleague on the case.

ADMINISTRATIVE RELATIONSHIPS BETWEEN THERAPISTS AND CONSULTANTS. While the referral relationship gives clinicians control over the treatment objectives for individual patients, it does not, by itself, give them influence over the general direction in which PT or OT is developed. To some extent, of course, the type and amount of work referred to PTs by consultants and GPs depends on their judgment of the quality and appropriateness of the PT or OT services available for their patients. The employing authority has the problem therefore of trying to ensure that applicants for PT or OT posts are as acceptable as possible to the clinicians who will be using the PT or OT services.

One possible solution to this question of acceptability which has been put forward for situations where a therapist or small group of therapists work very closely with a doctor or small group of doctors, is for the therapist to remain managerially within the therapy department, but to be attached to work within a monitoring and co-ordination relationship for the doctor or group of doctors.

In attachment with monitoring and co-ordination the clinicians would play a part in appointment but would not have managerial powers. In particular, if a therapist was to work full-time for a clinician, the attachment would take place only if acceptable to the clinician. Thus situations could be avoided in which the clinicians fail to get what they want for their patients and in which the PTs and OTs lack the conditions in which to develop their work.

Another possible solution is for the therapists to be organizationally independent of the consultant, and for the head of department to be completely accountable for the allocation of staff without reference to clinicians – but monitored perhaps by the DCP and DMT. Under these conditions it would be for the department head to provide an adequate service, and if the clinicians were dissatisfied they would take the matter up with the department head in the first instance, and if still not satisfied then to pursue it further through the usual channels. A variation on this arrangement could be to provide for the consultants to be involved in selection so that any major differences might be avoided.

STRATUM-3 PRACTITIONER WORK AND PRIME RESPONSIBILITY. Therapists working at Stratum-3 with independent practitioner status are increasingly to be found in a referral situation. It would also appear that there is a tendency for some OTs and PTs to be given *de facto* prime responsibility for patients under some circumstances of long-term psychological treatment, or of education for environmental adaptation, where after initial consultation and diagnosis, the case might eventually be transferred fully to the therapist – subject to referral back to a doctor in the normal way should complications of physical illness arise.

It is recognized that this last point about therapists assuming prime responsibility in work with patients raises very great issues. These issues will have to be faced up to in the NHS in the near future if many current difficulties are not seriously to fester. For the fact is that many situations now do exist in which in the absence of doctors, or infrequent visits, or changes in doctors, the therapist dealing with a case comes in course of time to take over prime responsibility by default. This situation exists in other fields such as speech therapy, psychotherapy, clinical psychology; or where there are graduate scientists. The problem may have to be tackled as a whole.[7]

THE RELATIONSHIP BETWEEN COMMUNITY PHYSICIANS AND PTS AND OTS. Against this background of referral and possible attachment relationships between clinicians and PTs and OTs, relationships between PTs and OTs and community physicians and employing authorities become easier to formulate. In their relationships with PTs and OTs, the employing authorities can assume that all is well if they get no complaints from the clinicians, since an explicit obligation on clinicians is to make their own judgments about general standards of work and report sustained and unacceptable deviations. In making appointments

[7] For discussion of the relationship of doctors to other professionals in different circumstances, see Chapter 9.

to its senior PT and OT roles and in deciding on resource allocations, authorities can control the kind and amount of PT or
OT available. But in the final analysis the definition of what
is good enough PT or OT for a district rests in practice with
those who require it (clinicians) and those who provide it (PTs
or OTs).

Given all this, the involvement of the District Community
Physician with PTs and OTs emerges as being no different, and
needing to be no different, from his involvement with anyone
else whose work contributes to overall health provision in the
district. The DCP *monitors* adherence of the therapist to AHA
policies and *co-ordinates* their contributions to total health care.
His responsibility in respect of PT and OT may be seen as the
same as his responsibility towards other district services such
as nursing, radiography, and diagnostic services.

Models of Department Organization

In this section, a number of alternative models of organization
for PT and OT will be presented. First the most common situation will be presented; namely, that of a full-scale department
with a work Stratum-3 manager, Stratum-2 therapists, in a
situation with medicine as the encompassing profession carrying prime responsibility for individual cases. A new small developing department will then be considered. Then, a number
of more complex circumstances, with higher level clinical therapist roles, and administrative and service development duties.

STRATUM-3 DEPARTMENTS. The Stratum-3 Department is one
with, say, four to ten fully-qualified Stratum-2 therapists who
may be in any of the several grades within that stratum. There
may be an additional complement of students, and perhaps one
or two newly qualified therapists. There may also be between
one and ten aides.

Such a department commonly warrants a Stratum-3
Superintendent or Head Therapist, who is a true department
manager, and who does some clinical work as well. This manager
would be a direct appointee of the AHA.

The Department Head could allocate therapists to cases on
referral from doctors. Or one or more of the therapists might

be specialized, or be designated to work with cases referred by particular doctors, and would receive *direct referrals*. Or some therapists might be *attached* to a doctor or doctors in a particular department, the doctors having a local monitoring or co-ordinative role, but the Therapy Department Head retaining. the full managerial responsibility.

The Department Head would thus be accountable for the work of all the therapists, including any who might receive direct referrals or who were attached to other departments, including accountability for maintaining professional standards. The Head would also be responsible for ensuring adequate induction of new therapists, training of students, and for the progression and upgrading of qualified staff.

The department would have its own budget for maintenance and minor equipment. For major developments, the Department Head would consult with the department therapists, and would formulate proposals for discussion with appropriate medical committees, and for final presentation to the DMT. The Head would be subject to the monitoring and co-ordinative activities of the DCP on service provision and development, and similarly to the DA on administrative standards for the department.

Where there is only one such department in a District, the Department Head would in effect be the District Therapist. Where there are two or more Stratum-3 Department Heads in a District, then one of the Heads would act as District Therapist in a co-ordinative relationship with the other Heads. Since the relationship is that of co-ordination among equals, the District role could, if desired, be rotated periodically, say every two years, among the various Heads.

VERY LARGE DEPARTMENTS. There may be some few situations in very large districts or single District Areas, with a large complement of therapists in many departments (for example, one District with some eighty qualified therapists in twelve departments and a training school with a total complement of nearly 200 staff) where it might be requisite to establish a Stratum-4 managerial role.

Such a role would be a District Therapist role with managerial duties which would include those of development of new types of service requiring perhaps several years to plan and to bring into being.

The organization of subordinate Stratum-3 departments would be as described above. There could also be provision in such large departments for Stratum-3 clinician roles, if such work were required, but not subordinate to the department head, since they would carry independent practitioner status.

VERY SMALL DEPARTMENTS. In smaller departments (or in some Districts with largely undeveloped services), there might not be the opportunity at the time to establish a Stratum-3 managerial role. The work of the department, say with a few therapists, and aides, could be organized by one of the therapists in a co-ordinative role. If this department were in a District with one or more Stratum-3 departments, it would be possible for the small department co-ordinator to be subordinate to one of the other Stratum-3 Department Heads, the small department being attached by this Department Head.

STRATUM-3 CLINICAL THERAPIST ROLES. Where there is work for Stratum-3 clinical therapist roles, research suggests that these therapists may act as independent practitioners, as indicated in earlier paragraphs. This independent practitioner work may be carried out in relation to referrals from doctors, where the doctors carry prime case responsibility, working perhaps as members of a co-ordinated clinical team.

Moreover, an emerging difficulty was described earlier in which some Stratum-3 clinical therapists are getting involved, *de facto*, in taking prime responsibility for patients. Such situations tend to arise, for example, in work with the mental handicapped, or in special schools, where a therapist may take on long-term treatment or educational responsibilities for particular patients, the doctor who initially was responsible for diagnosis and initiation of treatment either gradually withdrawing or perhaps handing over responsibility at an early stage. A doctor would of course always be available for consultation should medical complications arise, a new illness occur (as would be the case for anyone who becomes ill), but in the absence of such complicating factors, the therapist would be responsible for treatment.

Independent practitioner work at Stratum-3, if officially established, would call for direct appointment into non-managed roles, but with co-ordination by a District Co-ordinator or a Department Head. Eventually, there would probably emerge the equivalent of Cogwheel Committees, if and when there were a sufficient number of independent practitioners in a District.

These emerging *de facto* situations have not of course been officially recognized. The professions and the NHS will, however, sooner of later have to decide what to do about the matter. A wider spread of such developments is to be expected for two reasons: first, the larger number of more capable and more highly trained younger members being recruited and qualified; and the growing number of opportunities for independent practitioner work for therapists in psychotherapy and the services concerned with education in optimum use of physical and mental abilities.

This point is mentioned here, despite the fact that such roles are not officially recognized, because if nothing is done explicitly to deal with the situation, the fact that such work is going on may seriously distort the organization of PT and OT. The cause of this distortion would be the pressure by the extant Stratum-3 therapists for recognition of their higher level of work. There would then be difficult negotiations in which the demand of the Stratum-3 therapists would seem too great as far as most other roles were concerned (i.e., the Stratum-2 clinical roles).

In order to get such situations right, it may be necessary to make some special provision for Stratum-3 clinical roles under particular and specified circumstances, while maintaining the current Stratum-2 basic professional level of work, with opportunity for upgrading within the stratum, this latter work still constituting the backbone of the PT and OT services.

STRATUM-4 DEVELOPMENTAL ROLES. One possible type of Stratum-4 development role was described above in connection with the Head of a very large department. The possibility of similar responsibilities has also been mooted in discussion of the full role of Principals of training establishments, or in possible new types of roles at Regional level or in large complex Areas, concerned specifically with new service development. These possibilities have not as yet, however, been explored in detail.

Career, Grading and Education

Realistic career and grading structures can derive only from analysis of the work to be done. At the moment career opportunities for PTs and OTs are not the same throughout the country. Whether decisions on PT and OT organization in the reorganized NHS will lead to a general standardizing of the range and level of PT and OT in all districts is not known. Nor is it clear whether NHS decisions on PT and OT will increase opportunities for work at Stratum-4. Thus it is not possible in this part of the paper to detail any career and grading structures which would be applicable to all PT and OT work either now or in the future. But it is possible to make some general comments about the meaning of grading structures and their relationship to career opportunities and to note some emergent findings on the criteria on which some PTs and OTs feel grading structures might usefully be based.

GRADING IN STRATUM-2. Within Stratum-2 (the clinical practitioner stratum), at least three grading bands may be necessary if perceptions of the differences in responsibility carried by clinically based OTs and PTs are to be recognized. Such gradings within Stratum-2 would represent perceptions of stages of increasing confidence and competence in the way in which clinical therapists use their professional knowledge in practice.

Work done with clinically based PTs and OTs to elicit the criteria they use implicitly if they were asked to place themselves within one of the three grading bands postulated for work Stratum-2 has produced examples for each distinct grade.

In the lowest grade, the (c) grading, the sorts of characteristics associated with the work seem to include the PT or OT being able to work on her own case list unsupervised and having sufficient experience to be able to assess the cases and work on them accordingly and to know when to seek advice from others. But because she has not yet had enough experience to be able to consolidate and expand her theoretical knowledge, while she can demonstrate practically what she does, she cannot yet explain the theoretical principles underlying the practice. She cannot therefore be asked to supervise students but she can demonstrate techniques to them.

PT or OT work in the middle grading, the (b) grading, by contrast, seems to have to do with the ability to take on students to supervise because when the PT or OT is felt to carry a (b) grading she is able to envisage the place of her work within the general area of professional knowledge and make explicit the principles on which she is working.

And the characteristics of the work of those who are felt to command the top, or (a) grading, seem to include being able to undertake work which requires a full understanding of and confidence in the knowledge and techniques of their profession. This enables PTs or OTs to comprehend the boundaries and to help to develop knowledge and its applications.

The criteria given above are so far very tentative. On the whole therapists did not give detailed examples of specific techniques that are currently used at one grade rather than at another, because these can change relatively quickly. But given that people experience movement from a lower to a higher grade as bringing increased responsibility, the pay bands associated with each grade should not overlap, in the same way as should apply between work-strata.

No detailed work has been done on how many grades are felt to be necessary in Stratum-3. The only other grade that has been looked at in any detail is that proposed for PTs and OTs who have only just qualified. Because PTs and OTs feel that qualification does not necessarily mark attainment of competence to practise unsupervised at the basic professional level in PT and OT, many of them wish to see provision for a supervised grade for entry into Stratum-2. Newly qualified PTs and OTs in this grade would learn how to undertake Stratum-2 professional work, would make the transition between being a student and a practising professional by having case loads but working on them supervised by a senior therapist. This kind of practice would contrast with that in the bottom grade of Stratum-2 in which the therapist is expected to have enough confidence and experience to know when she has to seek help rather than, as in this supervised grade, having someone available to judge when she needs help.

IMPLICATIONS FOR CAREER STRUCTURE. There are three major implications for career structure of the developing grading structure described above and the assumptions on which it is based. The first is that gradings would not be tied necessarily to specific areas of activity – clinical, teaching, research or management for example. It is assumed that further work on the criteria for particular gradings would yield definitions which would allow the gradings to be applied to any PT or OT work. Thus if research posts were to be established in Districts and the definition of the research work to be done was in Stratum-3 terms (analysing present practice and formulating it so that it can be taught to others, say to members of the professions who have left working as PTs or OTs but who now wish to return), then these posts would be rated as Stratum-3.

Secondly establishments could be tied to a maximum financial sum, rather than to specific posts. This would make it easier for PT and OT managers flexibly to utilize the varying calibre and abilities of personnel. And thirdly, assuming the second implication were conceded and institutionalized, individuals could expect career progression without moving from post. For example, a (b)-graded PT attached to work with paediatricians could, with the personal capacity and scope in the job to develop new knowledge and techniques (and given the financial resources), be upgraded to (a).

RECRUITMENT AND EDUCATION. Recruitment and education levels are markedly affected by decisions about the level of clinical therapy work. Current clinical educational levels would appear to be pitched at Stratum-2 clinical work. Such programmes require a higher academic and conceptual level than would be appropriate for fields where the basic level of work was that of Stratum-1 technician. Thus, for example, if there were to be policies of more widely inter-professional basic education, it would have to be in conjunction with professions all of whose basic professional level was Stratum-2.

For Stratum-3 independent practitioner work, and the higher level Stratum-3 Department Head positions, post-experience training would be required in addition to the basic qualifying education.

INDIVIDUAL CAPACITY Finally, these grading and career issues may be connected with equivalent levels of work-capacity in individuals: capacity, that is to say, in the sense of *level* of professional or of managerial work which the individual is able to cope with successfully. Research currently being undertaken at Brunel would suggest that there are qualitatively different types of work-capacity associated with each work-stratum. This work-capacity is not static. It grows and develops throughout a person's working life, maturing with experience.[8] Thus, a person capable of working at the top of Stratum-1 by the age of thirty years, is likely to be able to progress to the *top* of Stratum-2. Or a person who is capable of working at the top of Stratum-2 by the age of thirty is likely to be able to progress to the top of Stratum-3. A systematic picture of the characteristics of these patterns of progression is available. It can be used both for individual career planning, and for the analysis of educational and training requirements at different career points.

There are a number of consequences which flow from this view of work-capacity. Thus, for example, if the basic level of professional work for a particular profession is, say, Work-Stratum-2, but the profession begins to recruit and train a significant proportion of members with Stratum-3 capacity, then these members will begin to seek professional work at the higher level, including higher degrees of professional independence: one result will be the development of stresses and strains in organization.

Another example of consequences would be that recruitment and training must be appropriate to the level of capacity sought for the particular professional work. That is to say, the type of training given would be different for a potential Stratum-2 professional group, from that for a Stratum-1 technical group, even though the 'same subjects' – say, anatomy and physiology – had to be taught.

Conclusion and Some General Implications
This chapter has attempted to face the full and real complexities of the organization of PT and OT in the NHS. These complexities are seen as an inevitable accompaniment of the professionalization and independence of these services. The point,

[8] See Jaques (1975), *A General Theory of Bureaucracy*, Chapter 10.

therefore, is not to try to wish away the complexities, or to seek for unrealistically simple solutions: but rather to recognize that professionalization can ensure better service for patients, and to seek to establish the various professions in their own right, and in effective working relationships with clinicians.

Without going into detail here it may be noted that some of the problems considered, and the concepts used for analysis and possible resolution of these problems, may be relevant to other professional groups, where very much the same difficulties and complexities are to be found.

Thus, for example, the possibilities of upgrading while remaining clinically occupied in Stratum-2 work may be relevant to such fields as nursing, where currently advancement cannot be gained while remaining directly in charge of ward clinical work.

Another instance would be that of some of the scientific and technical services, where it might be that the concepts of work-strata, grading, managerial organization, and referral work, might be of use as an approach to considering a range of problems concerned with departmental organization, relations between doctors and other groups, the position of graduate scientists, and related issues.

And finally, some of the problems associated with the emergence of *de facto* Stratum-3 independent practitioner work might conceivably apply especially in such fields as speech therapy, clinical psychology, psychotherapy, educational psychology, psychiatric social work, where independent work is being done increasingly in psychological and educational fields.

10

The Future of Child Guidance — A Study in Multi-disciplinary Team-work

Ralph Rowbottom and Geoffrey Bromley

The present time is one of great change and uncertainty for those in the child guidance field in Britain. Not only have major reorganizations occurred in health and social services, but these have been accompanied by, indeed have sprung from, radical reassessments of the functions that public agencies in these fields should be undertaking. In a Government Circular[1] of 1974, searching questions were posed about the future place for child guidance work in this changing scene.

Between December 1975 and January 1977 six conferences on the organization of child guidance were held at Brunel and attended by a wide variety of practitioners and administrators from the field. Discussions drew heavily upon a number of action-research projects undertaken in child guidance and other more or less closely related health and social services settings over the previous years by the Brunel research units.

[1] *Child Guidance*, a Joint Circular from the Department of Education and Science (Circular 3/74), the Department of Health and Social Security, and the Welsh Office. For an earlier view of the proper role of child guidance in Britain, and also a review of its origins, see: Underwood Committee (1955), *Report of the Committee on Maladjusted Children*; K. Cameron, 'Past and Present Trends in Child Psychiatry; *Seebohm Report* (1968), *Report on the Committee on Local Authority and Allied Personal Social Services*; W. Warren (1971), 'The Development of Child and Adolescent Psychiatry in England and Wales'; G. Rehin (1972), 'Child Guidance at the End of the Road'; DES and DHSS (March 1974), Joint Circular on Child Guidance; Court Report (1977), *Fit for the Future: The Report of the Committee on Child Health Services*; and K. Whitmore (1974), 'The Contribution of Child Guidance to the Community'.

What is offered here is a summary of the outcome of all this work.[2]

In the course of these discussions many reiterations of certain basic problems were encountered. For a start, child guidance was often seen as having something of an 'ivory tower' image. Its impact on the total problem of disturbed and maladjusted children in the community was often thought to be (for whatever reason) inadequate. There was seen to be a lack of effective machinery to allow those in child guidance to review needs more broadly, to evaluate existing services, and to join in comprehensive planning and the competition for additional resources.

Apart from this there were frequent references to confusions about the distinctive roles of each of the various professions involved, and about authority relationships between them. There was specific uncertainty, for instance, about the role of social workers in child guidance, about who should employ them, and about their proper relation to area-team-based social workers. There was specific uncertainty about the role of doctors and what 'medical cover' or clinical responsibility signified. There was much uncertainty about authority relationships between senior and junior members in any one profession, particularly for those in social work, psychology, and psychotherapy.

Generally, there was a major worry that gains and strengths that had been established in child guidance over the past years might be dissipated or lost completely in the various reorganizations contemplated.

Perhaps the most fundamental issue of all to emerge, however, was about the very nature and meaning of child guidance. Is child guidance to be conceived as a field of work of its own, distinct from child psychiatry, or school psychological services, for example? Is it a broader conception which embraces all these and other services for disturbed children as well? Or, is it (by contrast) the name for some particular method or approach which relies heavily upon, and is in effect defined by, multi-disciplinary teamwork?

[2] An earlier version of this chapter appeared in the form of cyclostyled Working Paper entitled 'Future Organization in Child Guidance and Allied Work', produced and published jointly by the Health Services Organization Research Unit and the Social Services Organization Research Unit at Brunel.

Our own line of attack on these last questions has been to start from a consideration of the whole range of possible responses to the needs of disturbed children and their families. Taking this broader vantage, it appears that there are in principle four main kinds of possible responses:

(i) those conceived primarily in terms of the prevention or cure of 'mental' illness, or the improvement of mental health – what might be called *health-centred responses*;
(ii) those conceived primarily in terms of the prevention and alleviation of social distress or breakdown: that is, in terms of improving the social functioning of disturbed children and their families in their permanent living environment – what might be called *social-services-centred responses*;
(iii) those conceived primarily in terms of dealing with educational difficulties (in their broadest sense), or with problems which immediately prevent or inhibit education – what might be called *education-centred responses*;
(iv) those concerned primarily with none of those above in particular, but with *all in equal combination*.

(That the first three, at any rate, of these conceptions link closely with existing major agencies in the British scene is a point to which we shall return.)

Now the term 'child guidance' might, with varying justification, be applied to any or all of these different responses. However, in the discussions summarized here it has tended to be used, for want of any better, as a specific label for the fourth approach outlined above. Without wanting to suggest that its use would be wrong for other approaches 'child guidance' will be used here then as the most convenient shorthand to describe any attempt to provide some combined or comprehensive response to the social, educational, and mental health problems of the disturbed child and his family, which is not primarily concerned with one of these same elements more than any other. (Whether or not any such attempt, defined precisely in these terms, is realistic is left as an open issue.)

We shall examine the various organizational models which flow from the four distinct conceptions identified above. Each of them allows the possibility of multi-disciplinary teamwork in the fullest sense. We shall see, however, that primacy (a concept carefully defined) logically rests with doctors, or perhaps a broader class of consultant therapists, in health-centred models; with social workers or other social service professionals in social-services-centred models; with educational psychologists or other educational professionals in education-centred models; and with the team as a whole in distinct 'child guidance' models. Before proceeding to this detailed examination, however, there are certain fundamental issues of relationships between and within the various professions that demand prior attention.

Basic Issues of Multi-disciplinary Teamwork
As we have said, the idea of multi-disciplinary teamwork is one which often is given prominence in discussion of the essential nature of child guidance or similar work. In its simplest form, a vivid image is frequently offered of the team as a group of equal colleagues, each drawing on different skills, each contributing freely to the common goal, and all sharing jointly the common burden of responsibility. Attractive though this picture may be, to take it as it stands is however to ignore or obscure a number of key issues which demand proper resolution (experience suggests) if amicable and productive relations between co-professionals are in fact to result.

IS IT REALLY 'MULTI-DISCIPLINARY' WORK THAT IS REQUIRED?
First, there is the question of whether 'multi-disciplinary' really means what it seems to. Is it really the work of those from a number of separate and distinct professions that is required? Here, account has to be taken of the considerable ferment and flux in which each of the four professions with which we are particularly concerned here – child psychiatry, educational psychology, psychiatric social work, and child psychotherapy – currently finds itself. There are large areas of potential, if not actual, overlap in role. It is not easy to establish with common agreement what is the distinctive competence of each. Some would even advocate a progressive merging of the four to reach an eventual 'child guidance professional'. Others would argue at least for the establishment of some composite professional

therapist, for whose practice a medical qualification, say, was incidental.

Of course, any complete merging of professions would logically destroy the very possibility of multi-disciplinary work. Only 'uni-disciplinary' collaboration could occur – though admittedly, some degree of systematic specialization within the generic profession might still be envisaged. However, on balance it seems likely that some variety of distinct professions or disciplines, whatever the overlap area of common training, knowledge or skills, will continue to exist in this field. This view is strengthened, the broader the range of possible services for disturbed children and their families that is considered. It is difficult indeed to imagine a future in which all social workers, psychiatrists, psychologists, and psychotherapists disappear into one new, common mould. We shall proceed then on the assumption of the possibility, if not the desirability indeed, of true multi-disciplinary work.

TEAMS OR NETWORKS? Even with this assumption, however, there are still some very real issues about the quality of the bonds or links between those engaged together in multi-disciplinary work. Should one be able to choose which individual colleagues to work with? Do they all have to work in the same clinic? Do they have to work there every day of the week? How far is the individual in multi-disciplinary work bound by the team approach? Exploration has shown that there is a major choice to be made in any setting as to whether it is really 'teamwork' that is required or some looser 'network' pattern.[3]

The significance of the distinction between the two models is this. In a team, practitioners are personally known to each other. They intend to work together face to face and frequently as a whole group, and to provide mutual support for an indefinite period. They are all able and willing to attend regular team meetings. They agree to conform to certain established

---

[3] There is a profound distinction here, one which goes far beyond the purlieu of child guidance or similar work to the very basis of social structure. It is that between the social *group* – a bounded entity with a clear division of members on the one side, from non-members on the other – and the social *network* – a pattern of social relationships whose links can be traced indefinitely in any direction.

common norms and procedures. It is desirable that they are all mutually acceptable as fellow members.

Teams can be built from direct appointments of members by their employers, on a full-time or sessional basis. They may also be added to by the specific mechanism of *attachment*[4] of different professionals by their immediate superiors, even where the attached members are employees of different authorities than those of pre-existing members. (An obvious example here is the attachment of community nurses or social workers to general medical practitioners.) Nevertheless, in both these cases a true team membership appears to imply the right of all pre-existing members (at least all those who are not in clearly subordinate positions, and perhaps only those with what will later be identified as having 'primacy' in the situation) to veto the appointment or attachment of new members.

By contrast, there are other situations of multi-disciplinary work where such strong personal links are not demanded. In a network situation practitioners work together who may or may not be known personally to each other, do not have to be considered for mutual personal acceptability, and do not necessarily work together face to face over extended periods of time. Good network relations can be facilitated, for example, by placing practitioners in close physical proximity in adjacent offices or clinics, or by the use of designated 'liaison' officers, or by aligning the boundaries of interacting administrative units, and so on.[5]

There are obvious pros and cons to either pattern. Teamwork tends, for example, to demand more resources of people; it assumes the need for constant interaction; and it may limit individual's opportunities for more varied experience. Networks, on the other hand, may be extended without limit; but they do not in themselves create the opportunity for such a rich interplay. Indeed, where boundaries between professions are ill-defined or in course of change, networks may fail to provide the kind of situation in which interacting participants are

[4] See Appendix B.

[5] It may be noted that 'network' is used here specifically of the relations of individual *practitioners*, wherever employed; in contrast to the reference in the Joint Circular of 1974 to 'networks of services'; though, of course, the one follows from the other.

enabled to develop better appreciation of what each has specially to offer. (The designation of specific, if temporary, teams for particular cases or projects may of course help to overcome some of these difficulties.) The choice between teamwork and network patterns is a fundamental one in considering any models for future child guidance work.

AUTHORITY RELATIONSHIPS IN MULTI-DISCIPLINARY WORK. Another idea that often appears to be taken for granted is that 'teamwork' necessarily carries with it the condition of absolute parity of status amongst members of the team, and more particularly that no one has authority over anyone else. But how far does equality really extend in the so-called equal team? Our own work has, in fact, revealed very considerable uncertainty and anxiety on this score amongst many of those working together in existing child guidance or similar teams. Often the myth of equality is confronted with the reality of the dominant role of one particular member, say the psychiatrist.

Of course, the effectiveness and morale of any team will depend on a number of things. There are the individual personalities concerned and their interplay. There is the compatibility of the theoretical approaches which various members adopt in their work. There is the collective 'style' or 'culture' that develops – formal, permissive, participative, and so on. But clarity about structural matters, like the authority, status, and responsibility, attaching to various positions, will play a major part as well. Moreover, complete parity of status with completely unstructured and spontaneous co-operation and consultation between colleagues is by no means the only possibility. Our own explorations in multi-disciplinary teams have led us to believe that what may be precisely defined as *managerial, prescribing, monitoring*, and *co-ordinating* relationships between various members all have their place in different situations.[6]

However (and it is a crucial proviso), as has been shown elsewhere[7] managerial and prescribing relationships between members of any one profession and another can only be justified in general where members of the first profession are agreed to

[6] See Appendix B for definition of these terms.
[7] See Chapter 5, 'Professionals in Health and Social Services'.

have by virtue of their training both a wider and deeper view of the issues involved.

We may here report that in no discussion undertaken so far in this particular field has any sustained case been argued on these grounds for any one profession, for example psychiatry, to have *prescriptive* authority over any other. It is assumed for the present that all the professions with which we are concerned here are to be regarded in this sense as independent, in whatever setting they may interact. At the most, therefore, we are talking about *co-ordinative* (or possibly in some specific instances, *monitoring*) relationships between members of these professions.

This would apply at any rate as far as any future models are concerned. For the present, it appears to be the case that because of considerable variations in the present extent, as well as the present level, of skills in individual social workers, psychologists, and psychotherapists, many individual psychiatrists carry something close to prescribing, if not managerial, authority to members of the other professions in existing teams. However, to repeat the point, our concern here is with models for the future.

PRIMACY AND PRIME RESPONSIBILITY. Prescribing relationships between these professions would appear then to be a non-issue, at least in principle. What has emerged, however, as a crucial issue, perhaps *the* crucial issue, is the question of where responsibility for individual cases rests in such multi-disciplinary work. The easy assumption that teams carry collective responsibility does not always survive the question of what happens when things go wrong. Here the view is sometimes expressed that it is the psychiatrist who takes 'final' or 'overall' responsibility (though this is not so likely to be said where the designated director of a clinic is, say, an educational psychologist).

In studying these matters, it has proved useful to employ the conceptions of *prime responsibility* and *primacy* where several practitioners are involved in the same case.[8] Thus, to ask in a particular case and in the setting of some given clinic whether, say, the psychiatrist carries *primacy*, that is the automatic assumption of *prime responsibility* (as we define it) in all new

[8] See the precise definitions of these terms in Appendix B, amplified in Chapter 5, 'Professionals in Health and Social Services'.

cases, is quite sharply different from asking whether he or she is simply the 'boss' (i.e. the manager, as defined here), or whether he or she is completely responsible for every decision taken.

Moreover, the carrying of prime responsibility does not deny the possibility of making referrals to other colleagues. In considering detailed organizational models we shall need in fact to take account of three distinct referral situations where one person X starts by carrying prime responsibility.

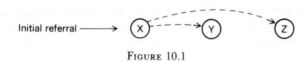

Initial referral ⟶

FIGURE 10.1

(a) *referral-for-collaboration*, that is 'consultations', requests for help in assessment, requests for specific kinds of treatment, where however X continues to retain prime responsibility;

(b) *referral-for-suggested-transfer*, where if Y, say, agrees to accept it, prime responsibility then passes to him (the initial referrer being informed presumably of this transfer);

(c) *referral-for-parallel-work*, where a new additional prime responsibility arises for some colleague working in parallel on a different aspect of the case, but in some clearly independent field (for example surgical treatment, police, or court action).

RETENTION OF SEPARATE RESPONSIBILITIES IN MULTI-DISCIPLINARY WORK. Finally, in this review of general issues in multi-disciplinary work, there is the question of the retention of separate, or basic, responsibilities by individual team members. What special responsibilities do social workers have, for example, on child-abuse cases? What special responsibilities do psychiatrists have by virtue of their medical qualifications?

Generally, it may be supposed that there is a fundamental obligation on any professional practitioner, by virtue of his professional membership, to act in certain ways in certain situations regardless of what others in the team might think. Thus, if a doctor sees signs which lead him to suspect organic illness (to take an obvious example), his professional status cannot allow him to ignore them, regardless of what his non-medical colleagues might think, or where prime responsibility might lie for the main run of work in the particular case concerned. Over and above this, if practitioners are clearly in *agency service*,[9] they will be bound as well by specific directions and policies laid down by their employees. (As in the case of suspected child-abuse, those are more likely to reinforce basic professional obligations than to run in conflict with them.) Thus, multi-disciplinary work can only ever take place within a free area bounded by various professional, agency, and legal requirements.

Intra-professional Organization

With some of the general complexities and choices of multi-disciplinary teamwork exposed, we may now complete our pre-paratory groundwork by turning to consider some basic issues of organizational structure *within* the various professional groups in child guidance. Here again, any simple notion of 'equal professionals' does not stand up to much analysis. There are obvious, and in this case specifically-designed, salary dif-ferentials. There can be little argument that there will in general be differences in individual skill, experience, and breadth of vision amongst members of any professional group, differences which salary differentials might well hope to reflect.

Using the conception of *work-strata*[10] on the one hand, and ideas of *agency service* and *independent practice* on the other,[11] let us examine briefly the situation within each of the four profes-sions with which we are chiefly concerned here.

ORGANIZATION WITHIN PSYCHIATRY. Within psychiatry there seems to be ready consensus amongst those with whom we have held discussions on what is the most appropriate model for internal structure, regardless of the setting in which work is carried out. The consultant psychiatrist is seen as in *independent*

[9] See Appendix B, and following discussion.
[10] See Chapter 7, 'The Stratification of Work and Organizational Design'.
[11] See Chapter 5, 'Professionals in Health and Social Services'.

practice and as expected to work at minimum at Stratum-3, that is as expected to make 'systematic provision' of psychiatric services. (The consultant grade is not seen, however, as limited to Stratum-3 work, but allowing within itself progression to Stratum-4 or 5 work, according to the spontaneous development of personal capability.)

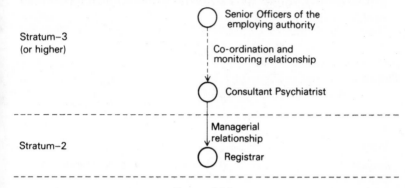

FIGURE 10.2

The registrar is seen as expected to work at Stratum-2 and subject to the managerial relationship of the consultant. Above the consultant there is no manager. Medical administrators, other senior officers of the employing authority, or medical chairmen, any of them in principle, may carry co-ordinative and monitoring roles in respect of particular issues, but they could not carry managerial authority without undermining the independent practice of the consultant.

ORGANIZATION WITHIN SOCIAL WORK. Within social work we have so far discovered no such clear consensus on either employment contract or work levels. Within settings that are clearly social-services-centred (local area social services offices or residential establishments for example), these and other discussions have suggested that the prevailing assumption is one of *agency service*.[12] Relations between social workers at successive strata are managerial, as here defined. On the other hand, in settings that are described as 'child guidance' or 'psychiatric',

[12] See Brunel Institute of Organization and Social Studies, Social Services Organization Research Unit (1974), *Social Services Departments*.

there is a tendency to move towards an *independent practice* model
for social work. Some would reinforce this idea by suggesting
that social workers in such settings were in any case more appropriately recognized and named as 'therapists'. Others would
argue strongly, however, that the presence of a generic social
work educational base was still of fundamental importance, and
a clear distinguishing mark from the basic training of the other
professions.

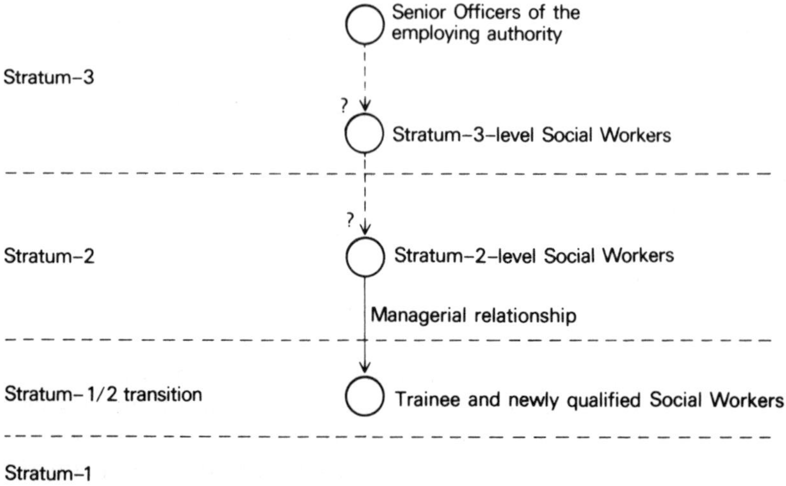

FIGURE 10.3

If this second assumption of independent practice in social
work is in fact taken, a difficult question then arises about the
proper level at which the practitioner should achieve full independence. It is generally accepted that the trainee and the
newly qualified social worker – both of whom can be located
in what may be described as the Stratum-1/2 'transitional
zone'[13] – should not have full independence but be subject to
'supervision' (that is, a *managerial* relationship in the terms used
here) by more senior colleagues. The real uncertainty arises for
fully fledged practitioners, well capable of Stratum-2 work, but
not yet (if they are ever going to be) capable of Stratum-3 work.
Should they be recognized as independent practitioners? If so,

[13] See Chapter 7, 'The Stratification of Work and Organizational Design'.

the relationship between 'principals' or other similarly designated social workers at Stratum-3 and such independent
Stratum-2-level social workers could not be stronger than monitoring or co-ordinating, without internal contradiction.

On the other hand, it might be argued that social workers,
like psychiatrists, should not be awarded full independent practitioner status until they had demonstrated a Stratum-3 level
of ability. In this latter case it would be difficult to see arguments against instituting clear managerial relationship between
Stratum-3 level 'principal' social workers of appropriate skills
and experience and such fully-fledged Stratum-2 level practitioners. Indeed, given the absence of such explicit managerial
relationships within the profession it might be that less explicit,
but nevertheless real, managerial links tended to develop outside the profession. Social workers within Stratum-2 might, for
example, see psychiatrists with whom they regularly worked,
of appropriate orientation and interests and operating at
Stratum-3 or higher, in something approaching a managerial
role.

ORGANIZATION WITHIN CHILD PSYCHOTHERAPY AND EDUCATIONAL
PSYCHOLOGY. With some of the general issues now exposed, the
situation within child psychotherapy and educational psychology can be rapidly summarized. Our discussions with child
psychotherapists have revealed that they clearly and strongly
see themselves as in *independent practice*. However, as far as discussions with educational psychologists have gone, it is still unclear
in which employment category they should be viewed. For both
these groups, if independent practice is assumed, exactly the
same question arises as for social work. Should full independence be achieved at Stratum-2 or at Stratum-3? According
to which answer is given, the same consequences would appear
to follow as for social work.

Models for Future Service
THE RANGE OF SERVICES UNDER CONSIDERATION. Coming now to
consideration of specific models for child guidance and allied
work in future, it is absolutely essential to take into account
the total range of services which may be provided for disturbed

children and their families. It has already been noted that
several fundamentally distinct kinds or conceptions of service
can be identified. Three of these – what we have labelled for
short as 'health-centred responses', 'social-services-centred responses', and 'education-centred responses' – are readily relat-
able to existing public agencies.

Now there are, and will continue to be, important arguments
about the respective functions of health, social services, and
educational agencies, and of distinctions between very general
ideas such as 'social distress', 'illness', and 'educational needs
and problems', which help define their respective roles. However, so long as these three different kinds of agency exist (as
is clearly the case at the moment in Britain, and also for the
foreseeable future) decisions are inevitable in practice as how
best to conceive or categorize the needs of any particular disturbed child or family, in terms of which one, or which combination of three different types of service, is required.

In making an approach for help to existing agencies, the
client or initial referrer will inevitably therefore have to judge
as best as he can which of three possible 'doors' he should knock
upon. (Furthermore, there may in fact be a choice of several
doors within any one major agency.) Moreover it is inevitable
that the person who responds will have to make his own best
judgment as to whether the approach is in fact appropriate,
whether it should be redirected to another agency, or whether
it should be accepted whilst attempting to involve another
agency as well. There is an obvious message here for professional training, but the hard fact must be faced that there
is an irreducible element of chance, or uncertainty, as to where
referrals or approaches are first made, and how they get subsequently dealt with, however well-organized and well-publi-
cized the agency arrangements, and however catholic the training programmes of various groups of professional employees.

Nevertheless, there are those who argue that a fourth 'door'
is vitally required in relation to the problem of disturbed children and their families. There is, therefore, in conception at any
rate, a fourth service which is specifically not labelled 'health',
'education', or 'social services', but which attempts (at least for
purposes of initial assessment) to avoid such premature labelling. In addition to the three conceptions of services for dis-

turbed children and their families just mentioned, there is what we have already opted to describe as a distinct *child guidance* response; that is one in terms of the combined social, educational, and mental health needs of the disturbed child and his family, at least (but not necessarily only) for the purpose of initial assessment. Several general points can now be made about these four possible conceptions of services, by way of clearing the ground.

First, it is obviously vital that the general public, including prime-referral agents such as schools, general practitioners, or the police, may see a clear label over each and every 'door' that may exist, and one which clearly distinguishes it from all other doors. Otherwise only confusion can result. Titles are important.

Second, the fallacy must be avoided of identifying any particular agency in principle, with a 'community' or 'institutional' approach (whatever may be the biases in their present provision). The new British Health Authorities, for example, are specifically not hospital authorities only, that is specifically not institutionally centred. Local authorities have both the power (and duty) to provide certain sorts of residential institutions as well as so-called 'community' services.

Third, it is an open question as to what range of functions any particular service or particular institution within it can most usefully undertake. At a minimum, assessment or diagnostic work will be expected. However, this may be extended if required to some direct treatment, training, or other intervention; to offering consultative or educative services to other professionals; or perhaps to various other forms of preventive work. Again, it is important to recognize that no one agency need have the monopoly of any one of these various kinds of activity.

Finally, even though a particular service is identified with, and made the prime responsibility of, one particular agency, this does not mean that it is impossible for employees of any other agency to be associated with that service. As will be discussed below, various *attachment* arrangements are possible in order to promote multi-disciplinary work in such situations. The deliberate establishment of a number of separate services, if that is what is required, does not necessarily imply the abandonment of all multi-disciplinary teamwork.

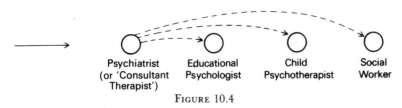

Psychiatrist	Educational	Child	Social
(or 'Consultant	Psychologist	Psychotherapist	Worker
Therapist')			

FIGURE 10.4

MODELS OF HEALTH-CENTRED SERVICES. It is clear that health authorities have the right, indeed arguably the duty, as part of their responsibility for the provision of comprehensive health services, to provide specialist services for children who may be described as 'mentally ill'. This they could do by employing in the first instance either consultant child psychiatrists, or possibly a broader category of 'consultant child therapists' not necessarily medically qualified, who in addition to being thought of as carrying consultant status, would also be considered to be able to take direct referrals in their own right. (In this second case the question of the necessary training, experience, and qualifications to fill such a position would need to be further explored, and also the minimum level of work required.)

Such health-centred services might naturally be referred to as 'psychiatric' or 'mental health' services rather than 'child guidance'. As we have indicated, they could include both services thought of as 'hospital-based' or 'community-based'; but in all cases it would be the responsibility of the Health Authorities to provide premises and supporting services.

Detailed features of the consequent organization might be as follows. For a start, all referrals would be directly to a psychiatrist (or, in the second possibility above, to a designated consultant therapist). Given the availability of other parallel services, the psychiatrist (or consultant therapist) in this situation might choose to refer specific cases to social services, or to school psychological services, or to other health services, either for proposed transfer or for work in parallel (see earlier discussion). In this way *networks* of practitioner relationships would be activated.

If it was felt desirable to build a more closely-working or extended multi-disciplinary *team* around the psychiatrist, this might be achieved by all or any of the following steps:

(a) the permanent appointment of child psychotherapists by the Health Authority, to work in conjunction with the psychiatrist;

(b) the *attachment* of educational psychologists by the Education Authority (or possibly the direct appointment of clinical psychologists instead?);

(c) the *attachment* of suitably-skilled social workers by the Social Services Authority or the Education Authority, whichever employed them.

To reiterate the point, it is assumed that the psychiatrist would possess *primacy* (as we have specifically defined it) in this situation, though he would not carry *managerial* or *prescribing* authority in relation to members of other professions. Where the psychiatrist spent a significant portion of the time away from the clinic, he would clearly need a deputy. It is doubtful if this role could be satisfactorily filled by a member of another discipline, let alone an employee of another authority. (What is at issue here is delegation of responsibility, not transfer.) Presumably only one of his own juniors, or one of his other psychiatrist colleagues, could realistically stand in for him.

The psychiatrist (or consultant therapist), assumed to be at Stratum-3, would naturally take the leading role here in system-development work, though other team members, particularly any who were also capable of Stratum-3 work, might be expected to play a very significant part as well. If a formally-identified 'clinic director' or similar post was required for internal or external purposes, it would in this situation also naturally rest with the consultant psychiatrist (or consultant therapist); or, where several were working in parallel in the same clinic, with any one of them. However, the authority implicit in such a role would be no more than *co-ordinative* (with possibly some additional *monitoring* component on such things as adherence to minimal standards of work or behaviour). Thus, whether the actual title 'director' would be the most appropriate is a debatable matter.

MODELS OF SOCIAL-SERVICES-CENTRED SERVICES. It is abundantly clear that many referrals or approaches concerning disturbed children are made directly to social workers employed as agents

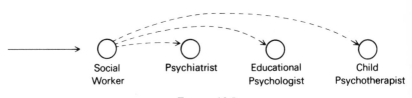

FIGURE 10.5

of the local social services authority, for example the countless referrals of children in need of care, protection, or control. In some situations, notably that of 'observation–assessment centres', psychiatrists, educational psychologists, and sometimes child psychotherapists are also regularly involved thereafter (whether or not as part of a team or simply a close-linked network). Nevertheless, it is the responsibility of the local authority to provide buildings and supportive services in such settings. Referrals by social workers to psychiatrists and other professionals in these particular settings are 'referrals-for-collaboration' (as we identified them earlier), at least whilst the child remains in the care of the local authority. *Prime responsibility* in such cases clearly rests with the social workers concerned.

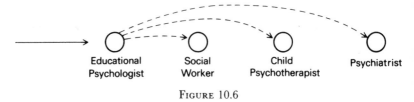

FIGURE 10.6

MODELS OF EDUCATION-CENTRED SERVICES. It is also apparent that Education Authorities have the right to establish services under titles like 'school psychological services' to cope with the educational, learning, or behavioural problems of young people discovered in schools or other educational establishments. Here referrals are directly to psychologists, more particularly educational psychologists. Sometimes the latter may then have the opportunity, if they wish, of referring-for-collaboration to a more extended team, including attached social workers, child psychotherapists, or psychiatrists who provide regular 'sessions' in the school psychological service. In this particular circumstance, however, prime responsibility remains with the educational psychologist. If there is no extended team, there is still the possibility of re-referring particular cases to specialist psychiatric services, or to social services departments (as described above), with either transfer, or work-in-parallel, in mind.

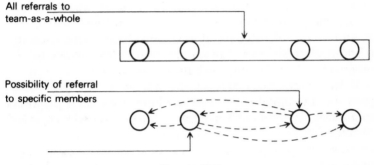

FIGURE 10.7

MODELS FOR A DISTINCT 'CHILD GUIDANCE SERVICE'. As we have seen, there is an important argument to be considered for establishing a 'fourth door' – a distinctive 'child guidance service' – in addition to whatever separate social services, educational services, and mental health services for disturbed children might exist. This fourth service might be expected to provide assessments only, or in addition certain specific kinds of further treatment, or certain kinds of consultancy or educative work. Such a service would call for very distinctive organizational forms. There is a strong implicit assumption that the close and regular collaboration of those from all four main disciplines is called for. That is, there is a strong assumption of teamwork, not just a network situation. However, there would be important differences according to whether all referrals were regarded, as a matter of principle, as being to the team as a whole (with perhaps some agreed pre-screening by individuals), or whether referrals to various individual members would be acceptable.

If the starting notion were one of referral to the team as a whole, no member or discipline could have primacy (that is, automatic prime responsibility). Each referral would be discussed by the full team, or a fully representative group, who would then agree who was to carry prime responsibility in the particular case concerned. A difficult issue would arise about action in disputed cases. What would happen when there was a real clash of professional judgments on appropriate action? Voting would clearly be inappropriate, but on the other hand, no one person would have an obvious right of final decision. Disagreements would presumably have to be talked through until some proposed course of action was reached which was, at minimum, tolerable to all members of the team. (Any distinction of those with 'consultant status' from trainees and others would, no doubt, have implications here.)

If, by contrast, referral to specific individuals was acceptable, then the individual concerned would clearly retain prime responsibility, at least until such time as he negotiated its transfer. Presumably, in this situation, each person would use team meetings as an opportunity to discuss their own cases, and to negotiate for the involvement of other team members in assessment or treatment, as required. It would need to be clearly established which team members were of 'consultant' status, and able to receive direct referrals in their own right. (If consultant status were achieved at Stratum-2 in some professional groups, and Stratum-3 in others, it might of course be wondered again how equal in reality were the so-called 'equal partners'.) Consultant status would imply the ability and willingness to take final responsibility for taking decisions about all or any issues, other than those of organic illness, which might arise. Trainees, for example, would clearly not be in this position. Presumably – in keeping with the spirit of multi-disciplinary approach – particular members would still retain distinct professional identities as psychiatrists, child psychotherapists, educational psychologists, or social workers, even though any might in principle receive referrals.

However, it must be questioned whether such a situation, where individuals from different disciplines could receive, and if necessary deal with, their own cases, as distinct from one in which the combined resources of the multi-disciplinary team was brought to bear automatically in each case, is really compatible with the basic assumption of this fourth approach. Would it be sufficiently distinct from a possible network of social-services-based, education-based, and health-based multi-disciplinary teams (as described above) to justify the establishment of a fourth service? Would, in other words, the ability to receive individual referrals not undercut the basic philosophy of a distinct 'child guidance service', which was intrinsically (and invariably) multi-disciplinary in its approach?

In any model which truly reflected the basic philosophy of this fourth approach it might be difficult furthermore to envisage a situation where any members were in an *agency service*, with strong, if not overriding, obligations to the specific needs of their employers. It seems probable, that is, that this model implies *independent practice* for all members, apart from those in a trainee stage. (Again, the question arises of whether this could properly be conferred at Stratum-2.)

As we have said, it seems clear that in a distinct child guidance service of the kind described here, there would be no fixed primacy for any one profession. It follows that no one profession would offer an automatic choice for the role of 'clinic leader'. Presumably, systematic development of services and clinic administrative matters would involve all the staff to some extent, but particularly any senior staff in Stratum-3. If a formally designated leader were needed he could be selected (by either election or appointment) from any of the more senior practitioners, whatever their professional disciplines.

Furthermore, there does not appear to be any general case (local circumstances apart) for any one of the major agencies regularly taking the prime role in establishing and fostering the service, and providing premises and supporting facilities. It is possible that the various professions could be employed by different and various agencies as at present. Provision of facilities and other general financial support, however, would logically be a joint matter for education, health, and social services. Thus, an effective joint planning mechanism would be required (see discussion to follow), and accountability for the adequacy of the service as a whole would inevitably be shared.

If this last situation of joint-sponsoring and joint-accountability were felt to be an unsatisfactory basis for any permanent service, then logic would appear to dictate the necessity of establishing separate 'child guidance' authorities – of appropriate scale – on a statutory basis. Such authorities would have to have their own powers to acquire or build premises, hire staff, and operate this special service, distinct from health, social, or educational services. One major question which would follow would be how to prevent professional employees of such an authority from getting cut off from the main body of their fellows employed in other agencies. More basic than this, however, is the very viability of such a conception of a separately-financed 'child guidance' authority in the public service world in Britain, as we know it and as it has developed. (Any who doubt the reality of such a proposition need perhaps to go back and examine again their own view of the validity of the basic assumptions which we have just explicated, for such a 'fourth service'.)

COMPREHENSIVE PLANNING AND DEVELOPMENT. This last question leads naturally to another topic identified at the start. Going beyond interaction in specific cases, there is the question of how adequate arrangements are to be made in any future disposition of services, for a more comprehensive evaluation of the basic needs of disturbed children and their families as a whole in the community, for a more comprehensive review of how well existing ranges of services are meeting them, and for more comprehensive long-term planning and development (with all its concomitants of staff establishment, buildings, and finance). Put another way, the question is how to establish mechanisms by which effective Strata-4 and 5 levels of response can be made in this broad field of need.

From what has been said already this necessarily means considering in conjunction the needs of not just one, but of a whole network of services. The activities of at least three agencies – health, social services, and education – are involved; and conceivably those of a fourth possible agency as well – a distinct 'child guidance' agency.

On the social services side prime responsibility for such higher level work obviously rests with local Social Services Authorities. Considering the level of work concerned, the direct involvement of the Director of Social Services or somebody of Assistant Director level is clearly implied,[14] although more senior social work practitioners might also be involved in the planning process. A similar analysis would apply to the comprehensive planning of education-centred services. For health-

[14] See Chapter 7, 'The Stratification of Work and Organizational Design'.

centred services, medical administrators and community physicians are expected to play a major role in planning at this level (though they do not, of course, carry managerial authority in such work). Child psychiatrists would obviously need to be involved through medical representatives, if not directly, in future planning of what would clearly be identified as 'child psychiatric' or 'mental health' services. Mechanisms would have to be explored to allow the involvement of other health-services-employed staff, particularly again the more senior practitioners.

However, leaving aside for the moment the additional existence of a distinct child guidance service, the inter-relation of health, education, and social services in meeting the problems of disturbed children is so clear that there appears to be the strongest case for introducing some regular *joint planning* mechanism, in addition to whatever separate planning is needed. This might best be undertaken by a joint officer planning group for services for disturbed children, established under the aegis of the Joint Consultative Committee (between Health Authorities and local authorities).[15]

Again, if effective work were to be done by such a working group, it would need to include officers of Stratum-4 or 5 level from all three services, as well as representatives of senior practitioners from various settings involved.

Given the existence of a distinct child guidance service, such a joint planning group at senior officer level would be no less necessary. Indeed, if such a fourth service were to depend on joint-financing by health, social services, and education, the formation of such a group would be vital. Even given control and funding by a distinct 'child guidance' authority, there would be the strongest case for a permanent joint officer working group to consider the production of co-ordinated plans for what would now be not three, but four, separate services.

MAKING CHOICES. Here then are a range of models of services of various kinds in the broad field of the needs of disturbed children and their families. The detailed models described all attempt to come to terms with certain fundamental questions, which demand some answers. For a start, there is the question

[15] See Chapter 17, 'Collaboration between Health and Social Services'.

of which agency or agencies are to carry prime responsibility for financing and developing the particular service. Beyond this, there are the questions of where responsibility for individual cases rests, of what authority relationships hold between members of different disciplines, and of what authority relationships hold within particular discipline groups. It is difficult to see how any adequate proposals for future organization can avoid some specific answers to such basic matters.

All the models described leave open, however, questions of another kind: the exact role and contribution of each discipline, the most appropriate technical modes of work to adopt (psychodynamic, behavioural, etc.) or the most appropriate range or mixture of diagnostic, treatment, and preventive functions to be undertaken. There is, and will likely continue to be, much discussion and indeed controversy about these latter issues. It is therefore important, whatever organizational frameworks are adopted, that they leave room for difference and spontaneous developmental change in respect of them.

Two practical issues face the service at the time of writing. The more immediate is consideration of the future role and organizational location of *existing* 'child guidance' clinic staff. Such existing multi-disciplinary teams are usually supported at present by either Health Authorities or Education Authorities. In the light of this analysis it would seem that the most obvious possibilities[16] for their future are:

(a) to recognize them explicitly as 'child psychiatric' or 'child and family psychiatric' teams (or some such name) of a kind precisely identified in the text above, with all that follows; or

(b) to recognize them explicitly as 'school psychological service' teams (or some such name) of the precise kind identified again, with all that follows; or

(c) to recognize perhaps that both kinds of team exist in embryonic form in certain given clinic sites, and to expli-

---

[16] Here of course, only general needs and characteristics can be considered. Obviously in any particular case, due weight will have to be given as well to a number of local and specific factors; the specific financial situation in each of the interested agencies, geographical factors, local interest groups, personalities, and so on.

citly distinguish and separately establish both in future;
or

(d) to move deliberately to the sort of distinct 'child guidance' team identified, with all again that follows (such
as all referrals being in principle to the full team, no primacy, independent practice perhaps, and the rest).

However, it would be a great mistake to see the only need
as one of specifying more clearly the identity and modes of
working of existing teams. The larger issue is what pattern of
organization of services is required to meet the needs in general
of disturbed children and their families more comprehensively
in future. Examining this broader question, it seems unlikely
that any decision could be taken *not* to develop health-centred
services of some kind (specifically mental health services), or
social-services-centred facilities, or school psychological services. And if these three kinds of services are to continue, an
adequate network of linkages must clearly be developed
between them.

Perhaps it is the case, then, that the most crucial issues for
the future all hinge around the development of multi-disciplinary teamwork, if indeed this is what is really needed. Should
each of these basic services be developing its own multi-disciplinary teams (using 'team' here as earlier defined)? Does the
ultimate logic of the full-scale multi-disciplinary approach lead
inexorably to the conception of the distinct 'child guidance'
team, oriented primarily to neither health, social, nor educational problems? If this latter development is what is really
required, how far could additional multi-disciplinary teamwork be justified in distinct health, social services, and educational settings as well? For the present, our own work leaves
all these questions quite open.

11

'Full-time' and 'Part-time' Patients: an Analysis of Patient Needs and their Implications for Domiciliary and Institutional Care[1]

Stephen Cang

Background and Summary

Looking after the sick at home has always been hard and demanding work. The technological, professional, and social changes of the last half century or so in medicine and related fields, coupled with massive changes in the form and functioning of centrally sponsored, or even centrally run, health services had together resulted in the virtual disappearance of domiciliary care. In recent years, concern over the impersonal character of large scale and institutionally based services, lately reinforced by the search for savings in outlay on buildings and maintenance, have provided the impetus for a fresh look at the nature and potential of health services brought to the patient in his home.

This chapter is based on an examination of one particular form of health service: what for example in the USA and Canada is called 'Home Care', in Adelaide the Domiciliary Care Service, in Auckland the Extra-Mural Hospital, in Finland the Home Care Scheme, and in France, 'Hospitalisation à Domicile'. The French services of this type have in particular proved worth consideration first of all because of the extent to

---

[1] Preliminary statements of some of the contents of this chapter have appeared in (i) Cang (1976/7), *Age Concern Today*. (ii) Cang (1977), *Lancet*. (iii) Cang and Clarke (1978), *Community Health*. Fuller discussion of the material contained in this chapter is to be found in Cang and Clarke (1978), *Hospital at Home*.

which their aim is to provide at home the kind of treatment (in the broad sense of the term) which is normally only to be found in a hospital, as against schemes which are in effect services to facilitate early discharge from hospital, such as the recent experiment in the Medway District in Kent. A second reason is that one of the services there, at Bayonne in S.W. France, specifically aims to offer the patient the choice of whether to be hospitalized at home or in hospital (given medical feasibility).[2] The idea of hospital as the only form of serious medical care has become so engrained that it is at times hard to recall that some 90 per cent of all work with patients is performed in general practice and without reference to hospital. Nevertheless, the expectation remains that serious medical conditions (using 'medical' throughout this chapter in its widest sense, to embrace not only surgery but also all other forms of professional help in the health field) can be dealt with only in hospital. It should be noted that what patients feel is serious is not necessarily restricted to what doctors or other professionals see as serious; for the latter seriousness is generally assessed in terms of the technical challenge offered to diagnostic, therapeutic, or rehabilitative skills; for the patient, however, technically quite simple conditions may be very serious in terms of disturbance to his way of life or emotional experience. I argue below that humanity in the provision of services will entail the recognition *in action* (i.e. in the form and manner of service provision) that it is how the patient feels that counts. The danger is always of basing organization on an insufficiently clear or accurate perceptions of patient needs, resulting in neat administrative categories which override patient-experience. The term 'patient-centred services' is indeed a curious one in the context of services whose centre or *raison d'être* should be the patient in the first place.

The possibility of patients having a choice as to where they are treated tends to arouse surprise or even ridicule, so usual has it become to picture the patient as the passive recipient of the fruits of expert planning and expert technology.[3] Our examination of domiciliary treatment for serious illness will

[2] Finanacial support from the Nuffield Foundation for examination of the French services in their setting is gratefully acknowledged.
[3] See for example: J. R. Butler and M. Pearson (1970), 'Who Goes Home?'

demonstrate how such a view of the patient helps to dehumanize him, his treatment, and the service which gives it.

We shall examine experience in the domiciliary context, i.e. where the institutional setting is withdrawn, and see the implications for him and his family, as well as further implications for GPs, hospitals, the nursing profession, and all health professionals whose work relates to people suffering from conditions which do not inevitably require to be dealt with inside hospital.[4] We shall also consider the implications for family life and for neighbourhood relationships.

Our review of the planning and organization of domiciliary health care will make it necessary to consider the absence of two concepts: that of a 'patient'; and that of the basic needs of a patient, distinguishing such needs from purely social ones. It will then be clear that because a patient does not cease to be a person his basic human needs remain part of his experience as a patient and indeed *a fortiori*. Using the two concepts mentioned we can then take account of the distinction between what I wish to call 'Full-time' and 'Part-time' patients, which seems to be essential for the planning and organization of requisite services, and which can help to clarify the proper meaning of hospital care as against out-patient care. This distinction is basic to the analysis of the position of the Primary Health Care Team and its relationship to the so-called 'Hospital at Home' schemes.

Before embarking on the detailed discussion of domiciliary care, it should be emphasized that what follows applies to somatic disturbances only, i.e. physical illness whatever may be its cause. The question of so-called mental illness is quite another matter.

The Meaning of a Full-scale Domiciliary Health Service

The existence of numerous schemes around the world suggests that there is no intrinsic difficulty about arranging for the treatment of many patients at home. The number of conditions which necessitate hospitalization is rather smaller than might be supposed, being limited to those requiring operating theatre facilities or other non-transportable technical equipment, and those in which the isolation of the patient is

[4] W. Holland and S. Gilderdale (1976), 'Principles and Policies'.

imperative. Home treatment services which have been in operation for between ten and twenty years in France may be taken as an example of how such schemes work. The account below covers the main points. Fuller description may be found elsewhere.[5, 6]

A patient falls ill and calls his doctor, who judges that hospital care is required. Medically it is no problem to carry out the work at home. The patient and family are offered the choice of hospitalization in hospital or at home. If they so wish, a request is made to the Home Service. A careful assessment is made of the physical environment, the psychological and social realities of the situation, the material and equipment necessary, and the kind and amount of staff time needed. This assessment is carried out in France by social workers, who until recently had always undergone nursing training before specializing in social work so that they were 'medical' social workers, specially familiar with the problems of looking after patients and versed in the often delicate psychological and social realities of patient-family relations.

It can be seen that a home treatment situation requires the active consent of several parties: the GP; the patient; his family; those responsible for providing the home service; and the hospital consultant if one is involved. The refusal of any one of these parties renders the home treatment infeasible. Many reasons of course might lead to such a refusal. The GP might not feel secure, fearing some major change in the patient's condition which would require technical and specialist attention leading him to judge that hospitalization in hospital was the only realistic choice; or the patient might prefer hospital – he might feel more reassured there, or not feel he wished to be in his home setting while ill; or the relatives might on reflection come to feel that they could not cope adequately with having the patient at home; or the service might judge that the physical conditions or the social ones were insufficient to allow them to do their work; or the hospital consultant might not feel he could contribute properly in a non-hospital setting. Each of these judgments is a matter for the individual or service concerned.

[5] Cang and Clarke (in press), *Hospital at Home*.
[6] Cang (1976/77), *Age Concern Today*.

Once established, however, the patient and family are assured of specified attention at given times and for given purposes. In some French schemes the GP is bound by statute to visit twice a week; the amount of nursing care of various sorts is specified; home help may be provided, and so on. This is the scheme in essence. Patients are admitted to it and discharged from it exactly as if it were a concrete hospital. The scheme in Bayonne recognizes that patients vary in the intensity of care they require and admits into one of three categories of amounts of care accordingly, varying the category as changes come about in the patient's state. The main reason for the categories, which specify the maximum number of hours of nursing time per day, relates to the French financial system for the funding of health care and does not bear on the main issues with which we are here concerned. Nevertheless, admission, discharge, and categorization lead on to a basic problem: how to ensure that neither too much, nor too little, attention is given to patients at home, whether in terms of the intensity of staff time or the overall duration of their 'stay' in hospital-at-home.

It is worth remarking that this question arises much more sharply in relation to home treatment than when hospital is the setting. This is partly because in hospital all the services are there anyway and no extra resources are furnished for each individual admission; and partly because whereas hospital is *only* an environment for the sick and which they leave as soon as they can, home in the case of a home care patient is *both* his hospital and his home, so that it becomes the more necessary to find a clear way of judging when he no longer needs hospital services in his home. In other words, the removal of the hospital setting raises the question of how a patient is defined, so that we can tell when he becomes and when he ceases to be a patient. What then is a 'patient'?

The Concept of a 'Patient'

Let us begin with a brief diversion into 'patient needs'. Because the status of 'patient' naturally arises with illness, it tends to be these aspects of a person connected with illness and its treatment that first preoccupy us when defining a patient. One thinks of doctors and nurses, drugs and dressings, sophisticated materials and equipment, specialized diagnostic and therapeutic activities of many kinds. In the hospital context, such an approach goes unremarked, because much is taken for granted. But if a home treatment is considered, the first issues to be settled are not to do with the illness but with the patient as a person: that is, we need to consider basic human needs and how these are to be met.

By basic human need is meant those needs which any normal human being in our social context would be held to require as a minimum, consistent with whatever norms operate at the time. There is thus nothing given or unalterable about them: in different societies at different times the very content of Basic Human Need, and certainly the level of provision, might be stated in quite different terms from those I now wish to discuss, and which might apply in Western Europe in 1978.

The proposition is that for a normal person Basic Human Need consists of:

(a) adequate food to live on, i.e. more than mere subsistence;
(b) adequate physical comfort: somewhere to live; something to sleep on; warmth; probably somewhere to sit;
(c) adequate contact with others, not in the psychological sense but simply in terms of seeing and being with others for at least some minimum amount of time per day or per week.

The content of this proposition is testable by asking whether or not someone lacking whatever is judged adequate in the respects mentioned would or would not be felt to be in some kind of 'social need'? In other words, in our present social context, it is assumed that there is something wrong if such minimum needs are not met. (It is not necessary to agree or disagree the proposed content of Basic Human Need; it is sufficient to my argument to agree that there is such a thing as Basic Human Need and that it is describable and definable in principle.)

If the existence of Basic Human Need can be agreed, it now becomes possible to state that in illness Basic Human Need (a) does not disappear and indeed (b) may be all the more important. Just how it changes will depend on the circumstances of each case – but any illness will make each component of Basic Human Need more sensitive. A patient does not cease to be a person, although not every person is a patient. Thus the next step in our analysis is the recognition that a patient must be assured of Basic Human Need, and at a level that takes account of his illness and treatment. The proposition is therefore that a doctor would seek to ensure that a patient had adequate food and other conditions *as part and parcel of being a patient* and undergoing treatment.

This seemingly obvious point does not emerge in hospital, where food, physical comfort, and other people are automatically to be found. (There are of course differences of view about the adequacy of such provision: the food may be judged poor, or the social isolation of hospital patients may be felt as too great; but *some* provision is assured under all the Basic Human Need headings.) It is quite otherwise in the case of home treatment. Here explicit checks have to be made about Basic Human Need: how will the patient be fed? Who will get the food in and prepare and serve it? Who will keep the sick room clean enough? Who will 'be around' to keep the patient company for at least a proportion of the time?

It may be noted in passing that when hospitals were first 'invented', what they provided was in effect Basic Human Need for those who could not furnish themselves – a clear recognition that in illness Basic Human Need is even more important than in health; that is to say, an ill person *must* be assured of Basic Human Need if possible, since Basic Human Need is the indispensable basis for healthy living. Of course it does not of itself ensure health; nor does it constitute all of the basic needs of patients (see below). Indeed, Basic Human Need under conditions of illness may well differ from Basic Human Need in health: food requirements may be special; the physical surroundings may need modification or some particular provision; and the company provided to the patient may not be just anyone – a dying patient for example may in certain cases need *not* to be with particular members of his circle.

As hospitals have moved towards more technical and specialized work, there has arisen a tendency to regard Basic Human Need as distinct from the work of health care and to label it as 'social need', giving rise to resentment at the hospitalization of so-called 'social admissions'. Yet if Basic Human Need is part of being a patient and not something split off from it, then hospitalization is logical for patients unable to assume responsibility for covering their own Basic Human Need – unless Basic Human Need can be provided outside hospital. The essential point here is that if the analysis of 'patient' as someone requiring provision for Basic Human Need is correct, then it becomes a health service *responsibility* to ensure that patients are so provided if need be, whether or not the health service in question itself does the providing. It would clearly be insufficient, however, to provide for Basic Human Need *for patients* by leaving it to the local authority to provide if they agreed to do so; since this would not be an adequate guarantee that what we may now term Basic Patient Need, which *includes* Basic Human Need, would be met.

We must now return to the definition of a patient, having established that Basic Human Need must remain at the core of the definition of patient need because ordinary needs form an integral part of being a patient. What distinguishes a patient from a person? It is evidently not the mere fact of being ill. There is reason to suppose that much illness never entails any professional intervention whatsoever.[7] For everyone who presents himself to a doctor there are likely to be several other sufferers from the same symptoms who might seek out respectively a chemist, a patent remedy, a friend, some unorthodox solution, or who indeed may take no action at all but simply trust that the symptoms will disappear as mysteriously as they came. A patient then is a particular kind of sufferer – one who seeks help from his own (or a) doctor, *and* who is accepted by the doctor as being in need of 'medical' attention of some kind. Both elements must be present: nothing arises if the patient fails to present himself; but equally no health care is provided if the doctor judges that no illness exists. (The reader is reminded that this chapter considers only those whose complaint arises in somatic form.)

Basic Needs of Patients
We can proceed to consider next what the basic needs of any patient are. Indeed, it might be asked whether such a notion is likely to have reality, given the enormous diversity of human

[7] See e.g., G. Stimson and B. Webb (1975), *Going to see the Doctor*. N. Kessel and M. Shepherd (1965), 'The Health Attitudes of Persons who seldom consult a doctor', pp. 6–10.

constitutions and the ills that can afflict them? I believe that a concept of basic patient need does underlie our experience and our thinking about patient care. The proposition can be stated as follows.

Basic Patient Need for any patient (as defined above) is as a minimum:

(i) the surveillance of a doctor, covering diagnostic, therapeutic, and rehabilitative activity;

(ii) 'looking after' – what may be called nursing (with a small 'n'), which is discussed more fully below, but which may be taken to mean general care for the patient and his comfort, including whatever is necessary for his ordinary physical and emotional well-being, keeping him clean and attending to wounds and medicaments etc.;

(iii) active co-ordination of his experience as a patient. By this is meant *not* the co-ordination of services for the patient: a function which those responsible for his care must of course also carry out. We mean here, however, a different function; one that relates to the patient's state of mind rather than to the services he may be receiving. It is the function of meeting a patient's normal concern about his condition and its prospects. This function may be carried out by the GP, or in hospital by the ward sister and consultant between them; or it may not be explicitly provided for or met at all, in which case patients feel anxious and not adequately 'treated' as patients. Further analysis of the medical role might show that this co-ordinative responsibility requisitely belongs to the doctor and that in pre-technical days doctors did indeed carry it out. With increasing specialization and technical activity, this same work has become both more necessary and harder to carry out;

and, of course, at the core of it all,

(iv) Basic Human Needs, modified as may be judged necessary in relation to the illness.

It should be emphasized that the proposition simply states what any patient's needs are. It makes no assumptions about *how* these are or should be met, though ordinary illustrations have been given.

The argument so far can be summarized diagrammatically as in Table 11.1 thus:

TABLE 11.1

Basic patient need
{
1. Doctoring
2. nursing
3. co-ordination of illness and treatment

and

4. Basic human need – Food
                 – Physical
                   environment
                 – Social
                   contact
}

For completeness, we may add that of course for many patients a variety of special needs arise, depending on their diagnosis. Special Patient Needs will be needs for medical specialties (e.g. surgery, cardiology, radiology, pathology, *et al.*), for other specialties in the field (e.g. remedial therapy, chiropody, medical social work) and for any materials and equipment that may be needed. But these will be *ad hoc* – many patients will have no need of anything beyond Basic Patient Need.

'Full-time Patients' and 'Part-time Patients'

We are now almost ready to return to that consideration of domiciliary care which first showed us the need to define 'a patient' and what patients need. Before doing so, we must take account of one further characteristic of patient experience – its variability in terms of the extent to which a patient is rendered incapable of looking after himself. I find it convenient to distinguish between 'full-time' patients and 'part-time' ones, a distinction which seems readily enough perceived by patients, GPs, and nursing staff both in France and here.

Since the distinction has nothing to do with ordinary *clock* time, either the patient's or that of the service caring for him, more logical labels might be 'Fully-dependent' and 'Partly-dependent' patients; such terminology is however cumbersome.

Two reasons are therefore advanced for retaining 'full-time' and 'part-time'. First, they are easier terms to use. Secondly, they reflect an underlying sense that in *psychological* time[8] one may feel 'full-' or 'part-time' and that this feeling is generally related to the degree of dependence involved. The two types of patient may be described as follows. A *part-time patient* is one who, while a patient as defined above, is nevertheless not in need of overall care from others. He can still 'look after himself' without serious shortcomings in relation to Basic Patient Need which includes Basic Human Need. This radically affects the form which medical attention can take, and its delivery in time and space can be planned in the context of the patient's co-operation: he can attend his doctor, or an out-patient clinic if specialist work is needed; or even if he cannot leave his home for some reason, the provision of the necessary discrete procedures of medical or nursing help by a primary care team are quite adequate. An example might be an otherwise healthy person with a poisoned finger or toe, living in normal social circumstances, i.e. where neither Basic Human Need nor nursing are issues by virtue of his complaint.

By contrast, a *full-time patient* is an individual, let us say with the same complaint, but for whom the effects are much more serious; as they would be for a small child who might be quite unable psychologically to cope with such a problem without a lot of 'looking after'; or as they might be for someone who already has an arthritic other arm and for whom a poisoned finger on the good hand means an inability to cope alone with the preparation of food or simple toilet tasks. He cannot 'look after himself'.

The Full-time Patient needs help with Basic Human Need and with nursing, not because of the diagnosis but because the realities of his position result in a different level of need: he cannot meet all his own Basic Human Needs, nor all his own Basic Patient Needs. Help therefore is required. This time different consequences arise for the form, content, and organization of health care. Such a patient's needs can either be met by taking him into hospital or by providing for them at home.

It may be seen that the distinction between Full-time Patient and Part-time Patient is independent of diagnosis. How then can it be known whether a given patient is full-time or part-time? The answer is that an assessment requires to be made

[8] E. Jaques (in press), *The Form of Time.*

in each case – in itself already a humane proceeding – and that the outcome will depend on many factors. Among these we may number such facts as: the extent to which the patient is able to 'cope' with the illness emotionally – X is able metaphorically to take a poisoned toe in his stride while for Y it is much more of a personal burden – he has never been particularly good at coping with adversity; the realities of the individual's social context – X lives with an energetic spouse, well able to supply Basic Human Need and some of the less specialized elements in 'nursing' while Y's spouse is crippled or blind or very anxious or dead – he therefore needs the 'looking after' as well as the specialized nursing procedures involved; X lives on the ground floor and can hobble about, while Y's dwelling has stairs and no lavatory on the bedroom floor. And so on: it is the need to judge each case individually which offers the possibility of an increased humanity in dealing with individuals' problems.

The work of such an assessment requires skill in gauging what patients, relatives, and neighbours can actually do in relation to what needs to be done. The conceptualization of Basic Human Need and Basic Patient Need may help to clarify what should be assessed.

We may note briefly here that one reason why elderly patients (whatever their medical situation) constitute such a problem to the NHS is that it is in this group especially that one finds difficulties in covering Basic Human Need and nursing. These difficulties appear to come about for a number of reasons, such as: relative poverty in old age; smaller social circle and/or family; changes in content of Basic Human Need (e.g. more warmth may be needed as people get older), and Basic Patient Need so that the content of nursing (though not Nursing) may be more comprehensive, and the co-ordinative function more important. The combination in many elderly people of more prominent Basic Human Needs and of more obviously straightforward medical problems brings out especially clearly that hospitalization is undertaken *only* because *that* is where such Basic Patient Need and Basic Human Need can be provided, which in turn tends to reinforce irritation that hospitals are meeting 'social needs'. The various 'half-way' steps which have been devised, such as day hospitals of various kinds, can be seen as attempts to provide Basic Patient Need and Basic

Human Need. There remains, however, the idea that such 'social' activities are not truly part of NHS provision. The real question is whether those so served are or are not patients.

The reader will have realized that apart from the question of how Basic Human Need is covered, two elements in Basic Patient Need become crucial in the Full-time patient/Part-time Patient distinction: the question of 'nursing' and the work of 'co-ordination'. Each of these needs to be discussed, following which the question of domiciliary treatment can be reopened, when it may be found that several organizational problems will appear less obscure than when we began.

The Meaning and Role of Nursing

The fastidious reader may have noticed (and the pedantic will certainly have done so) that nursing has been spelled with both upper and lower case Ns. This is no printer's whim: the use of Nursing and nursing is intended to reflect what many people (nurses, other professionals, patients, and the public at large) are increasingly beginning to notice, both here and in other countries. The French report the phenomenon and it is well advanced in the USA. The matter concerns the increasing tendency of the nursing profession to disown what might be called Basic Nursing (nursing) in favour of the specialized and more technical work (Nursing).

The well-known phrase 'non-nursing duties' has opened the way to a split between tasks thought not to require specialized training and those which have been judged as more in line with professional aspirations. This is not the place to pursue the logical consequences of such thinking. Its effects however are serious in that there is increasing difficulty over the proper structuring (i.e. recruitment, training, control, and normal working) of what used simply to be called nursing.

The basic work of caring for the sick has acquired the status of less important, menial work, unfit for true professionals and something of an embarrassment, therefore, to an aspiring profession. At the same time, the work remains to be done and those who have ever had need of nursing might not agree so readily that it is menial and unskilled work. Part of the difficulty in achieving clarity in this area is that in relation to the sick the term 'looking after' appears to cover *both* activities which any normal person could be expected to perform, such as fetching a glass of water, plumping up the pillows and so on; *and* the rather more specialized work of taking temperatures, attending to basic toilet needs, and generally keeping the patient comfortable in bed.

The way forward would appear to lie in recognizing the distinction between professional work at Stratum-2 and above and skilled work at Stratum-1. (See Chapter 4.) Once this is clear the field of nursing could be recognized as including the ability to attend the sick with an acknowledgedly higher degree of skill than is had by the ordinary commensensical and sympathetic relative, and its identity might be both clearer and more soundly based in experience and work.[9]

Once more, the situation is less sharply evident in some ways in hospital than it is in the home. In hospital the attending to patients' wants, while admittedly split between fully qualified Nurses, nursing aides under various labels, ward aides, housekeepers, and (as is commonly acknowledged) ward orderlies and domestic staff, is nevertheless accomplished somehow. There is usually someone around, and patients of course often also contribute to nursing one another. In the home, what is to be done if the Nurse refuses to empty the commode, or to tidy the sickroom, or to pull together a meal for the patient, or indeed to do anything other than those increasingly specialized procedures which her training has led her to expect and to which her rate of pay is geared? But the non-Nursing duties (a more accurate typography), remain to be done nevertheless. And while practice varies greatly from one person or team to another, it is common for those trying to keep a sick relative at home to find that since none of the health professionals is *charged* with such work (although many do it out of common humanity and common sense) it falls to the family to cope. Where the family cannot in fact do so, hardship arises and hospitalization of the patient (and often also of exhausted relatives) can follow.

In France, home hospitalization makes much use of the Caring Aide (Aide Soignante) to fill this gap. There is nothing new about the role except the recognition of the field of activity and

[9] This point is pursued *in extenso* in Cang and Clarke (in press), *Hospital at Home*.

the naming of those who work there. The point again is that the work exists and has to be done whatever the nomenclature employed. It is the Caring Aides, working under the supervision of higher-qualified Nurses, who supply the nursing which is part of Basic Patient Need, and who in France do this both in hospital and in the home hospitalization services. It is they who become essential when a patient enters Full-time Patient status, and it is in work of this kind that those who enter the field of nursing out of a desire to look after the sick may find their satisfaction.

Co-ordination

It may be assumed that co-ordination as we have defined it becomes more important once a patient becomes full-time. A measure of co-ordination exists in even the most trifling illness (because of the potential deterioration of any trouble) but the ability of the part-time patient to 'look after' himself appears to encapsulate something of this work as well. It is as though the occasional contact with his doctor, or the nurse, or the specialist, can supply enough guidance to enable him to cope.

In the same way, the inability to contain the illness 'on a part-time basis' so to speak, implies a corresponding increase in the need for help in carrying out the co-ordinative work. In the hospital, the co-ordinative function is most clearly seen in the patient's relationships with both the ward sister and the consultant: between them they contribute the most important information that helps to create the patient's sense of security about his illness and what is being done about it for him.

Providing co-ordination to a Full-time Patient in a domiciliary situation however requires other arrangements: in France the work rests mainly with the GP, with contributions from the supervising nurse and the Caring Aide, who, being regular attendants on the patient, supply him with an important element of co-ordination through their continuity. We can further consider how this function in the domiciliary situation might be performed in the National Health Service in the following section on organization.

Some Organizational Aspects of Domiciliary Health Services

What now can be said about how domiciliary work is organized, and how it relates to such existing activities as those of the Primary Care Team? Analysis of the needs of patients shows that questions of the organization of domiciliary health services cannot be discussed without specifying whether it is part-time or full-time patients who are to be cared for, because what has to be provided differs in each case. Part-time patients do not need Basic Human Needs *as patients*, and have no need of nursing, although they may require specialized Nursing. This helps to explain why the Primary Care Team models (since there are considerable variations in the composition and work content of PCTs, so that generalization is not helpful) usually cope adequately with Part-time Patients and less so with Full-time Patients. The PCT is organizationally so to speak the obverse of the out-patient clinic: a particular activity is to be performed, and then on to the next patient.

No problem arises when the need is of just this kind (the changing of a dressing, the giving of an injection and suchlike); but patients, relatives, and PCT staff begin to feel less comfortable when the 'nursing' area of work presents needs, i.e. when the patient has, or is entering upon, full-time status. Thus the giving of a bath on the 'giving a procedure' model is often experienced as inappropriate – it properly belongs to a more extended looking after (=nursing) form of need and therefore plan of work.

The delineation of Basic Human Need may prove helpful in sorting out individuals in social need, who then fall ill and become Part-time Patients, and who in that context will have needed Basic Human Need provision from social services plus health service help (whether domiciliary or not); from those who, having fallen ill and become Full-time Patients, need Basic Human Need because of their Full-time Patient status, and for whom the meeting of Basic Human Need is a health service responsibility.

The role of the doctor in deciding that Full-time Patient status is no longer required then becomes socially more significant, since in withdrawing Basic Patient Need which includes Basic Human Need, the patient is left to cope on his own, or else the assumption is made that social services are adequately capable of meeting Basic Human Need for non-patients.

One implication of this analysis is that if too large a gap exists between the standard of Basic Human Need as supplied by the health service and social services respectively, a more primitive attitude to patients may be expected. An example of this attitude may be seen in the view that since all patients are people, every person should have the same as all patients, whether that person is a patient or not.

A major organizational question arises in the UK: whether the existing Primary Care Teams can form a basis on which domiciliary care for Full-time Patients could be structured. This question is pursued at length elsewhere[10] but two main problems may be briefly mentioned here.

The first is that in the case of PCTS based on a GP practice, there arise questions about the efficiency of arranging for Full-time Patient care, when any one GP might have perhaps three or four patients at most in home hospitalization at any one time. Related to this is the point that home hospitalization requires the rapid (within hours) availability of a substantial range of equipment which it might be uneconomic to maintain on a practice (as against a district) basis. There is also the major question of managing the service and responsibility for doing so, which a GP would be unlikely to be able to take on without a major change in role.

The second problem is that of nature of work and the associated staffing, including training, morale, and maintenance of the organization. There is quite a difference between caring for Part-time and Full-time Patients. Many of the latter need substantial amounts of nursing over a long period. It would have to be seen whether the mixing of both kinds of work was organizationally realistic.

There is also the question of how the work of co-ordination might best be achieved for the patient in the context of the NHS. Further work remains to be done on the relationship between medical responsibility and where co-ordination of the patient's experience lies but it would seem likely that the GP and the supervising nurse could together fulfil the same work on this aspect of Basic Patient Need as their counterparts in France – provided that the GP–patient relationship under NHS conditions was sufficiently personal to enable such co-ordination to be carried out meaningfully.

The overall organizational picture can be illustrated by

[10] Cang and Clarke (in press), *Hospital at Home*.

reference to the treatment of cancer. For many cancer patients, the course of their illness is by no means steady and linear. There can be markedly better and worse phases, resulting in what may be several moves between Part-time Patient and Full-time Patient and *vice versa*. It is striking that this analysis fits the range of organizational solutions independently adopted by St Christopher's Hospice, London, by the Macmillan Unit at Christchurch in Dorset, and by the Leclerc Centre at Dijon in Burgundy.

Each place specializes in the treatment of cancer and each has hospital, hospital-at-home, out-patient, and PCT-equivalent forms of service, thus enabling their patients to be treated at home or at the hospital whether PT or FT at any given time. Each centre appears thus to be able to allow its patients to receive their services in the most appropriate setting according to the patient's state and his own preference. Such freedom depends of course on having the means to provide hospital-at-home services; it also results in the avoidance of hospital admissions for those who neither want nor need them.

Wider Implications of Domiciliary Health Services
In conclusion, I wish briefly to adumbrate some further points which domiciliary health care helps to bring out especially for Full-time Patients. There are several matters to consider, namely: the question of cost; the implications for hospitals; for GPs; for nurses; for other professional staff; for families; for neighbourhood relationships; for the creation of work, and of course for patients.[11]

So far as cost goes, it is not part of our concern to try and reach a conclusion on the relative cost of domiciliary as compared with other forms of care. Nor is it our concern to press for any particular type of service. The literature on domiciliary health care in the USA, France and other countries argues that savings of around 60 per cent or 70 per cent are achieved with domiciliary as against hospital care, but these figures are in doubt in the UK where studies of comparative costs are currently under way. It is sufficient for the present discussion to note that there seems no reason to suppose that domiciliary care

[11] Each of these is considered in greater detail in Cang and Clarke, op. cit.

would cost significantly *more* than institutional forms. The detailed exploration must be left to the techniques of health economists. A useful discussion of the basic methodological problems in pursuing this extremely complex issue is the contribution by Wright in Cang and Clarke.[12]

What would be the implications for hospitals if the alternative of home hospitalization were available?[13] First of all, it needs to be recognized that the two forms of care would not be in competition: Full-time Patients who had the choice (i.e. where all the other parties agreed) would not all want to be ill at home. It seems reasonable to assume that some people would prefer hospital anyway, while others would never feel that a home hospitalization bed was really the equivalent of one in hospital. Hospitals would remain centres of specialization and a major form of service appropriate to Full-time Patients, quite apart from their training, research and out-patient work. Consultants in certain specialties might become involved in more domiciliary consultations than now, but that is scarcely new. Then what of the work of the GP? Taking on responsibility for a home-care patient would mean the GP visiting the patient, possibly quite often during the course of his illness. This would imply the development of a different relationship between GP, patient, and family from that which exists when the patient is only seen in the surgery: a far more comprehensive knowledge of the patient will be gained by the GP from seeing the patient in his home. For some GPs, this increase in clinical relationship with patients may be welcome, for others the reverse. There is also the greater part played by the GP in the medical management and surveillance of a wider range of conditions than can obtain when the only facility for Full-time Patients is hospital. This might increase the medical interest of the job for many GPs, and enhance the opportunities for continuing medical education and for research.

[12] op. cit.

[13] A full-scale 3-year pilot scheme to explore the potential of such a service, and to put to practical test the analysis adumbrated in this essay, is now being mounted in the Peterborough Health District of Cambridgeshire Area Health Authority. This pilot scheme, and the researches on organization and on standards of care which form an integral part of it, are made possible thanks to the generous initiatives of the Sainsbury Family Charitable Trusts.

Administratively, the NHS contract for GPs with the FPC might need review if a GP found he had so many patients in home hospitalization that he could not manage them all and serve the rest of his list properly as well. This is unlikely to arise, but there may be a general point here about the possible conflict between working on an individual basis, such as home hospitalization implies, and a much less personal one embodied in the GP's list, the capitation fees and the generally pre-arranged nature of doctor–patient relationships which the present structure in the NHS is tending to foster.

For the nursing profession, as has already been mentioned, domiciliary treatment of Full-time Patients in particular highlights their problems *vis-à-vis* the content of Basic Patient Need and Basic Human Need. Other countries have no problem in recruiting and retaining Caring Aides of all ages, which suggests that here is a kind of work which many wish to do without seeking any different kind or status of work. Domiciliary work with Full-time Patients also offers to Nurses the kind of continuity of relationship with a patient which many wish for even though engaged on more specialized Nursing work.

For other professionals, such as physiotherapists, speech therapists or occupational therapists, for instance, a similar chance exists in domiciliary work to enrich the clinical and individual character of their work with patients. Many are already finding that domiciliary work brings greater clinical satisfaction, and the needs of domiciliary care so far as specialist services are concerned can readily be accommodated by staff also working in a specialist centre, thus affording them the benefits of each.

There are also implications for families and neighbourhoods. If a modern Western family is given the kind of support which it tends to need if one of its members is (full-time) ill at home, it is possible for them to look after their sick member to a considerable degree. Under such supported conditions, which implicitly encourage families to help themselves, it seems likely that much could be achieved to strengthen family ties, and on the basis of a kind of work that particularly binds together those who undertake it because it is work in the service of health and life.

Much the same can be said for neighbourhood links, which

play a part in home hospitalization in several ways. First, because neighbours are often a useful support to patients in a variety of ways. Secondly, because home hospitalization schemes seem naturally to be organized best in small staff groups (up to about fifty people, excluding GPs) and serving a locality, so that the major staff groups – nurses, Nurses and home helps – tend to be drawn from that area. Over time such a pattern would create a palpable degree of local acquaintance, and an awareness that important and personal services were provided not by unfamiliar officers of a service but by local people.

There would thus also be a potential for the creation of work in inner-city areas, work which elsewhere has been found to appeal both to young women (and some men) who do not feel drawn to Nursing training, but who want to nurse; and to older women who enjoy looking after people, sometimes on a part-time basis, and who equally do not want to undergo, or do not feel themselves cut out for, full Nurse training.

We may conclude with the most important implications, those for patients. It is now recognized that near the beginning and towards the end of life it is especially important not to remove people from home. The consequences of a hospitalization for a young child or an elderly person may be extremely serious; if hospitalization is unavoidable on medical grounds then on balance that may be judged the only course to follow. But for Full-time Patients whose admission is simply the result of an absence of organization to enable full-time illness to be coped with at home, the position is different. Anyone who has experienced the agony of patients or families over separation in illness or when the last weeks of life are being lived will know what is at stake.

There is also the sizeable group of people for whom hospitalization is especially difficult, namely those who are already handicapped by such conditions as blindness or partial paralysis, and who cannot therefore transplant to hospital without a major upheaval in every aspect of their living.

Finally, there is that group of unknown dimensions containing people who simply have a deeply rooted preference for staying at home when ill, and for whom to do so is very probably a positive aid to recovery as well as a humane form of help.

12

The Role of Departments of Geriatric Medicine[1]

Tim Packwood

Once recognized, demographic change is one of the most potent influences upon social policy. Over the last half century the increase of the elderly, both in terms of absolute numbers and as a percentage of the total population, has been dramatic. In 1901 the elderly represented 6.8 per cent of the total population of the UK; by 1971 they represented 16.3 per cent.[2] Despite the warnings of commentators such as Townsend,[3] the implications of this change for society, and for the welfare state in particular, have only belatedly been realized. In some cases the resulting policies have been relatively consensual and direct, as, for example, in attempts to relieve some of the financial inequalities of the old. In the provision of personal services, however, the response has been more tentative, reflecting not only the economic crisis and the organizational complexities involved but also the deeper ambivalence towards the elderly that exists within our society. Indeed, it must be doubtful how far there is any meaning in attempting to think of the elderly as a unity in social policy terms.

The needs of the elderly are now seen as a priority in the Health Service, which, in 1976, deployed a third of its expenditure on services for those over sixty-five. Community care has

---

[1] The substance of this paper was published in the *Health and Social Service Journal*, 25 March 1977.

The issues raised have emerged from field-work and conferences undertaken by the Health Services Organization Research Unit over the last three years.

[2] *Social Trends*, 1974.

[3] See Townsend's (1976) comments on 'Local Authority Plans for Social Services for Old People in 1963', included in *Sociology and Social Policy*.

become the new orthodoxy: but it is advocated as a valve, with surprisingly little hard evidence as to its costs and benefits. And, paradoxically, while community care largely depends upon the decisions of individual local authorities, the centrally controlled NHS continues to devote the lion's share of its resources to the hospitals where the elderly occupy nearly half the available beds.[4]

All these ambiguities are central when considering the role of geriatric departments. Their development may have been late but it has been striking. Whereas in 1963 the whole-time equivalent of 329 hospital medical staff were working in geriatrics, the figure for 1974 was 914.[5] And it is clear that the trend is to continue, *Priorities for Health and Personal Social Services in England* suggesting the provision of around 1,150 additional geriatric beds.[6] Yet geriatric medicine remains an oddity. Straddling the boundaries of treatment and care, its scope withstands precise definition. Are geriatric departments indeed part of the NHS at all? Why should the elderly require a 'general purpose' medical specialty? The relationship of geriatric medicine to other hospital specialities and to the whole web of community services is somehow more crucial, and fraught with difficulty, than is generally the case with hospital services.

In considering the special nature and problems of geriatric medicine and its organization it is first necessary to briefly place it in context. Geriatric medicine in the hospital setting is generally concerned with the medical, as opposed to surgical or psychiatric,[7] and rehabilitative needs of those over retirement age, although, as discussed later, the orientation of service offered varies from one department to another. It has been defined as the branch of general medicine concerned with the clinical, preventive, remedial, and social aspects of health and disease in the elderly.[8] Patients reach the department by referral from a GP, by referral from other clinical specialists in the hospital,

[4] DHSS (1976), *Report of the Hospital In-patient Enquiry for 1973, Preliminary Tables.*

[5] DHSS (1976), *Health and Personal Social Services Statistics for England, 1975.*

[6] DHSS (1976), *Priorities for Health and Personal Social Services in England.*

[7] In practice, however, the distinction between confused geriatric and psycho-geriatric patients is not always clear cut, and facilities for the latter are not always available.

[8] Definition by the Royal College of Physicians, 1972.

or as emergency admissions. Many of the elderly with medical problems will initially be referred to that specialist appropriate to the particular illness rather than to the consultant geriatrician, so the total number of elderly patients in hospital considerably exceeds the number in geriatric departments.[9] The department, too, is likely to be geographically divided. Geriatric medicine has its origins in the poor law and developed separately from the main stream of acute medicine. This isolation persists today, although the DHSS recommends that 50 per cent of geriatric beds should be located in a District general hospital. Indeed there are advantages in having rehabilitation and long-stay cases located in local community hospitals. The environment is likely to be less frenetic and relationships with relatives and friends are that much easier to maintain. This division does, however, represent a cost in terms of management and medical supervision. Geriatric departments are led by consultants, perhaps by consultants in general medicine with a special interest in geriatrics but increasingly by doctors who specialized in this field of work from early in their career. To date geriatric work has proved one of the less popular fields for native-born junior doctors and as a consequence departments rely heavily on immigrants. These doctors are likely to have grown up in societies with very different attitudes to the care of the elderly from our own, compounding the familiar problems of language and social attitudes.

A major difficulty experienced in geriatric departments is the feeling of being pulled in different directions by demands from the community and hospital services. Orientating the department too far to one rather than the other must significantly alter its role. The differences can be brought out by using two, admittedly extreme, models.

[9] Green states that geriatricians, in fact, deal with less than one-fifth of the over-sixty-fives admitted to hospital and that only two-fifths of over-sixty-fives in hospital, are in geriatric beds. M. Green (1975), 'Services for the Elderly'. The Hospital In-patient Enquiry for 1973 also showed that in 1973 the elderly occupied approximately 92,000 beds daily, of which just over 49,000 were in geriatric departments, 13,500 in general medicine, 9,500 in general surgery, and 6,500 in orthopaedics. Many of those in geriatric departments are, of course, long-stay cases.

Model One – The department exists as an independent speciality in the hospital

The department will take a full range of patients – acute and chronic, young, elderly and not so young – from the district it serves as well as some referrals from within the hospital. It will provide diagnosis, medical treatment, and rehabilitation and, wherever possible, return patients to the community as quickly as possible. Such a department will need a high proportion of general to long-stay beds. It will also need access to sophisticated diagnostic and treatment facilities which means that the general beds, at least, need to be located in a DGH. Many referrals to the department will come direct from GPs and the staff will need to create strong links with Health and local authority staff working in the community. The department needs to develop procedures to put it in touch with patients early in an episode of illness so in addition to providing out-patient clinics staff are likely to become involved in domiciliary assessment visiting and in the provision of day hospitals.

Model Two – The department exists as a supportive speciality in the hospital

In the main the medical needs of the elderly are catered for by the general physicians with their organ-based specialities but the department provides for those needing long-term rehabilitation and medical supervision who cannot be adequately catered for in the atmosphere and environment of surgical and medical wards. Such a department requires assessment beds, a rehabilitation unit, and a large proportion of beds for chronic cases. The first category, at least, should be located in the DGH.

As might be expected, each model has its strengths and weaknesses. Model One sees the geriatric department somewhere near what is currently advocated by the DHSS. As a speciality in its own right it is thought likely to prove attractive to staff and to raise the status of work with the elderly. In treatment terms it is aiming to provide a comprehensive service, meeting the various medical needs of the elderly as they arise as flexibly as possible. By its attempts to keep people in the community as long as possible through timely intervention, such a service may eventually reduce costs – for the Health Service – by reducing the need for lengthy hospitalization.

For this model to work the geriatric department must be treated equally with all other hospital specialities in terms of resource provision; and in the geriatric context equality often means positive discrimination to make up the backlog of past neglect. Nevertheless, the model is grounded on the assumption that, as a group, the elderly are different from the rest of the population in that they require their own branch of general medicine. Thus the expansion of geriatric departments in the Model One mode may be reinforcing the way the elderly are labelled in our society and provide another example of selectivity in social policy.

Model Two is more traditional and its attraction to many non-geriatric orientated clinicians is obvious. The long-stay patients who 'block beds' are taken off their wards, freeing them to devote their skills more productively. The medical needs of many long-stay patients are slight, and appropriate rehabilitation can be organized more effectively in the environment of a geriatric department than in surgical or medical wards with their wide range of acute cases. However, this policy is condemned by the DHSS as misguided. It is likely to result in the geriatric department becoming full of the more intractable cases and, as this happens, waiting lists will increase and the service available to other specialities must inevitably diminish. The model also assumes a gradient of institutional care with the geriatric department at the bottom. This will inevitably affect the morale of both patients and staff, the former feeling stigmatized and the latter seeing the work as less interesting and of lower status.

It is argued, then, that both models of the geriatric department cause problems in social terms. Do the elderly really require their own all-purpose medical speciality? Some would argue that the medical needs of the elderly are distinctive because of the frequent need for multiple diagnosis and emergency treatment and the requirement to understand and assess the social background. Others feel that the elderly could be catered for by the same range of NHS services as the rest of the adult population. Clearly if this were to be the case some fundamental changes would be needed.

First it would be necessary to assume that all hospital clinicians were interested and prepared to work with the elderly.

Patently this is not currently the case. The elderly frequently prove to be most difficult patients and the work does not offer the same scope for medical interventions and applications as other areas. The presence of geriatric departments in the teaching hospitals may help change medical attitudes and develop necessary skills, but it hardly solves the problem of differentiation. An alternative strategy might be to move away from the medical model altogether, recognizing that rehabilitation and care of chronic cases, while a necessary part of the health service, do not necessarily call for continuous medical direction and responsibility. These services could be set up under the control of nurses, rehabilitation specialists, or some new, emergent caring discipline. There would then be no need to cajole hospital clinicians into performing, what appears to some, inappropriate work.

Secondly, GPs would need to provide a complete primary care service to the elderly, whether they were in their own homes or in a residential home. Many already do this, but overall, and despite higher capitation payments, the past decade has seen the terms of trade moving against the elderly as far as GPs are concerned. Investigations of the elderly are always potentially time-consuming, playing havoc with an appointments system. They cannot always be surgery based, yet home visiting by GPs has fallen by about 60 per cent over the last fifteen or so years.[10] Perhaps the best hope here lies in the development of the primary care team. A number of studies have demonstrated, for example, that health visitors can accomplish a great deal through regular domicilary screening.[11]

Thirdly, rehabilitative and supportive services in the community would need to expand, and some more than others given the variation between local authorities. The continuation of the present financial situation obviously limits what can be done, but unless constant nursing care is required chronic geriatric cases might be far more appropriately cared for in the community by social services staff, than in hospital by the Health Service. Their medical needs, which frequently require

[10] Royal College of General Practitioners (1973), *Present State and Future Needs of General Practice*.

[11] See, for example, J. Barber and J. Wallis (1976), 'Assessment of the Elderly in General Practice'.

monitoring rather than intervention, could be initially covered by GPs in the same way as for the rest of the population. Hospital staff are increasingly likely to take the home environment, both physical and emotional, into account in their treatment programmes. A successful outcome, however, depends on continuous support and co-ordination from the community services which, at present, are fragmented and incremental, split between different Authorities, different disciplines from the same Authority and voluntary bodies. When people are being treated or cared for in their own homes the general assumption is that they, or their relatives, are capable of co-ordinating the application of welfare services. Many elderly, however, find this impossible. The current policies to shift more and more care into the community surely make vital both rationalization of services,[12] and the provision of a clear locus of responsibility for the comprehensive and continuing care of individuls.

In the meantime the geriatric department, whether orientated towards Model One or Two, is under pressure from both directions. In mediating these demands the quality of working relationships is crucial, and the consultant in charge of the department needs to be a skilled diplomatist. In the hospital setting clinical policy is not defined through a managerial hierarchy but rather emerges from the negotiations of a collegium of senior staff. Decisions taken in any one area are likely to have important repercussions on the collective. Policy as to priorities by the department of physical medicine, for example, will clearly affect what the geriatric department can achieve. Given, too, the demands on the hospital system from the elderly, the consultant geriatrician is likely to have greatest effect if he, or she, can be accepted by colleagues as an adviser (which is perhaps the true meaning of being a consultant) and not just a point for referrals. In this way all elderly patients in the hospital and the staff who treat and care for them can benefit from specialist knowledge. Clinical skills, then, are not sufficient. The consultant must possess the capability to negotiate, and to teach as well as learn.

The same requirements exist in reference to relationships outside the hospital where the geriatric department needs to be

[12] It is significant that there has never been an official review of the totality and interrelationships of welfare services required by the elderly.

involved in the wider organization of patient care. The sphere of inter-organizational involvement is vast and complex and the potential work load enormous. Even in a small health District the department may be dealing with seventy or so GPs. Links with social service departments are important and this can mean relating to field social workers, residential staff, and the various supporting services such as home helps and occupational therapy. Clearly there is a strong case for the attachment of a social worker to the geriatric department. Health-care planning teams, and the broader liaison committees concerned with current problems that some health Districts still maintain, provide an opportunity for working relationships to be developed and approaches agreed. If the geriatric department is to make the most of these possibilities, and since reorganization they have partly become institutionalized into divisions, committees, or teams, the consultant in charge, and perhaps other members, must again become involved in the processes of negotiation and education. These are increasingly time-consuming and do not directly utilize expensive professional skills.

So here, then, is a dilemma. Both negotiation and teaching require skills which may be completely foreign to Health Service practitioners, never having figured in the training syllabus. The assumption is, perhaps, that such skills can best be acquired by experience, but if the success of our welfare services is now so dependent upon its practitioners being able to negotiate and educate each other this may be too great a risk to take. At the same time, if these skills are pursued at the cost of the primary work with the patient or client they become meaningless and the practitioner becomes out of touch. The balance between clinical practice, administration, teaching, and research is always delicate in medicine. In geriatric departments where the consultant is likely to be responsible for the treatment and care of large numbers of patients, and probably in mental handicap and illness as well, this balance is particularly crucial. Since it is the demands and conflicts inherent in the work that largely differentiate geriatric medicine from most other hospital specialities, it would be helpful if the pressures were made more explicit. At least staff, thinking of going that way in their careers, would then know something of what was required.

13

The Organization of Care for the Severely Mentally Handicapped[1]

Tim Packwood and Ian Macdonald

Services for the mentally handicapped are a 'grey area', although their improvement is a declared government priority. Currently the severely mentally handicapped are largely provided for in residential institutions, the majority of which are located in the NHS and titled hospitals.[2] However local authority education and social services are also heavily involved in work with the handicapped, the former through its responsibilities for children and the latter through its social work with individuals and families, both within and outside the hospital, and through its provision of residential and adult training facilities. Voluntary agencies represent another input.

Some consider that defects in the services are, at least in part, attributable to divided responsibilities.[3] Is this so, and, if it is, what is the way forward? What would be the rationale for placing an unequivocal responsibility with any one of the current partners, or with a newly created service? What would the service look like? Would it be able to satisfy demands for clearer national recognition for the mentally handicapped while also recognizing the importance of local communities in service organization? Would it be able to meet the needs, which are now being more clearly enunciated, for safeguarding individual

---

[1] The substance of this paper was published in *Social and Economic Administration*, Volume 10, Number 3, Autumn 1976.

[2] In 1973 there were 51,747 mentally handicapped in-patients in hospital. DHSS (1976), *Health and Personal Social Services Statistics for England 1975*.

[3] See, for example, W. Harbert, Director of Social Services for Avon County (1977), in 'The Hospital Anachronism'.

rights and quality of service? And how would the necessary specialist contributions from other welfare services be arranged? These are the concerns of this chapter, but before examining organizational problems and possibilities it is first necessary to show briefly how the current position has evolved.

Antecedents

Traditionally mental handicap was seen as little different from mental illness or other forms of 'deviant' behaviour, and the all inclusive umbrella of stigma, with its associated fear and typification, made the subject unattractive both for research or resource provision until the last decade.

The first real attempt to systematically examine the nature and treatment of mental disorders was made in England by the work of Lord Shaftesbury in the first half of the nineteenth century, culminating in two Acts of Parliament in 1845. These broadly attempted to set out regulations for the treatment and provision of care for 'lunatics'. But the asylums created in the nineteenth century for those of 'unsound mind' virtually treated the mentally ill and handicapped as one. Some trends towards separate provision were even reversed. Thus the Lunacy Act of 1890 was conceptually at variance with the Idiots Act passed four years previously and ignored a reform movement which had existed for almost half a century. Such policy reflected a lack of resources as well as conceptual unclarity.

Although the eventual recognition of the need for separating mental illness and handicap may in one light be seen as potentially beneficial for the handicapped, at the time its implications were less obviously so:

> The old, easy optimism – the belief that almost all defectives could be cured, given time and patience, had vanished. In its place grew a profound pessimism, a conviction that mental deficiency was hereditary, insusceptible to treatment and training, and a growing danger to the whole of society. Life long segregation, and a public policy of sterilisation of the mentally unfit, were seen as the only useful principles for action.[4]

[4] K. Jones (1972), *A History of the Mental Health Services*.

Despite this mood, the 1908 Royal Commission made a significant attempt to produce a moderate and practical solution to the problem of caring for the handicapped.[5] Their recommendations that the handicapped should be protected and not regarded as animals were influential in affecting the underlying attitude towards the handicapped. The eventual administrative solution offered was to set up 'colonies' for the mentally deficient, first under the Poor Law and then under local authority control, where 'patients' were cared for by the medical profession. Admission to these institutions was not always determined by certain or rigorous categorization founded on systematic assessment procedure but could be on the grounds of 'moral danger' (largely for females) or 'excessive aggression' (males). They came to be filled with rejects from the community.

The combination of nature of the work, type of patient, societal attitudes, and geographic isolation resulted in the staff of the institutions becoming somewhat detached from the mainstream of their professions. The unpopularity of the post of consultant in mental handicap illustrates the problems. Not only were working conditions all too often impoverished but the duties of the post were something of an anomaly in consultant medicine compared with its traditional emphasis on treatment, research, and cure of illness. The role became translated into care and maintenance, embodied in the post of medical superintendent.[6] This isolation was reinforced in 1946 when separate HMCs were set up for subnormality hospitals.

These, then, were the difficulties that the NHS inherited. And although there was some alternative provision from other sources, such as local authorities and voluntary bodies, the history of philosophical confusion and decisions of administrative convenience generally failed adequately to solve the problem of how best to provide for the mentally handicapped.

The 1959 Mental Health Act,[7] while attempting to delineate between whether the mentally subnormal should be receiving treatment for a condition or punishment for an offence, did not

---

[5] *Report of the Royal Commissioners on the Care and Control of the Feeble Minded* (1908).

[6] Medical Superintendents were designated chief officers of mental deficiency hospitals in 1948. This was rescinded in 1960.

[7] Mental Health Act of 1959 (HMSO, 1959).

totally clear up historical anomalies. Despite increased awareness of clinical differences between mental illness and handicap
there was still a tendency to act as if they were one group, for
example sharing sheltered accommodation and training facilities. The new term 'severe subnormality' was linked with mental illness and called 'mental disorder':

> Some people objected to this on semantic grounds, pointing
> out that 'dis-order' implied a prior state of order, which was
> patently not the case with the mentally handicapped, but
> the joint term was convenient and came into use.[8]

Once again convenience rather than clarity won the day. But,
almost incidentally, the Act did undermine some of the assumptions for provision of care within the Health Service. The
emphasis given to the potential role of 'the community' left
it open to the local authority social service and education departments to take over some of the responsibility from the
Health Service. Ironically, however, the 'open-door' policy
(later reiterated in 'Better Services for the Mentally Handicapped')[9] could become a 'revolving-door' policy as the handicapped pass from hospital to a community that cannot
adequately care for them and hence come back into the hospital
again. This was largely because the policy was founded on
medical advances, the use of tranquillizers for example, and
was unaccompanied by adequate increases of resource allocation in alternative spheres. In fact, since the 1959 Act there has
not been an enormous reduction in mental subnormality beds.
This is not solely due to the failure of the 'community' to respond, for in the last three years home and hostel provision has
increased by 25 per cent, but is because of, first, a failure to
analyse systematically the appropriate placement of care, and,
secondly, the increased use of antibiotics and higher hygiene
standards which have increased the life-expectancy of the mentally handicapped to be almost equal to the rest of the population.

The 1959 Act also tackled the problem of patients' rights and
by re-examining grounds for compulsory admission brought

[8] K. Jones (1975), *Opening The Door.*
[9] DHSS (1971), *Better Services for the Mentally Handicapped.*

into discussion the attitudes of society to problems of mental handicap and mental illness. One major problem was that through the combination of increased physical isolation with the social isolation due to societal confusion and the defensive labelling of the mentally handicapped as 'sick' which is reinforced by their presence in hospitals, 'patients'' individual rights had been eroded. The Act removed the judicial role in compulsory admissions procedure, which required the involvement of a magistrate,[10] but the medical role was strengthened. This role in turn was, and still is, frequently over-emphasized, and has been exercised too vigorously,[11] to the detriment of the intention of the Act. Under the terms of the Act hospitals are required to have Managers to preserve the interests of the compulsorily detained. Others, the informal admissions who make up the majority of in-patients, presumably do not require such formal safeguards since they have the right, like any patients suffering from a physical illness, to discharge themselves from medical care. But in the case of the mentally handicapped it must surely be asked how real is this distinction? The rights of informal, as well as detained patients, can be fully respected only if the role of the Managers is interpreted to mean they are responsible for actively monitoring the overall condition of both patients and hospitals. For although medical knowledge is assumed to be necessary, it is not officially decisive in determining the lives of patients.

But it is clearly difficult for a lay body to maintain such a role in a hospital setting, traditionally the domain of the medical profession, in which context by implication the clinicians have the last word. This may be an example of dysfunction arising from the application of the medical model.

Historically, then, the development of services has been sporadic and the rationale for location generally pragmatic.

Current Difficulties
Locating responsibility for treatment of the most severely handicapped in the Health Service also implies the possibility of cure. But mental handicap is very different from mental

[10] Although the involvement of the Sheriff in cases of compulsory admission continues in Scotland.

[11] DHSS (1974), *Report of the Committee of Inquiry into South Ockendon Hospital.*

illness and the general range of physical illnesses in this regard. Clearly many of the most severely handicapped require care and medical support, for handicap is often accompanied by other medical complications, but generally medical treatment can only ameliorate handicap, not cure it.[12] However, the involvement of the Health Service brings with it the aim of cure. This provides hope. As the mentally handicapped lack a sense of personal drive the presence of hope may provide them, and their families, with motivation and reduce stigmatization.

The hospital presents a further problem when treatment is organized on the medical model. In NHS terms this implies clinical autonomy and prescription. The mentally handicapped become the patients of a particular clinician who determines their treatment requirements and prescribes for them accordingly. But the treatment requirements of the mentally handicapped are very broad indeed. The environment supplied by the hospital may be more important than the application of drugs. Given this importance of the non-medical, caring components of treatment, is the traditional medical model applicable? Examples abound of problems arising from differences in perception of need between clinicians and members of other caring disciplines. The multi-disciplinary approach stressed by the Hospital Advisory Service cannot easily contain clinical autonomy unless all concerned are prepared to give a lot of time to communication and are willing to abandon established attitudes.

Further, the medical model may hamper training in social competence for the severely mentally handicapped, for there seems little reason to assume that this figures prominently among clinical skills. Because of their location, mental handicap hospitals do not fit easily into the structure of the District-based operational Health Service that has been developed with reorganization. One institution is likely to serve a number of health Districts and, perhaps, health Areas. The problem can be tackled by special arrangements, such as dividing the hospital into divisions each of which is linked to a catchment District, but DHSS proposals appear to see mental handicap insti-

[12] Illich (1975) points out, in *Medical Nemesis*, how according to many authorities mental deviance is primarily non-clinical, not susceptible to either the language of natural science or to operational verification.

tutions as having long-term independent life.[13] As a result the hospital is usually run by the health District in which it is sited, often as a separate administrative sector, and its facilities are made available to patients from other Districts on a service-giving basis. Inevitably then, the hospitals tend to remain organizationally isolated in the Health Service. District-based health care planning teams and Community Health Councils have to make special arrangements to work with them. This organizational isolation, often compounded by geographic remoteness, carries important implications for patients' attitudes, staff motivation, and resource allocation. There are signs, however, that this problem has at last been recognized in health service planning. When addressing a conference of the National Society for Mentally Handicapped Children on 26 February 1975, the Secretary of State, Mrs Castle, announced that she would be asking Health Authorities to appoint new consultants in mental handicap to health Areas or Districts rather than par-. ticular hospitals, which will help break down this isolation.

With the current division of accountability for the mentally handicapped between Health Authorities and local authorities, no one service can provide comprehensive care and treatment. The various services, as well as the disciplines within them, must collaborate. Now different disciplines and services clearly have their own values and policy objectives, which makes it difficult to secure a truly integrated service. Thinking becomes compart-mentalized. The discharge of patients from hospital to com-munity care demonstrates the problem. For the hospital this may represent a successful outcome (although a long-term evaluation of the quality of the discharged patient's life would be desirable), for the social services an additional responsibility is incurred. Thus policy divisions between services must hinder the attainment of policy objectives for a multi-serviced client group. At the individual's level they become translated into the all too familiar problems of lack of communication, consistency, and coherence between professional staff. The dangers have official recognition! In her address quoted above, the Secretary of State expressed her fear of misunderstandings arising from the lack of congruence between hospitals and local authority

[13] DHSS, 'Management Arrangements for the Reorganised NHS – Defin-ing Districts', HRC (73)4.

policies and indicated that things had been made worse by the reorganization of the NHS. She went on to announce that integration would be encouraged by the allocation of money for joint projects and by the creation of a multi-disciplinary development team to assist Area Health Authorities and local authorities in the planning of comprehensive services.

Another aspect of this problem can be seen in regard to staffing the services. Work with the mentally handicapped is particularly demanding and is unattractive to many. Its division among different welfare services, each of which includes other, higher status, branches of work, means that career opportunities are limited. Humanitarianism is, of course, a powerful value, but how significant can this remain, even where bolstered up by special incentive payments, in an age of materialism and economic inflation?

The operational effect of divided accountability has given the mental handicap services a low visibility in policy-making. Health, education, social services all have other priorities to meet; priorities which apply to their major service commitments in terms of health facilities for the physically ill and schools for the 'normal' child, etc. Consequently these needs have taken precedence while mental handicap services have suffered, and still do suffer, from a lack of resources.[14] Latterly the service has become more visible, but has done so through its Elys and South Ockendons, becoming a special case in an era of cuts and restrictions. Additionally, it can be argued that resources given are applied too indiscriminately, without taking sufficient account of particular service developments. The emphasis on community rather than hospital care has, for example, not been accompanied by appropriate resource allocations to local authorities.

And finally what of societal attitudes? Mental handicap is natural, but the present organization of competitive, urbanized society often precludes the luxury of expending resources on 'inefficient' members of that society. Mental handicap appears to share the stigma carried by mental illness although its etiology is different. Permanent hospital residence appears to reinforce the labelling process, keeping the recognition of stigma

[14] See DHSS (1975), *Facilities and Services for Mental Illness and Mental Handicap Hospitals.*

damped down by removing the problem from public view. However, the issue of the mentally handicapped has been aired more in recent years, both from a theoretical standpoint and through the activities of promotional groups such as MIND. The increased involvement of community-based services is likely to produce a testing and clarification of societal attitudes and values.

Possibilities in Provision
Given that the existing organization of services to the mentally handicapped poses such problems, is it possible to develop a better system? The remainder of this chapter takes up this question. In all of the possibilities discussed, however, it has not been possible to think of provision as the sole and independent responsibility of any one service. Different Health and local authorities' disciplines must be involved! The development of complementary policies, of continuity of treatment, and of adequate communication remain as inescapable necessities for improved provision. Given the persistence of this multi-disciplinary factor, significant implications follow from the location of prime responsibility for those 'in-patient' services required by the severely mentally handicapped. In turn this paper briefly considers what might be involved in reorganizing and placing such responsibility with: the NHS; the social services; the education service; a newly created specialist service; no particular service at all.

1. UNDER THE NHS
Provision for the severely mentally handicapped in NHS hospitals could be more definitively divided to recognize that only some patients have a prime requirement for medical treatment, either because of the nature of their mental condition or because of associated physical malfunctions. The need of the others is for care and social training. The former would be placed, as now, under the charge of consultant specialists. The care of the latter group would be the accountability of either specialist nurses or, as is more likely with the present trend in the health service, a multi-disciplinary team (nurses, psychologists, remedial therapists, etc.). In the longer term this function might fall to the new professional group of care staff predicted

in the Briggs Report,[15] although this could well shift the caring unit out of the NHS. The Association of County Councils advocated such a single caring profession in evidence to the Jay Committee, but felt it should have a social work rather than a nursing bias. Medical support for those receiving care would come from GPs.

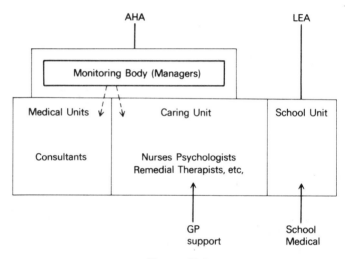

FIGURE 13.1

Decisions as to the appropriate provision for any one individual would depend on multi-disciplinary assessment and agreement, although the initial assessment unit in which an individual was placed on entering the hospital would be under consultant control.

The organizational structure would be more in keeping with the needs of the handicapped. Its adoption would also allow some freedom for expensive and scarce specialist medical resources to be applied in the wider community rather than being tied up, often inappropriately, in the hospital. The opportunity could also be taken to strengthen public control. Accountability for the maintenance of adequate standards of individual treatment and care would lie with the Area Health Authority. Given the formidable work-load facing this body it

[15] *Report of the Committee on Nursing* (Briggs Report) (1972).

would seem sensible to extend the current role of Hospital Managers in mental hospitals and set up a body to monitor the work of the hospital on behalf of the AHA.

Initially it might prove more convenient to organize this model on an Area basis. The AHA would find this easier in exercising its managerial role and the non-medical staff in the hospital could be 'latched-on' to the management of appropriate Area officers. Over a period of time, however, the situation could be assessed and if necessary the hospital could be integrated into a health District and thus move into the mainstream of operational health services.

Such a mental handicap hospital would, in fact, be more like a residential community than the traditional concept of a hospital – a community with its own specialist hospital facilities, a community with its own educational facilities, which as far as children are concerned, would be the accountability of the local education authority. As a possibility for change it would disturb existing arrangements least, keeping provision of mental handicap services within the NHS, but moving away from the medical model, with its many attendant difficulties, towards a more caring orientation.

2. UNDER THE SOCIAL SERVICES

If the problems of the severely mentally handicapped are not seen as essentially medical, the 'caring' institution replacing the 'curing', then this could point to local authority social services departments (SSDs) being allocated the responsibility for the organization of services. This would meet the case stated in 'Better Services for the Mentally Handicapped' but would do so by removing all responsibility from the NHS for hostel provision. 'Hostels' or 'homes' would be a demand on LA resources rather than those of the AHA and it would be for central government, as a partner, to ensure adequate provision by each local authority.[16] Such a move would be consistent with the philosophy that a welfare agency, here the SSD, provides alternative homes in the community where for one reason or another the real home situation is inadequate. The argument

[16] In 1974 local authorities provided 6,473 places in homes and hostels and 31,604 places in Adult Training Centres – DHSS (1976), *Health and Personal Social Services Statistics for England, 1975.*

of the Campaign for the Mentally Handicapped against invest-
ing in new hospitals would be supported. The SSDs would be
providing homes, and thus need not provide education or
health facilities. The latter could well be provided by GPs, and
education is already the LA's responsibility.

The relationship between social services residential staff and
field workers would need to be clarified, especially if it is considered that the handicapped person may not need to continue
in residential care. The presumption would be that the prime
need of the severely mentally handicapped is for operational
social work. This would include basic social work with individuals but, where needed, would also include the provision of
basic services, such as accommodation, food, and the provision
of social and cultural life, and of supplementary services, such
as occupational training and sheltered employment.[17] If these
services are provided then the severely mentally handicapped
will be in a position to benefit from other services, such as education and health, and to become less isolated from the pressures
of society but rather guided through them. The organization
of provision of services could be along the lines shown in Fig.
13.2. This outline would be compatible with existing SSD
organizational structure: the Director of Social Services being
accountable to the LA for the work performed. In this model
there is a specific post for a manager of all homes for the mentally handicapped in the SSD; he or she would be accountable
to the Assistant Director, Residential Work. This manager
would carry overall responsibility not only for the day-to-day
functioning of the homes and the co-ordination of residential
services for the handicapped but would also be accountable for
liaison with other relevant service providers. In the longer term,
however, many of these current distinctions within SSDs would
be lessened if the proposals in the Briggs Report were implemented. Members of the new caring profession would work
with the mentally handicapped both in residences and outside.

The councillors would be ultimately responsible for ensuring
an adequate local service but given the notorious history of lack
of provision there may well be a role for a national lay body,

---

[17] For a fuller discussion of these distinctions see Rowbottom *et al.*, (1974),
'Analysis of the Present Functions of Social Services Departments in SSORU'
Social Services Department, Chapter 3.

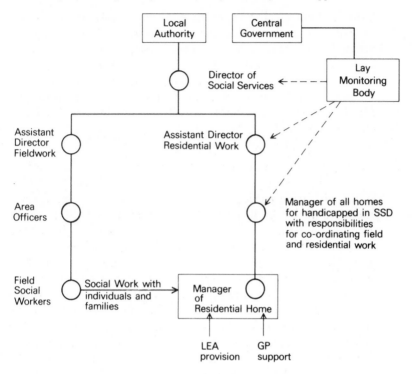

FIGURE 13.2

accountable to central government for monitoring the mental handicap services of local authorities throughout the UK. The body could consist of members who have interest and involvement in both the nature of mental handicap and in the development of policies to meet needs. This would be not only a 'watchdog' function but would include a positive input (perhaps annual reports) into central government's overall policy and planning of service provision. The monitoring process would give a check on the service being provided by the various local authorities and would also supply a mechanism through which the managers of homes could influence overall policy in the light of their specific experience. Such a body would be less appropriate at a local level analogous to the LEA Board of Governors, or the AHA sub-committee. First, because such a local body would be less able to present suggestions for overall, national policy on the experience of one SSD, and secondly because there is a clearer line of accountability for the provision of services within the SSD, uncomplicated by issues such as clinical autonomy.

3. UNDER THE EDUCATION SERVICE

Since mental handicap may be defined on the basis of intellectual performance one should consider seriously the claims of the education service to organize provision. The main argument would be predicated on the prime need of the mentally handicapped for social adequacy, and that this can be taught. A consideration of the numbers of mentally handicapped in the population as compared with those receiving significant help appears to support this assertion. This is not to deny that a specialist form of teaching would be required. Social adequacy would have to be made central and explicit. It could not be left to be acquired as a by-product of academic education. The teaching role, as it is commonly perceived, would diminish, and the new caring profession might well emerge in its place. But then it must be remembered that the education service is already heavily involved in work with the mentally handicapped.[18] Since 1971 all children of school age, institutionalized or not, are the educational responsibility of the relevant local authority. This is an acknowledgement of the fact that no child is so handicapped that he, or she, cannot benefit from education. Education staff in special units have long experience of the demands of this work and have become used to liaising with GPs and other supporting services. Teachers in hospital schools have found it desirable to become involved in the total life of their charges and to work with nurses and psychologists. And as a result of this increased commitment there are some signs that the status of these 'special teachers' within their profession is, at last, beginning to rise.

[18] In 1974 local authorities provided special school education for 87,173 children deemed educationally subnormal of whom 7,435 boarded. A further 8,923 children were being educated in hospital schools and 9,851 were attending special classes in maintained schools.

Many education authorities, too, have already amassed considerable experience in the provision of residential education. They have staff who are familiar with the necessary organizational arrangements and, more important, with the demands for caring that must be satisfied. Unfamiliarity comes in respect of supplying permanent, life-long care, for children who grow into adults. Clearly the teachers who worked in these educational communities would need to be specialists, trained to socialize and care for the mentally handicapped. The institutions would need close support from the school medical service, but for routine illness would draw on the services of the local

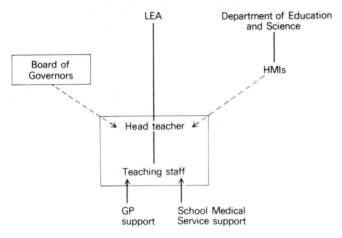

FIGURE 13.3

GPs. They would, however, require easy access to more specialist health service provision. Since the objective for each community would be to 'graduate' its students out to lead useful, satisfying lives, with a minimum of support, in the community, it would also need both good links with social workers and an organization flexible enough to increase or diminish the degree of institutional involvement as warranted.

Public control of the service would be divided. While the operational control would remain local, under the direction of the local authority and open to scrutiny by elected members, national interests would become the responsibility of the Department of Education and Science. The latter has a strong tradition of being being ready and willing to set the limits for local discretion. Its inspectorate has a monitoring role and HMIs have proved an important source of innovation into the service. Even so, it might well be desirable to provide for more intensive lay scrutiny on behalf of those who lack the capacity to safeguard their own rights. This would seem appropriately to be the role of each institution's Board of Governors, although it is accepted that currently the accountability and authority of these bodies in the education system is by no means clear.

4. UNDER A NEW SERVICE

This possibility is frequently suggested as desirable. See, for example, the Labour Party's pre-election survey of the health service.[19] Unfortunately, and all too typically, the authors were not able to enter into any detailed discussion as to how a national mental handicap service might be organized.

The arguments in favour of separating mental handicap services from their present multi-purpose locations and fusing them together in a single specialist service are appealing and would go some way to meet the current problems outlined earlier. A single mental handicap service could certainly gain a much greater visibility in terms of resource allocation. Its very creation would signal a new emphasis in social policy. The service could have its own spokesman, or woman, in central government able to battle for its needs. Advantage could also be taken of the act of creation to organize a service in such a way that problems of control and clinical autonomy would not occur. Medical services, if not provided by GPs, could perhaps be provided on an agency basis, as is the case with the school health service. Staff morale, too, might well increase with independence. Mental handicap work would no longer be just one among other, often more glamorous, specialities. But questions abound. What kind of discipline, or disciplines, would work in the new service? If it were created, as seems most likely, by 'creaming off' those staff presently working with the mentally handicapped, would existing inter-disciplinary differences be perpetuated? What type of unified career structure could be offered?

Alternatively, if the service were to comprise a new 'caring' discipline, concerned with social training and the creation of a

[19] The Labour Party (1973), *Health Care: Report of a Working Party.*

supporting environment, the dependence of the new service on contributions from the health and education services would be enormous. Very sophisticated collaboration arrangements would be required. And what form of organization would be requisite? The Social Security model, with control by a minister down through a department that covered the nation through a regional and district hierarchy? The NHS model, with control exercised through a hierarchy of statutorily appointed bodies? The local authority model, with more or less guidance and finance being dispersed from a central government department and operational accountability vested in the local councils? Control by a commission hived off from direct government control? One can only speculate on the possibilities. In each case the organization has got to be capable of providing an individual service within local communities. Remote management would be dysfunctional.

It must also be asked whether the creation of a new specialist service would not significantly worsen societal attitudes to the mentally handicapped. Could it exacerbate their stigmatization, with the new institutions becoming seen as dumps?

In the face of these particular difficulties, which would be compounded by the economic crisis and the reverberations of recent NHS and local authority reorganization, it is hardly surprising that the Labour Government has, for the time being at least, abandoned the idea of separation.

5. UNDER NO SERVICE
It may be felt that all the above discussion merely boils down to the most superficial social engineering, tinkering with the problems of the mentally handicapped in our society but fundamentally leaving them untouched. Certainly the possibility can be visualized of ceasing to provide any specific service for the mentally handicapped in terms of special in-patient or residential facilities. Instead they would be absorbed within the general hospital, the educational system, the community supporting services and, particularly, within the community at large, drawing on both formal and informal sources of voluntary effort. Their general interests might be watched over by a National Council which, although in no way accountable for providing services, could recommend necessary developments

to the various agencies involved. This possibility, more in keeping with the views so ably expounded by Ivan Illich,[20] would require an abrupt change both in the direction of social policy, channelling resources more towards individuals and families than to agencies, and in the way in which we choose, or have been required, to live. Nuclear, mobile families are not well adapted to either autonomous or mutual care. The argument might be that such a *volte face* would be part of a wider change in life style, forced upon us by economic and environmental pressures as the cost of survival. From the standpoint of the mentally handicapped, the possibility of divesting ourselves of permanent, full-time institutional services appears retrograde unless accompanied by such a comprehensive societal change.

Conclusion

Unquestionably if the severely mentally handicapped require, and are going to continue to require, medical treatment, social work, and education, it follows that a variety of inter-agency collaborative and co-ordinative mechanisms are needed to involve those concerned with individual cases, those who are organizing services and those who are planning future provision. But in this chapter it is argued that the prime need of the mentally handicapped is for adequate care – care that can provide them with an appropriate living environment that can develop their range of social competences, and is sensitive enough to call in other specialist services when they are needed and to co-ordinate their work with, and for, the individual. Given the problems of the present divided situation, the question posed in this chapter is which, if any, of the services cur-

---

[20] The argument that institutional health care (remedial or preventative) after a certain point ceases to correlate with any further 'gains' in health can be misused for transforming clients hooked to doctors into clients of some other service hegemony. The consumer is encouraged to ask himself where health services should end and where other social services would contribute more decisively to his health status or that of his group. What begins as consumer protection quickly turns into a crusade to transform independent people into clients at all cost. Any kind of dependence turns into an obstacle to autonomous mutual care, coping, adapting, and healing and, what is worse, into a device by which people are stopped from transforming the conditions at work and at home which do make them sick. Illich (1975), *Medical Nemesis*.

rently involved with the mentally handicapped is best equipped to provide such care and to take prime responsibility within our society?

Whatever solution is favoured, or, indeed, whether any problem is perceived, depends essentially upon perceptions as to the nature of mental handicap and the role of the handicapped person in society. Can handicap be treated and its sufferers returned to some kind of 'normality'? If so, a medical model would seem most appropriate. Must handicap be accepted, its sufferers humanely cared for and guided to live with their difficulties in the best possible way? This would seem to shift accountability towards the social services or to a new service. Can handicap be surmounted through education and the handicapped educated and trained to fulfil socially acceptable roles? This implies that the service is a function of the education system. The problem is that attitudes towards the mentally handicapped in our society are by no means clear enough to give a definitive answer. The divided and multi-disciplinary nature of the current service inevitably blurs the issue through the lack of congruence between professional objectives, and it renders that much harder the implementation of even favoured treatment in social policy terms.

14

Assessment of Mental Handicap: The Leavesden Project

Ian Macdonald

In the previous chapter some of the historical problems of understanding the nature of mental handicap were outlined. It can be seen that the realization that mental handicap is not an illness brought with it a deep and lasting sense of pessimism. The assumption was that if mental handicap is not curable then there is not much that can be done apart from segregation and containment. However this pessimism is only justifiable if 'cure', in the sense of being able to live a normal, independent life, is still taken as the criterion of success. Therefore it is important to clarify the nature of work with the handicapped. The purpose of the chapter is to explore the relationship between the level of care provided for the mentally handicapped and their level of capacity. By specifying the various levels of opportunity it is possible to use those levels in the design of institutions.

This chapter concerns a research project which assumes that the handicap is a particular level of capacity, and that those people working and living with the mentally handicapped have the same task as many others in society: to allow and enable those in their care to express their capacity, at *whatever level* that capacity might be. There is a need to clarify not only what a person's capacity is, but also how it is possible to provide full opportunity for the expression of that capacity. This chapter does not attempt, as the previous one does, to analyse which particular professional groups of people might requisitely carry out this task, or certain aspects of the task-teachers, nurses, social workers, or others. It is based on work with health and social services staff who, whether requisitely or not, are at present taking the responsibility of caring for a large number of the mentally handicapped people in our society.

The results of the research project at Leavesden Hospital and in three London Boroughs so far indicate that there are qualitatively different ways in which mentally handicapped people perceive their worlds and there are consequently different ways in which staff can organize their work. What was required from the research was an assessment procedure to look, not only at the capacity of the handicapped person but also at the level of opportunity offered by the staff and the context they work in and with.

Assessment of the mentally handicapped in residential situations is crucial for all those concerned. Depending upon the outcome of assessment is usually the total life situation for the handicapped person and a large part of the working lives of staff. The project reported here grew out of the establishment of a new unit which was set up at Leavesden Hospital, Hertfordshire, in 1973. Its aims were to 'de-institutionalize' patients so that they might return to life in 'the community'. The nursing and medical staff were naturally concerned that the unit achieve its aims. As a result nursing staff at Regional level, along with the nursing and medical staff at Leavesden, worked on a research proposal put forward by the Regional Nursing Research Liaison Officer, Miss A. Lancaster. The purpose of the proposed research was 'to design a tool for the recording of the social behaviour of "low dependency" mentally handicapped adults which will provide information on which to base decisions regarding their readiness for transfer from hospital wards to intermediate units, and from intermediate units to hostel accommodation'.[1] Social analysis[2] was chosen as the research because the initiative for the research had come from the Health Service staff. Social services staff had also been consulted, and indeed had themselves requested to be included in the project, which they now are. The method of working was therefore consistent with that of the HSORU. The only unusual aspects were, first, that there was a specific time constraint of two years; and, secondly, that the subject of the research was

[1] I was seconded from HSORU as Research Fellow, when the project was funded by the Small Grants Committee of the DHSS.

[2] R. W. Rowbottom (1977), *Social Analysis*.

an assessment method which, however, had implications for organizational relationships in identifying the nature of the staffs' work. These apparent differences do not significantly change the actual research relationship.

Once the project was funded this fact was communicated to staff both within Leavesden Hospital and the Boroughs which form the catchment area. From the requests which followed work began in five field sites: two wards within the hospital and one hostel in three London Boroughs.[3]

Discrete Stages in Progress
One of the major problems that emerged in the field-work was to define the meaning of 'progress'. It is a common assumption that there is a line of progression from *'hospital'* to *'intermediate unit'* [both usually Health Services] to *'hostel'* [Health, Social Services or Voluntary organizations] to *'group home'* [usually Social Services or Voluntary] to *'independent living in the community'* (usually including the categories of bed-sitters, unstaffed homes and return to family life). However the scale upon which this continuum is based is somewhat tenuous. It carries with it a sometimes unwritten but usually felt assumption that a hospital admission is a retrograde step from the home or hostel. A re-admission from a hostel can be seen in terms of a breakdown in the person; an incapacity. This is a particularly narrow view of both the health services and local authorities spectrum of provision of services. It is possible for health services to provide for a very high level of independence and social services for a low level. A confusing factor which blurs this possibility is a posited 'need for nursing care' being equated with low capacity. The argument runs as follows: because people who need *nursing* care are sometimes the most mentally handicapped, and because nurses are in hospitals, then hospitals con-

[3] A Steering Committee was set up with representatives from the interested health and social services staff. The wards were the 'de-institutionalizing' ward mentioned above and a 'home management' ward, which runs a four-month residential course in shopping, cooking, cleaning, etc. These with the three hostels all provided for adults generally regarded as 'low dependency'. The 'low dependency' category being quite broad and part of the subject of the research was to clarify its boundaries. The wards at Leavesden being 'Willows' and 'Heather'. The hostels being 'Bessborough Road,' Harrow; 'The Retreat', Hillingdon; and 'Parkhill', Ealing.

tain only the severely mentally handicapped people looked after by nurses. This is neither logical nor consistent with the feeling of staff involved in the project. Also the *nursing* care can in many cases often be, and is, provided in local authority hostels by residential social work staff. Hostels, group homes, and family life may requisitely have far more rules and extensive supervision than some wards.

This is not to argue that the continuum from hospital to social services should be reversed, or that the policy of more 'community care' should be abandoned. Rather it is arguing that a more logical and coherent continuum could be used to express the progress towards independence without assuming the above argument. Transfer decisions based on the existing assumptions may not only be ineffective but would cause considerable distress to the individuals whose expectations have been raised as a result of 'de-institutionalization' programmes.

Apart from descriptive labels such as 'hostel', 'group home' etc., one *concept* being used to differentiate between these residential situations was that of the amount of 'supervision' that had to be given to individuals. However this was too broad a notion. It could mean: supervision because of policy or legal restrictions; or supervision because of lack of capacity, or supervision because of expediency, perhaps due to lack of time on the part of staff. Also the concept of supervision was inadequate as it was usually described in terms of 'more' or 'less' of the same rather than recognizing the possibility of qualitatively different types. Essentially the initial phase of the research found the need to develop more clear concepts to provide an assessment tool which would chart a person's capacity and range of behaviour within a specified context.

If the meaning of supervision could be clarified it seemed possible that this would provide a framework within which level of opportunity and capacity could be assessed, and the design of institutions improved.

From the discussions with staff it emerged that what had been called supervision might be divided into qualitative, developmental stages. These stages were observed to relate to reported 'significant' changes in behaviour. Staff reported these significant changes in terms of qualitative jumps in the *initiative* shown by an individual. This notion can be illustrated by an example from the Willows. Lunches come in on a trolley from the hospital kitchens, and staff usually serve them. One lunch-time the staff were delayed so that they were elsewhere on the ward when the lunch arrived. After a few minutes of the residents sitting waiting for the staff, one man went over to the trolley and began to serve the food. The staff observed this and noted, with excitement and pleasure, that this man was one of the most reticent on the ward. He had never shown this sort of behaviour before. It was further noted that he not only tried to serve himself but also the others. This was considered by the staff to be a significant breakthrough on the part of this resident. It had occurred because, almost by accident, the level of opportunity had changed. The usual level of 'supervision' had been temporarily suspended and the opportunity for initiative, in this activity, increased.

Further, the important part of this behaviour for staff was *not how well* the fellow actually served the meals; (proper portions, correct order, etc.) but that he interpreted a need and acted on it without, as far as could be observed, waiting for external sanction or command. The subsequent development of a skill, i.e. learning to serve meals better, *does* suit a comparative description; an additive process. This is similar to the differentiation between strata and grades, made in Chapters 6 and 7. The person's initiative in the serving of the meal is akin to a change in stratum, any improvement in the actual serving being akin to changes in the grades. It also was important in terms of a change in relationship on the part of staff.

The Five Stages in Capacity Progression
Therefore the task of the research became to identify how many of these qualitative changes would be needed to describe the progress of development from 'high dependency' to 'low dependency' and eventually to a stage where a person could be described as 'independent', or capable of living without continued, active 'supervision'.

A further distinction was made between the outcome of behaviour and the method of obtaining the outcome. This distinction was made because many assessment forms concentrate almost exclusively on outcome, and this was one reason why they had not been regarded as fully relevant. For the purposes of the research we called the *outcome* the *goal*. That is a desired state, to be realized in the future one way or another: a cup of tea, a purchase, going to see a film. The *method* of achievement we called the *plan*.

Using these two concepts, goal and plan, the possible developmental stages were explored: five emerged, which are now described in detail.

The five stages were concerned, as stated above, with significant changes, and are described in terms of initiative. For the purposes of the research these stages are called *modes*, as they are concerned with the ways in which a person approaches and achieves a task and how far staff encourage or limit this initiative. They form a logical progression: and the basis of the Assessment Chart of Initiative and Independence developed at Leavesden Hospital.[4]

Mode 1: is where there is no goal or plan initiative. Thus for goal-directed action to occur, both the goals *and* the plans (mentioned above) are externally set, i.e. by someone *other* than the patient/resident. It is thus a situation of virtually complete dependency.

Mode 2: is where the action to achieve a goal depends on that goal being set by another person. It is a situation of dependency; but the plan involves initiative; that is, once the goal has been set action occurs to realize the goal.

Mode 3: is where there is goal *and* plan initiative but not toleration of variation. The plan is repeated, as exactly as possible, to achieve a goal which is, as far as possible, an exact replica of the previous goal which was successfully achieved. There is no flexibility without considerable anxiety.

Mode 4: is where, again, there is goal *and* plan initiative. However in this case although the goal remains fixed (as in Mode 3) the plan can be altered. Thus there is a possibility of trying new ways to achieve the goal: new plans. Anxiety arises if these new plans do *not* actually lead to the goal.

Mode 5: is where there is not only goal *and* plan initiative

---

[4] For a more detailed account of the project work and the actual chart itself contact I. Macdonald, at BIOSS, Brunel University.

but also when, on trying a new plan, the goal does *not* material-
ize there is not the frustration and anxiety that arises in Mode
4, or 3.

Indeed there may be a substitution of an approximate goal
or new goal which satisfies the person.[5]

The Five Levels of Opportunity

These modes relate the capacity of the mentally handicapped
person. However they are also intrinsically linked to the relationship between staff members and the handicapped person
in terms of the level of opportunity offered. The different
models of relationship corresponding to the discrete stages in
capacity were formulated as follows:

Mode 1 level of opportunity: is where the person is not *allowed*
any discretion. The goal and plan are so prescribed as to pre-
clude feasible alteration; for example a staff member requires
a person to wash and the procedure is given as an instruction:
'You wash when I say, and you wash like this ...'[6]

Mode 2 level of opportunity: is a situation where staff are prescribing the 'what', but not the 'how'. The similarity between
this and Mode 1 is that in terms of goals, the handicapped person is dependent on *external* sanction and stimulation.

Mode 3 level of opportunity: is one of *monitoring*, not goal or plan
setting. Therefore the staff member would *check* on the goal *and*
the plan. In effect it is as much a monitoring of the context
as the actual goals and plans: 'Are they realistic given facilities?' However if the monitoring does not lead to the introduction of a Mode 1 or 2 level of opportunity the person can
be said to have completed the action himself.

Mode 4 level of opportunity: takes flexibility into account. Like
Mode 3 the relationship is one of monitoring, not goal and plan
setting. There is no monitoring of the *plan* however. Therefore
the staff member may check where a person is going: to the
shops, for a drink, etc., but *not* how they are going to get there,
whether they are going by bus or train, etc.

[5] For a fuller explanation of the five modes, see Jaques (1978), *Level of
Abstraction in Logic and Human Action.*

[6] A most explicit example comes from the game of Monopoly: 'go to jail,
go directly to jail, do not pass go, do not collect £200': there is not really
much room for manœuvre.

Mode 5 level of opportunity: is one where the staff member is available on request. No active goal or plan setting or even monitoring is done *unless* at the request of the patient/resident. Thus the staff member assumes that the patient or resident is capable of *interpreting* need for themselves even if they do not have the skill or expertise to answer the need independently. An example of this relationship is typically the GP–patient relationship. It is assumed that when a person feels a need, illness, etc., he or she contacts the GP. Further, that if dissatisfied with treatment it can be terminated by the patient. The GP does not call in to see his or her patient just because they have not been to the surgery for a few months, i.e. he or she does not check up to see if those people on the list are ill but have not realized it.

Capacity and Opportunity

The reason for the close relationship between these levels of opportunity and the capacity of the mentally handicapped people lies in the nature of the concept of capacity being used in the project. Throughout the discussion the term capacity is used in the sense of a 'creative capacity'. It is the perception of one's self in an environment in particular 'ways' or perspectives. These 'ways' open up various possibilities for action. It is these 'ways' which are described by the five modes. Thus it is neither a purely cognitive capacity nor an emotional capacity. In the case of the assessment chart the measurement of capacity is concerned with describing an approach to life, taking into account the extent to which a person can and does *act on the environment*;[7] using specified activities as examples,[8] or the extent to which a person is *dependent on the environment* for instructions for action.[9] Another way of describing this capacity is using the concept of *'psychological ownership'* developed in the research. This psychological ownership of action refers to the

[7] See related discussion of this example in Chapter 4, 'Structural Aspects of Doctor–Patient Relationships'.

[8] For example going shopping, making a bed, having a bath.

[9] This concept has been more fully developed by G. Stamp, 'Assessment of Individual Capacities' in E. Jaques *et al.* (1978), *Levels of Abstraction in Logic and Human Action*; in the same book Jaques also compares the concept with other similar approaches.

extent to which a person feels they own or are responsible for what they are doing or for problems they have. If a person feels his or her actions are prescribed by others (as in the case of Mode 1) then, to that extent, the other person has claimed the psychological ownership.

There is a relationship between this psychological ownership and initiative. If a person initiates an activity he or she is more likely to 'own' it. There is a difference between the original psychological ownership of action and the subjective experiences according to different types of relationships subsequently entered into.

For example a person may be capable of perceiving and acting to solve a problem: it is felt to be their problem, and the inclusion of others is in a mature, collaborative relationship. In such a relationship both parties have and feel the right to withdraw. In this first case there would be no change in psychological ownership.

However, it may be that in attempting to enter into this collaborative relationship the new person begins to take over: lay down conditions, and structure situations, even deliberately to mystify the first person. The first person's experience is one of loss. The ownership in one sense remains with the original person but, in effect, action has been so circumscribed as to frustrate this ownership. The person is alienated from the action, or a part of him may be split off and dealt with as if it is separate, no longer legitimately within the domain of the original actor, e.g. treatment of a 'heart' condition. Conversely the problem may be projected onto the collaborator. A 'disowning' takes place and the collaborator may be seduced into assuming, manifestly, the ownership.[10] This concept is not only relevant to the relationships between the staff and patients/residents but also the on-going research relationship between staff and myself. It is not possible in this chapter to enter into a fuller discussion of the concept. However the question in the field of mental handicap is not only concerned with the extent to which this psychological ownership is denied, by one party or another, but is concerned with whether some people *do not have the capacity*

---

[10] Such mechanisms are described in the theory of Melanie Klein as splitting and projection. See also the discussion in Chapter 4.

for psychological ownership with regard to certain, basic activities necessary for survival. This would seem to be the case in Modes 1 and 2 (see above), and still to be problematic in Modes 3 and 4 if frustration cannot be coped with, with the consequence that a more structured goal-and-plan-setting relationship may be requisite.

Capacity and the Design of Organizations

From the above analyses the five levels of opportunity offer an alternative to the inadequate concept of a continuum from hospital to community, mentioned at the outset. It must be stressed that there is no assumption that any level of opportunity is intrinsically better or worse than any other. The relevance of each level will depend upon many factors: the person's capacity, available facilities, and wider constraints such as legal restrictions. Nor is it assumed that all mentally handicapped people will or should progress through *all* the stages.

What is assumed is that where a person is judged to have a certain capacity, services will as far as possible be provided to allow the person to express, legitimately, that capacity. In the course of development, mentally handicapped people may move from one mode to another. The important thing is to note that there is discontinuity, qualitative change points or jumps, in this development, each jump involving a complete reorientation for the individual concerned. Thus, for example, progression from Mode 3 to 4 involves the person for the first time, in modifying his own needs to those of others, at his own initiative. Such a reorientation may be interpreted as a crisis, due to the increase in level of anxiety. It will be important to distinguish these *constructive crises* from anxiety due to an incapacity (for example offering a Mode 5 level of opportunity to a person of Mode 1 capacity). In the event of the constructive crisis it would not help a person's development to lower the level of opportunity as a result of the anxiety. The effects of wide differences between opportunity and capacity have not yet been adequately analysed.[11] This is partly because the assessment method itself is still, as yet, developmental.

[11] A study of these implications is part of a new proposal for the continuation of the research.

In summary, from the research a five-level model of residential services is offered:

Mode 1 where staff are expected to be setting goals and plans;
Mode 2 where staff are setting goals but allowing discretion in plans, which are monitored;
Mode 3 where staff are allowing discretion in goals and plans but monitoring both;
Mode 4 where staff are allowing discretion in goals and plans but monitoring goals only; and
Mode 5: where staff are available only on request. They are not actively setting *or* monitoring goals or plans made by residents.

It is this final level which corresponds to effective independence. The person now has complete psychological ownership.

It is of note that where level of opportunity and capacity correspond at Mode 5, staff in practice no longer use the terms 'mentally handicapped patient or resident'. The reticence to use the term does not seem to stem only from a general dislike of 'labels', but whatever the IQ score or other assessment, if a person shows capacity and is given opportunity at Mode 5 it seems inappropriate to use the term whether the person is present or not. At 3 and 4 'resident' is more usually used (whether in hospital or social services). This seems to reflect the lack of direct dependency for action. The person is resident, living his or her life and needs rather to be monitored or checked, rather than being subject to a series of rules and regulations. In Modes 1 and 2 'patient' is more usually used although patient and resident are fairly interchangeable at Mode 2 depending on health or social service setting. This may also give some insight into the meaning of 'patient'. Rather than being defined in terms of specific ailment it rather reflects the degree of dependency: the need for a particular relationship to ensure survival or avoidance of severe distress (even if for a temporary period).[12]

Although services could be organized designing residential establishments in terms of one predominant mode, this is not a necessary result of the analysis. It may be preferred policy to have establishments where it is policy for staff to offer several

[12] See Chapter 11, 'Full-time and Part-time Patients'.

modes. Also individual mentally handicapped people do not necessarily require *one* mode of relationship only. The relationship may well vary according to activities and individual inhibitions: a person may also have a physical handicap necessitating a 'lower' level of opportunity in certain areas. The analysis does provide a conceptual framework which can be used, according to policy, so that it is at least possible to specify what level(s) of opportunity *are* provided.

The assessment technique has been developed with and for staff working in daily contact with mentally handicapped people. It seems most applicable at the level of officer in charge/ward sister/charge nurse, each being accountable for the assessment and ensuring staff contribution. Assessment at this organizational level enables the information to be brought to discussions where decisions are made concerning both the immediate future of the mentally handicapped and general policy. It is a model, a framework for organizing observations and on-going assessments being made in residential establishments. Thus a plan of action can be outlined, put into operation and tested.

At present the results of assessments in the five field placements have helped to formulate the following basic hypotheses, which it is hoped to test more rigorously in the future:

that there is a qualitative developmental scale which includes five stages (the five modes) to independent living and social survival in the community, and that this scale can be meaningfully used to assess the progress of mentally handicapped people;

that there is a complementary level of provision of service according to a person's capacity;

that if the opportunity and capacity are not complementary (again expressed by the five modes) behaviour problems result;

that both level of service and level of capacity can be expressed in terms of the amount of discretion allowed to express initiative in decisions concerning social functioning;

that the length of 'institutionalization' is not significant in determining the rate at which a person can re-adapt to take opportunities which are consistent with his or her capacity.

The research has attempted a first formulation of an assessment technique which charts capacity and level of opportunity simultaneously so that staff can make decisions based upon information regarding a total situation. The validity of the concepts, as always, needs further testing. One result reported by staff to date is that the assessment is helpful to them in focusing their observations. It requires staff to discuss their work and to question assumptions made in the course of that work. It requires a questioning of whether level of opportunity is compatible with capacity. Staff can then possibly alter the level of opportunity and further test their assumption about a person's capacity. The long-term aim is thus to enable mentally handicapped people to contribute to a society which in recent history has found it difficult to appreciate handicapped people's abilities as well as their inabilities.

Part Three

Participation and Collaboration

15

Community Health Councils: Intentions, Problems and Possibilities

Stephen Cang

One of the most novel elements in the reorganized Health Service has been the attempt to build 'public participation' into its running. In many ways the setting up of Community Health Councils (CHCs) exemplifies the way in which, in social as in personal matters, it is easy enough to have aims and ambitions while at the same time having no really clear idea as to what would be involved in translating such aims into practical reality.

The present chapter makes no attempt to deal with the broad issues of public participation, nor to enter the political debates now under way about the pros and cons of having CHCs. The aim here is restricted to the much more modest objective of reporting some detailed work which may contribute to a fuller understanding of the nature of CHCs and therefore to a clearer view of how they might fit into the larger NHS picture. One of the main questions thrown up by the creation of CHCs is how their functions relate to those of the governing authorities in the Health Service, especially the AHA. Examination of several practical problems which have been raised with the Unit in the course of field-work, and in conferences with a total so far of some 500 CHC members and secretaries, together with NHS officers and Authority members, may serve to put that question into sharper focus.

Before turning to specific problems, however, it is worth recalling that participation by the public in the running of health services must be understood to include any means by which people at large can affect the way the services function. Included among them, therefore, would be the people's collective voice speaking through Parliament and government;

the same at local level insofar as local government policies may influence the workings and aims of local AHAs through collaborative mechanisms; complaints by members of the public; the activities of a large variety and number of associations of all sorts, such as groups seeking to improve the lot of a particular category of patient, for example, or pressure groups seeking the adoption of particular policies; and, not least perhaps, the effects on the service of direct interactions between individual members of the public and individual members of the NHS.

Each of these channels affects the service. Yet the current usage of 'public participation' does not normally refer to any of the above. Instead two other ideas may be discerned in the discussion: first, the notion that additional, specifically 'participative' machinery is needed as part of the structure, and with the avowed aim of producing an identifiable impact on decisions taken by or within the service; and secondly the notion that the service must be responsive to people *personally*, leading to the desire to ensure that each individual should have some means of making his own mark on the service somehow.

Just what these ideas could mean in reality is discussed below; for the moment it is enough to note that, assuming they have been correctly stated, their meaning is far from clear.

The alternative to these ideas is felt to be an impersonal impenetrable and inappropriate entity, altogether out of touch with ordinary people and their concerns. The pressure has been and is for greater political control and a more 'open' service, less in the grip of the professionals and more under the sway of those who use it. It is striking to note (even though we cannot here pursue the theme) that this general movement is not confined to the NHS, nor even to state-run health services: one of the chief spokesmen of this outlook is Illich,[1] and the malaise is not confined to non-professionals.

Within the medical profession similar expressions of doubt and loss or error of direction are now audible,[2] forming part of a larger debate about how far the views and expectations

---

[1] I. Illich (1973), *Medical Nemesis*. See also M. Wilson (1975), *Health is for People*.

[2] See for example R. Carlson (1975), *The End of Medicine*, and P. Rhodes (1976), *The Value of Medicine*.

of patients, clients, and the public are reflected by officials and professional workers in the service.

What the instrument should be whereby participation by 'the public' takes place is, however, by no means a matter of general agreement. Here again there is a broad area which we cannot discuss, but which would include, among other matters, such debates as that about privately-financed, as against public, services, where the degree of personal control by the patient and the public at large is sometimes claimed to be greater.

So far as CHCs are concerned, however, the fact is that they are a given; they exist; and the meaning of their existence can be examined. This we can now proceed to do.

The CHC

Discussions of the CHC so far published have concentrated on two areas: surveying the characteristics of CHC members, comparing such matter as their age, political affiliation, attitudes, opinions, and activities; or else taking the CHC as a point of departure for more general discussions about the problems of participation, national public services or organizational structures. Most studies contain both.[3] The approach followed here is neither of these, though it is more closely linked with the general discussion of issues than with the gathering of survey data. The discussion which follows is based on the examination of specific problems raised for discussion by CHC members or secretaries, or by NHS members. By specific problems is meant problems in day-to-day conduct of business, which if examined and analysed for meaning lead rapidly to the general underlying features of the situation – such questions as what the work of the CHC should be, who is entitled to decide what, and so on. Consistent with the approach reported in other chapters in this book, our work has been directed to the construction of testable formulations about these underlying features.

Major Problems

Both in field discussions and in conferences, problems have consistently been reported under three heads: problems to do with CHC/NHS relationships; problems to do with CHC/public

[3] See R. Klein and J. Lewis (1976), *The Politics of Consumer Representation*; J. Hallas (1976), *CHCs in Action*.

relationships; and problems to do with the structure and functioning of the CHC itself. This grouping of issues seems to fit experience readily enough. It should therefore serve us as a framework here.

Problems of the CHC's internal organization and working must initially derive from what the CHC thinks it is doing; since this point can be illuminated, if not actually determined, by reference to its relationships with the public and the NHS respectively, it seems logical to leave the internal problems till last: if clarity on the other fronts can be reached much of the internal picture might fall into place.

Research to date has brought out the existence of a continuum of possibilities for a CHC identity, with consequent clarifications of policy on all three matters; public, NHS, and internal relationships. We now briefly review the problems under each heading and can then consider the analysis.

The CHC and the Public
The relationship between the CHC and the public seems the most important point to start from. Four main questions have arisen in CHC members' experience:

  (i)   in what sense does the CHC speak for the public?
  (ii) how can the public be involved by the CHC?
  (iii) what can the CHC do to become aware of what people really think about health services in the district?
  (iv) should the CHC give a 'balanced view' of public feelings and opinions, or should it concentrate on particular issues?

The questions tell their own story. For they contain a number of unresolved difficulties, to which no solution has yet been reached.

In the first placed, it has proved *impossible to find a single 'public'* where matters of health (or illness) are concerned. The contrast may be made with such other issues in daily life as environmental factors: pollution, aircraft noise, green belts, and so on. Everyone feels himself affected to a greater or lesser degree by the single issue. But there seems to be no such single issue so far as health/sickness is concerned. Instead there are a number of sub-populations, whose members share some common experience by virtue of suffering the same complaint, and which therefore may shift with time.

Secondly, a *general* involvement of the public in health matters has proved somewhat hard to achieve, with the exception of the issue of local hospitals and closures. Again, involvement is according to experience. Where no particular experience exists (i.e. among those generally healthy) there is no great incentive to become even active enough to signify one's existence to a CHC.

The third question brings out even more strongly what is already implicit above: the existence of a very particular difficulty in the field of health (i.e. sickness) services, and one which research in the field has ignored to its cost. The problem is that it is very difficult indeed to gain access to what people really think about the services they depend on when ill. The reasons are that if you are healthy the experience of sickness is far from consciousness and there is nothing much to report. While if you or a relative are ill, then you are too anxious to risk antagonizing the very people on whom you depend for help. Figures from patient-satisfaction surveys, regularly showing 90 per cent plus of satisfaction with the way things are, need to be interpreted in the light of this consideration. They also need to be contrasted with conversations commonly overheard in shops and buses, where health services and those who man and run them seem to attain a lower figure of satisfaction.

Finally, even if the CHC makes successful contact with the problems of the sub-populations, a major basic issue in representative government still arises: what is the CHC's position when it finds, as it inevitably would, that the wishes and pressures of the divers populations either bear no relation to each other or else carry contrary implications? Should the CHC pass on the raw material to the AHA via the DMT? Or should it somehow 'integrate' them into a balanced statement of the District's needs? And if in the course of 'balancing' the views of a section of the public get forgotten or squeezed out, where does the CHC stand then?

The CHC and the NHS
Failure to resolve the questions about its position *vis à vis* the population does not put the CHC into an easy position when

it comes to the NHS. (By relationships with the NHS is meant the whole spectrum of links with officers, teams, working groups, Authorities, and, in this context, the DHSS.) The main questions confronting CHCs have been:

(i) whether to act as a channel of information from the NHS to the public;[4]

(ii) what information about the NHS to obtain, and how to go about it;

(iii) whether to inspect the NHS and if so in what sense.

Each of these questions contains in turn a mass of practical uncertainties. CHCs have on occasion been seen by politicians as a useful channel for the conveying of health education propaganda, acting for the Secretary of State; or by NHS Authorities and officers as the PR wing of the service; both suggestions leading to discomfort in some CHC members at selling the public down the river.

The issue of information similarly poses basic practical uncertainties: does the CHC want all it can get? If so what does it do with it? If not, how to select? What rights has it (apart from the stated right of access and of obtaining information from the AHA) in practice to press the NHS, and what happens if the CHC gets unduly unpopular with the NHS for pressing a point – does the ill-feeling rebound on the CHC only or does it sour the whole feeling of the relationship between the local hospitals, clinics, and staff and the ordinary people?

In acquainting themselves with what goes on in the NHS and in the treatment (in the general, non-clinical sense) of patients, just what is the CHC doing? An inspectorial job? If so, how does this square with keeping up a useful interchange with the NHS? And how does it leave the CHC in relation to the public, since inspectors must be fair to those they inspect, partly identify with them and take account of their problems. Is this what the public wants of its CHC?

The Internal Workings of the CHC
Uncertainty on the above issues in turn again feeds uncertainty in the area of the CHC's own working arrangements, which

[4] Government policy has always included this view of CHCs. See, for example, Department of Health and Social Security (1977), *The Way Forward.*

of course directly depend on who it thinks it is and what it thinks it is trying to do. The main issues experienced are:

(i)   does the CHC function as a corporate body, with one voice; or is it a collection of independent subgroups which arise from such factors as the voluntary bodies represented, or from the interests of sub-populations in the district, or from other affiliations of CHC members?

(ii) should CHC members be experts on the NHS, and perhaps even members of the NHS?

(iii) is there an optimum structure of working groups of CHC members to deal with CHC business?

(iv) should CHC members have personal links with associations such as voluntary bodies with particular responsibilities for given groups in the community?

These are not 'nice' questions. In the case of one CHC which sought explicit clarification of such issues in collaboration with the Brunel Unit, the impetus behind its search was the finding that a proportion of members was becoming increasingly worried about the ineffectiveness of the CHC and the feeling that no real work was going on while at the same time a great deal of paper flew about and many evening hours were passed in talk. Conference discussions confirmed that this CHC was by no means alone in its experience.

An Underlying Polarity of Meanings
Preliminary analysis suggested that the uncertainty and consequent paralysis of action sprang from the co-existence in the CHC of two distinct and incompatible views of what the CHC was; and that these divergent views did not simply divide the members, but that some members were themselves divided. (This hypothesis, though of course not proving anything, was at least compatible with the reported experience of the CHC.)

The two views were broadly identified as follows. According to view A, the CHC was fundamentally a pressure group. It did not seek to run the NHS, nor to assume responsibility for its actions. Such a CHC, and its members, were first, foremost, and last identified with members and groups in the community who had need of health services and who wanted improvements in those services. According to view A, there was no sense in seeking 'The Public'. It did not exist, but its absence was no problem. The CHC merely got on with exploring the problems of the various 'publics' that did exist.

The questions posed above (p. 270) about relations with the public would be seen as follows: there was no speaking for the public, only the presentation of various pressures and opinions; contact with the public was all-important, and one of the major tasks of CHC members was to undertake the technical problems raised by such an aim; the balancing of views was for the AHA to do.

In other words, type-A members saw themselves as active in the community, carrying out explorations to determine the pattern of views on specific issues, fighting battles with the NHS as the need arose and generally gearing themselves to whatever was currently of importance among people in the District. The job of reconciling conflicting wishes and priorities was seen as belonging strictly to the AHA: the CHC's task was to help people who felt concerned to express to the AHA the full import of their experience.

Those who saw the situation this way often belonged to particular voluntary associations; but there were also independent members, unaffiliated to either such bodies or to local political structures, who simply had an interest in health provision and felt that much could be done to improve the services by paying greater attention to the views of those who received them.

View B by contrast was more identified with the NHS. Type-B members saw themselves somewhat as a constituted alternative AHA, an opposition or shadow body attempting to make itself felt as such. Inherent in this view of the CHC was the idea that the CHC should act as a corporate body. This implied that the CHC could realistically agree on a single view of conflicting interests and outlooks, and that if necessary it would be possible to settle matters by a vote. According to the view-B outlook, the purpose of the CHC was to transform public views, as expressed through the medium of CHC members themselves, into a balanced, single view which the whole membership would be prepared to stand by, and which they could be held responsible for having put forward to the AHA. In other words, CHC members spoke 'for the public' in something of the same sense that elected councillors or MPs spoke for their constituents – there was therefore little need to go among the people and discover the details of their views, since the fact of being on the CHC itself conferred representative status. By the same token, the task of balancing conflicting priorities could be confidently undertaken. View-B members tended to feel that the maximum of information was to be obtained and that the programme and structure of work would be significantly affected by that of the AHA and the Health Service, whereas view-A members felt less constrained by what the NHS was doing and more under the pressure of what was being felt by consumers.

In contrast to A-views the B-type outlook saw no great difficulty about promulgating official information and policies in such matters as health education.

Such an analysis, crude and exaggerated though it was, nevertheless served to clarify matters to some extent. It appeared that the choice was not either A or B, but that there might be a continuum between the two, allowing individuals and CHCs to locate themselves where they felt it appropriate.

In saying that for the time being these are questions of politics, what is admitted is that the principles underlying these choices remain obscure. It is hard to believe that none are there to be found.

The question of information provision is interesting in this connection, for it shows how underlying principles can begin to show through experience, if experience can be inspected closely enough.

CHC members and others had raised the problem of how to handle requests from the CHC to the NHS for information. In discussion, four separate problems emerged:

    (i) requests arising from NHS initiatives; e.g. where the DHSS seeks CHC views, and where the CHC needs information from the local officers before responding to DHSS (such as on the question of fluoridation of water supplies);

    (ii) requests arising from expressions of feeling among the public, which have become CHC projects (such as whether there exist plans to develop given services);

    (iv) requests from individual members of the public but conveyed through the CHC.

Discussion quickly resolved that the first two types of requests would reasonably entail the NHS providing the information – in the first case because it was an NHS sponsored matter, and in the second because the principle of answerability (in this quite concrete sense of providing answers) to the public presented no difficulty. The work of the CHC in relation to this, second, category of request was in effect to confer on the request the status 'of public concern' (i.e. not just an individual matter). The principle of the jury could thus be seen at work: the group of 'ordinary' people (i.e. not NHS members) deciding what was of concern to ordinary people.

This clarification answered the third kind of question: it would not be a legitimate request unless converted (by CHC ratification) into a second-category request. Thus where a CHC member with local knowledge of people's concerns could convince his CHC colleagues, his request became an 'on behalf of the community' request and moved across the boundary from merely being personal to him.

The fourth type of request would also require CHC judgment: it might or might not be pursued.

Analyses such as these open up the possibility that clarifying and creating appropriate mechanisms for getting the 'views of the public' on health (or any other service) matters back to those running the local service, whether it be locally or nationally funded, is likely to depend on a clearer understanding of how local communities are structured. For the moment we do not know enough about that question: but it seems that issues of 'local' response require more understanding of people in the context of their locality.

What Future for CHCs?

The main outstanding question is whether there is really a future for CHCs, at whatever point on the A–B continuum they put themselves. For if the choice is nearer to Type-B, then the range of conflicts which have arisen in some places between CHC members on the one hand and either AHAs, or teams, or individual officers (or all three) on the other may finally resolve themselves by formal incorporation of CHC members into the NHS structures. At this point the possibilities of hearing the ordinary voices of ordinary people might have faded.

Indeed, it is striking that already CHCs have on occasion been regarded with suspicion by pressure groups, or even by-passed by them altogether in the latters' dealings with the AHA, because of the feeling that 'the CHC is really too much a part of the NHS'. Such developments as the drawing of future AHA members from the CHC may be expected to reinforce these views of the relationship between the work of the CHC and AHA respectively.

However, if activity remains close to Type-A, it becomes hard to see the need for so elaborate a structure as the CHC. A federation of voluntary associations in the health field would do as well, and would reflect the state of local pressures. The CHC's right to be heard by the AHA is important, however, and it may be that this right would have by some means to be given either to the federation or to all pressure groups.

The natural wish of AHAs is to have one view put to them by one voice. This may, however, be shirking the main issue: which is precisely that *someone* has to judge the relative merits (in terms of current resource possibilities) of many pressures, all of which are deserving. The question is where *that* decision (and that responsibility) should lie? With the appointed-cum-elected AHA? Or with the less clearly chosen members of the CHC Type-A?

The present structure of the NHS makes it clear that responsibility for such decisions lies with the AHA. It is the membership of the Authority that is collectively charged by the Secretary of State, directly and through the RHA, with ensuring the provision of services. This must include decisions about precisely which services, the level to be achieved in each, and so forth.

In making their decisions on these issues, AHAs are subject to pressures and views from numerous sources, including for example higher level policies and recommendations, and the views of professional bodies and of staff groups. The setting up of CHCs in no way alters this state of affairs: it merely adds one further channel through which information and opinion can reach the AHA.

There is no reason, therefore, why the CHC should

necessarily present a single balanced view to the AHA. It may choose to do so, but that choice would be governed by CHC judgments about the best way of handling each particular issue.

The problem posed by the creation of CHCs remains: what are these groups? They are not corporate bodies, speaking with one voice; nor are they 'polyvalent' committees[5] bringing together clearly represented interests. Put in other terms, in what way can a community express its views? Neighbourhood councils, community councils, parish councils all share with CHCs the job of expressing local views. The important issue is how such communities are defined, because size and boundary play such a large part in facilitating or hindering the sharing of common experience and the gradual crystallizing of broad opinions.

Thus it may be that the formation of natural health care communities is necessary if the intentions behind the CHC are to be fulfilled. If such entities were set up, and the confusions attendant upon present districts and areas reduced, with better links made possible between the Health Authority and the staff of the service, and between the staff and the local population, then the growth of local opinion might become correspondingly easier to observe and make explicit. This would be the work of the CHC.

[5] This term is used by Brian Parkyn of Glacier Institute of Management, Cawston, Rugby.

16

Employee Participation

Elliott Jaques

The problem of employee participation in the NHS will not be resolved if it is constrained within a narrow industrial relations context. It must be seen as part of a much broader issue: that of the constitutional question in Britain as a whole of the dispossession of 23 million men and women from the right to take part in setting the policies which affect them in their work – as manual workers, office staff, managers, nurses, civil servants, scientists, social workers, local government officers, specialists, and so on.

A person's work is of enormous psychological as well as economic importance to him. If he has no constitutional right to take part in determining the long- and short-term policies which have such a bearing on his work and career, he is resentful, hostile, and suspicious – all readily predictable reactions of sound and sensible human beings feeling imposed upon by forces outside their control. Suspicion starts the process of alienation from work and withdrawal from reasoned argument; if things go wrong, even with well-intentioned management, withdrawal increases in the form of low motivation in work, or absenteeism. Finally, in the event of strong disagreements, collective withdrawal results, leaving management in an impotent position and with reasoned debate difficult to re-establish.

Bitterness and resentment are particularly acute in Britain compared to any other industrialized democratic nation. Britain was the first to industrialize; over 90 per cent of its citizens who earn a living do so in employment for a wage or salary – a higher proportion than any other nation; over 11 million of the 23 million employed are collectively organized in trade unions.

It is for this reason of the scale and age of its industrialization that Britain is experiencing particularly difficult problems of industrial relations. Other industrial nations will encounter similar difficulties in the coming years. It is because of their seeming intractability that the problems of industrial relations – not only in industry but in the public and social services as well – have moved into the position of the most important issue for the survival of Britain as an efficient and prosperous community, with humanity, democratic cohesion, and justice. Investment, production, exporting, innovative new products, are all of great importance. But effort in these directions is increasingly thwarted because of nascent industrial tension and unrest.

In their role as citizens, the employed men and women in Britain enjoy universal suffrage. Legislative policies are not imposed. They are arrived at by the power of persuasion – by argument, pressure group advocacy, and Parliamentary debate. The important feature is the constitutional setting – of Parliament and local government – in which this rational power can be freely exercised. A framework of rule of law exists which can be relied upon and which by and large allows reason to hold sway.

In contrast to the political life of the nation, in the large employment systems – and the NHS is one of the largest – in which so many are engaged in so many occupations and professions and at so many levels, there is no constitutional setting which allows citizens to have the same involvement in making the policies which affect them in their working lives. This state of affairs is democratically unacceptable and economically ruinous. The urgent constitutional task of the late twentieth century is to extend the democratic idea into the work setting.

Greater opportunity for open and constitutionally established rights must be provided. Every private or governmental employer must realize that in taking up such a role he is accepting responsibility for helping to tackle the single largest problem in the whole employment zone. The way in which he deals with employees adds its cumulative contribution to what the work force – from managers to shop and office floor – thinks about Britain today.

At the same time, many employees want very rapid change. They must be given the opportunity to express their desire through constitutional channels of participation. Those channels do not exist. Until they do there is no outlet other than for varying degrees of non-co-operation or disruption. By contrast, in the presence of constitutional channels, radical thinking can become a lively stimulus to effective change.

Power and Participation
The basic need to work out new institutions for constitutional participation arises from the dramatic changes in the distribution of power which have taken place since 1945. These changes are not yet complete.

Up to 1939 power had been steadily migrating from individual employers and employers' associations to trade unions. Since 1945 this migration of power has accelerated until today the potentiality of employers to resist demands from individual trade unions has radically diminished. This change is dramatically evident in the relationship between government itself and trade unions of government employees, as in the NHS itself.

Alongside this migration of power from employers to trade unions another migration has been taking place. This is the migration of power from the central organization of individual trade unions down through their hierarchies of officials to shop stewards. And the process does not stop there. A third movement of power can now be discerned: a migration of power from shop stewards and other elected representatives of employees down to the grass roots – to groups of individual employees.

This on-going process of growing power in the shops and offices can be readily seen in industry, in commerce, in the Civil Service, in public and social services, in education – in short everywhere where people are employed, and in particular in the larger enterprises. And here is where the big problem arises: in contrast to our historical national shift to the universal franchise in government, there are no adequate constitutional means by which employee power can express itself through shop steward representatives and other representatives, as a matter of right, in order to take part in setting the policies which govern the enterprises in which they are employed.

It is just such a constitutional right by which we shall define participation in this paper.

Consultation and Participation

A number of processes, commonly referred to as consultation, must be sharply distinguished from constitutional participation as we shall define it here.

First there is the normal everyday consultation between a manager and his immediate subordinates – briefing groups, as they are often called. Such consultation, in which a manager keeps his subordinates informed and seeks their views and advice, is a fundamental requirement of effective manager–subordinate relationships. There is a regressive trend in some enterprises to refer to this ordinary activity of any good manager by the title of 'participative management' and, because they believe that this is what participation is about, to think no further.

Second, there is the process – which may be termed *consultation* – whereby a manager will consult with elected representatives – for general discussion, usually excluding what are termed 'negotiation issues' (that is to say, payment and conditions). In this process, the manager remains free to take his own decisions after consultation. What is less commonly noted is that the representatives and their constituents, if dissatisfied, are also free to take the matter further, the mechanism being to issue threats or actually to exercise power by withdrawal in one form or another.

In this process the manager often sincerely believes that he remains free to take his own decisions after consultation. If differences of aspiration are small or the issues trivial the manager may get away with it. But where interests really diverge, a manager's decision to proceed without agreement appears to representatives as lacking in integrity. It throws up the question 'Why consult with us if you intend to proceed anyhow?'

This sort of consultation, well-intentioned as it may be, breeds feelings of cynicism and distrust. As a reaction to this felt authoritarianism on the part of managers, the thoughts of the work force turn to consideration of the need to use its power to withdraw. Is it to be a work-to-rule, a go-slow or a down-tools? Morale is debased and active co-operation is at a discount.

If active use of power to disrupt the enterprise is threatened, then – win or lose – attitudes emerge which for a time will in-

hibit the ability of all parties to the conflict to debate it rationally – the essential prelude to effective agreement.

In short, consultation procedures of this kind – while un-
doubtedly well-intentioned – are nevertheless in the final analysis built upon the very uncertain foundation of the power of
withdrawal from a reasoned argument and then from work
itself. Resentment, touchiness, unease, are never far away –
these are the feelings which breed distrust, make for unreasoned
resistance to necessary change, and lead to explosive reactions
to stress.

Managers and subordinates alike try to maintain the surface
appearance of goodwill and reasonableness. But these attitudes
do not strike deeply. Underneath there is little room for patient
and rational work. There are too many unanswered questions
surrounding the issue of 'What if we – or they – do not agree?'
The answer – either swallow it or fight – does not make for
long-term progress in sound working relations.

The Conditions for Constitutional Participation

We wish, therefore, to set out what we believe experience will
increasingly come to show to be the absolute requirements of
constitutional participation.[1]

There must be provision for a Negotiating Council in each
Health District. A Negotiating Council is a negotiating body
which would take part in determining policies and procedures
for the site it covers, within the constraints of such external
policies as the law, national agreements between employers and
trade unions, and agreements arrived at in the enterprise as
a whole.

Councils would of course not take part in negotiations on Parliamentary legislation. Everyone must work within the law –
including employee representatives in whatever enterprise,
public or private, they may be employed. But within the law
there is massive scope for discussion and negotiation, on local
establishment and conditions, differential investment in various

---

[1] Much of this analysis has been drawn from experience at the Glacier
Metal Company, described in a more general context in Jaques (1976),
General Theory of Bureaucracy, Chapters 12 and 13, and in Wilfred Brown
(1971), *Organization*. The conceptions have been checked in field discussions
in the NHS, and in HSORU conferences on participation.

services, and on all the other varied means of implementing legislated enactments.

These Councils would comprise one or more members of the DMT meeting with representatives of all staff in the District. Not only the 'shop floor' staff, but each of the nationally recognized negotiating bodies with members in the District, must be able to have its own representative in the policy-making processes. Many of these groups are union-organized, and many are professional but not trade unions. Mixed union–non-union representation on Councils is thus called for.

The role of the DMT member(s) is to express the view of the AHA and top management, to seek change, to give information to the Council members, and to keep the AHA and higher management informed of the views and attitudes of employees.

No subjects would be excluded from Council agendas, although decisions would have to have regard to the higher policy constraints already referred to. The point is to be able to consider all issues in their interrelationships, especially the explosive issue of differential entitlements. One of the main reasons why this issue of differentials is so difficult nationally is because of the failure of enterprises to handle their own internal differential problems adequately.

The Council members must be kept fully informed about all matters: work prospects, plans for new services or new methods and developments, income, transfer of activities to other sites or departments, and so on. Where release of confidential information might be damaging to the enterprise, the Council could be informed of the subject in general terms, so that no questions of secrecy could arise.

Because the Councils would not only represent all groups in the District but also all levels, they would give opportunity for interaction between representatives at lower and higher levels up to the level of the DMT and Department Heads.

Decisions on Negotiating Councils should be by consensus. That is to say, discussion and debate could continue over more than one meeting if no clear consensus had emerged. Discussion and work can go on between meeting, new possibilities explored and considered, with a view to working through to a negotiated decision in which all are sufficiently in accord to make for a workable policy when adopted. During such a continuing negotiation process, all must accept the continued operation of the *status quo*.

The decisions of Councils would have to be binding upon all the members represented, including the Authority. Equally, where trade unions are represented by their shop stewards, the unions would be committed: it would therefore be necessary for there to be wide circulation of agendas and minutes, not only within the enterprise but also to the local trade union offices so that no agreements would be negotiated which were unacceptable within the unions.

It would be useful if at least some of the staff from the District were enabled to attend as observers. This would give those represented on the Council the chance to know at first hand what was going on.

The process described will be seen to be precisely the opposite of the common pattern of fragmented negotiation in which each power group negotiates separately and confidentially with top management. The result of such fragmented negotiation is the familiar leap-frogging, together with an avoidance of face-to-face debate among the negotiating groups. Thorough-going consensus is not achievable by these means.

Decision by Consensus in Negotiating Councils
The principle that decisions of Councils must be by all-round consent (that is to say, no decisions must be imposed by out-voting a protesting minority) is fundamental. The status quo would obtain until change had been agreed by all Council members. To be absolutely specific: management would not impose unacceptable change upon employees; nor employees upon management; nor – and this point warrants reflection – employee groups upon one another.

The basic concept here is that no significant power group shall be coercively overridden by the imposition of a change to which it is determinedly opposed. The reality of power in these circumstances is the precipitation of industrial action, per-haps short of strike at first but by strike in the end. What people fail to see is that, once the strike has occurred, all round agree-ment must certainly then be discovered by some means before work can be resumed.

The process of constitutional participation described has the effect of absorbing the physical conflict into due constitutional process around the conference table while work goes on. That is what due process is about. And paradoxically, far from slowing the process of decision-making and preventing change, experience shows the opposite to be the case: decisions are not only reached more quickly, but they are better, more carefully thought-out, and less patched up to reach desperate last-minute compromise.

The reason for these apparently paradoxical outcomes is not far to seek. They arise because once coercive imposition has been constitutionally debarred, it becomes possible for everyone to listen to other arguments and to give consideration to them; and it becomes essential to present rational arguments not just on a personal basis but on behalf of one's real constituents – the employees in the enterprise. The fact that sound constitutional arrangements give the greatest chance for rational argument and debate to take place (even though they cannot guarantee it) is one of their most constructive features.

It is the opposite arrangement – fragmented negotiations even if combined with consultation – which is destructive of sound decision-making. Fear of coercive imposition leads to suspicion, uncertainty, and to everyone's 'Playing it close to the chest'. Authorities and their DMTs are unwilling to be too bold for fear of unknown employee reaction. Employees are unwilling to give too freely for fear of setting precedents that will be regretted. In such influences are the real sources of indecisiveness, unnecessary delay and stagnation.

Apart from Acts and Regulations agreed by Parliament it is improper for central government simply to impose its will on public and social service employees. The decisions which Authorities make in the course of implementing legislation must be subject to participation by employee representatives as are the policies of the Board of an enterprise. The principles of participation must apply.

For government and its Authorities representing the people, to reject employee participation in the name of the people would be to turn the democratic community into an autocratic management seeking unquestioning obedience to its decisions from its public servants.

17

Collaboration Between Health and Social Services

Ralph Rowbottom and Anthea Hey

Although controversy still lingers on whether the provision of health and social services should be combined within one public agency,[1] the issue has been largely decided in practice in Britain[2] at least for the immediate future, with the creation in 1971 of unified social services departments (SSDs) under local authorities, and the separate creation in 1974 of unified Area Health Authorities (AHAs) under direct government control. From the time of their separate conception, however, it was recognized that close collaboration between the two services would be crucial for a mass of people whose ill-health or handicap was combined with vulnerability in their everyday living situation.[3] Even so, the attempt to engineer close collaboration has not proved easy. Some of the difficulties have stemmed directly from the specific administrative changes just mentioned. Others are more deeply rooted in different modes of professional practice and organization.

In exploring this subject further we draw material from two main sources. The first is a series of six conferences on various aspects of collaboration between health and social services, held at Brunel between 1974 and 1977. The second is a number of different field projects in health and social services, which took place at about the same time, also concerned in various respects

---

[1] The controversy is still lively, for example, in the field of mental handicap. See Chapter 13.

[2] Excluding Northern Ireland, where combined health and social services agencies do exist.

[3] See Government White Paper (1972), *National Health Service Reorganization: England.*

with collaboration, including three projects in the specific field of health social work.

One whole group of problems which was encountered concerned the relationships of doctors, nurses, social workers, and other practitioners interacting in particular cases, and how they might be strengthened and improved. How could social work best be provided in hospitals? How could closer links be made between social workers and general medical practitioners? How could better co-ordination in the provision of health care and social services be achieved for the chronically ill or handicapped; or, for example, for the elderly person living at home? And (most generally of all) how could social workers and other social services staff on the one hand, and doctors, nurses, and other health staff on the other, better understand and appreciate each other's distinct competences, outlooks, and contributions?

A second group of problems which was encountered concerned collaboration in broader development and planning. What, for example, were the proper functions of the so-called Health Care Planning Teams, conceived as part of the original design for the new Health Services, whose constitution specifically allowed for regular social services representation?[4] What, by contrast, were the proper functions and relationships of the so-called Joint Care Planning Teams and District Planning Teams which were introduced at a later point?[5] What specific role should be played in planning and development by those community medicine specialists who were given particular responsibility for liaison with social services?[6] And from the social services side, what should be the specific role of the variously-named 'health service advisers' and 'health services liaison officers'.[7] What should be expected from the Joint Consultative Committees, the bodies which brought elected members of local authorities (the providers of social services, education, housing, etc.) face to face with appointed members of corresponding

[4] Department of Health and Social Security (1972), *Management Arrangements for the Reorganized Health Service*, Chapter 2.

[5] DHSS Circular HC(77)17 (1977), *Joint Care Planning: Health and Local Authorities*.

[6] DHSS Circular HSC(IS)13 (1974), *Community Medicine in the Reorganized Health Service*.

[7] DHSS Circular LASSL(73)47 (1973).

Area Health Authorities? Should these joint bodies attempt to foster or finance schemes of their own? Was it in any case really possible to combine joint planning either with existing corporate planning processes in local authorities, or with the complex national planning process which was being developed in the National Health Service?[8]

Looking overall, problems arising from lack of conterminosity and the absence of clear counterpart units in the two services were constantly posed. How did one cope where several social services authorities related to one Health Authority, as in London? Should senior officers of the SSDs be looking primarily to officers at Area level or at District level in Health Authorities, for their natural counterparts? How could health services like those for the mentally ill and handicapped, which were often supplied on an Area-wide if not a trans-Area basis, be brought into the collaboration framework? What was to be done where the geographical subdivisions of SSDs did not correspond to the boundaries of Health Districts?[9]

Further problems were raised about such things as intrinsic difficulties in current health services planning procedures; about the excessive demands for consultation with staff unions and other public and voluntary agencies, on both the health and the social services side; about the very reality of undertaking so-called 'planning' in times of acute economic stringency; and so on. Many of these problems too were seen to bear indirectly, if not directly, on issues of collaboration.

It is apparent, then, that the problems that can arise in connection with collaboration are many and varied indeed. What

[8] For official reports on these various matters, further to those already quoted, see DHSS (1973), *A Report from the Working Party on Collaboration between National Health Service and Local Government on its activities to the end of 1972;* DHSS (1973), *A Report from the Working Party on Collaboration between the National Health Service and Local Government on its activities from January to July 1973;* and DHSS (1974), *Social Work Support for the Health Service – Report of the Working Party.*

[9] Because of their very local and particular nature, problems of geographical overlap and lack of conterminosity are not further explored here. Nor, in spite of their more general nature, are specific problems of collaboration arising in multi-district Health Areas since these are so contingent upon the whole conception of the possible separation of District and Area functions (see below) the adequacy of which comes increasingly in doubt, as discussed in Chapter 2.

we shall try to do, drawing from our research, is to highlight what we see as some of the main issues, and to reveal the prime factors that appear to have to be taken into account in trying to get to grips with them. It is not our aim here, however, to explore all or any of these specific problems in great detail, let alone to offer a full range of possible model solutions.

Intrinsic Features of Present Health and Social Services Which Make for Difficulties in Collaboration

For a start, if we take a closer look at the field in which collaboration is to take place, it appears that there are (at the time of writing) a number of prominent features of health and social services which present intrinsic obstacles to easy collaboration.

First and foremost there is the striking difference in the fundamental shape and kind of organization in the two services, as illustrated in Figure 17.1. (We shall contain our discussion and analysis to local level, leaving aside, that is, Regional Health Service organization and central government.)

The organization of health services exhibits, even within the AHA, a most complex pattern.[10] The main outlines are shown in Figure 17.1. There is a mixture of medical staff in *independent practice*;[11] nurses, administrative, and other related staff in a series of separate but parallel *managerial*[12] hierarchies according to occupation; and paramedical and scientific staff (not shown in Figure 17.1) whose exact organizational situation is still somewhat unclear.

The lead in the general planning and control of health services within each District is expected to be taken not by one chief executive officer, but by a team, the District Management Team (DMT). The DMT is itself a complex mixture of appointed officers and elected representatives of medical consultants and general medical practitioners, in which no one person has managerial authority (as here defined) over any of the others. The DMT may enlist the help of Health Care Planning Teams (HCPTs)[13] in various special fields in its work of

[10] See Chapter 2, and also DHSS (1972), *Management Arrangements for the Reorganized Health Services.*

[11] For the definition of *independent practice* see Appendix B.

[12] For the definition of *managerial* roles, see Appendix B.

[13] To be renamed 'District Planning Teams' in the light of DHSS Circular HC(77)17 (1977), *Joint Care Planning: Health and Local Authorities.*

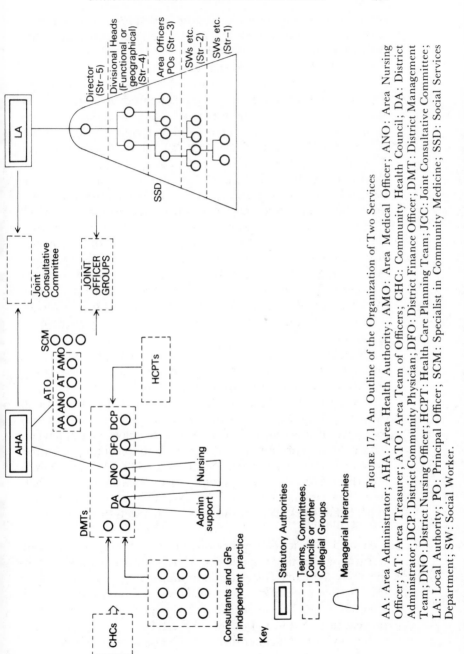

FIGURE 17.1 An Outline of the Organization of Two Services

AA: Area Administrator; AHA: Area Health Authority; AMO: Area Medical Officer; ANO: Area Nursing Officer; AT: Area Treasurer; ATO: Area Team of Officers; CHC: Community Health Council; DA: District Administrator; DCP: District Community Physician; DFO: District Finance Officer; DMT: District Management Team; DNO: District Nursing Officer; HCPT: Health Care Planning Team; JCC: Joint Consultative Committee; LA: Local Authority; PO: Principal Officer; SCM: Specialist in Community Medicine; SSD: Social Services Department; SW: Social Worker.

comprehensive planning. Again, the fundamental relationships of the members of any HCPT are (in general) collegial rather than managerial, one to another.

Since the optimum size of the Health District as the basic unit for the comprehensive provision and development of integrated health services has been estimated at roughly one-quarter of a million population, a large proportion of Areas (which were by specific ruling to be coterminous with either non-metropolitan counties or with one or more metropolitan district local authorities) have had to be split into two or more Health Districts. This leads to the unusual conception of a Health District organization which is not a separate and lower tier to be administered by Area Officers but a primacy manifestation of the executive organization of the Health Authority. DMTs have direct access to the membership of the Authority itself. Chief officers at District level are not (manifestly at any rate) accountable to their Area counterparts, but directly to the AHA. The ostensible role of the Area Team of Officers (ATO) in a multi-district Area is not to *manage* District Officers or District organization, but to *monitor and co-ordinate* them on behalf of the AHA.

Using the idea of *work-strata* described in Chapter 7, it seems implicit in the very idea of the Health District that the DMT as a body is intended to consider matters of 'comprehensive service provision' (Stratum-4). Indeed, it is not unreasonable to suppose that they are intended to go a stage further, in considering ways of meeting health needs in the most general terms within their given territories, that is of undertaking 'comprehensive field coverage' work (Stratum-5). Thus, both the DMT and the ATO as bodies (though not necessarily each of their individual members) might be assumed to be working, or expected to work, at essentially the same level, that is Stratum-5.

Health Districts do not of course have their own separate statutory governing bodies. The AHA is the immediate governing body for each District. To enhance the responsiveness of the District to public needs and views, a Community Health Council (CHC) has been established in each with considerable powers to monitor, comment, and advise.

By contrast, the general shape of SSDs is relatively straightforward, being that of a single managerial hierarchy headed by the Director of Social Services.[14] Moreover (and in contrast to health services), it is not too difficult to identify the different broad levels at which various categories of staff are expected to work, although of course detailed organization within these levels varies considerably. Using the concepts of *work-strata* described in Chapter 7, the Director of Social Services, for example, may be expected to be concerned with 'comprehensive field coverage' (Stratum-5). Immediately below him various Deputy Directors, Assistant Directors, or in some cases heads of large geographical Divisions, may be expected to be concerned with 'comprehensive service provision' (Stratum-4), each in his own defined field. Various Area Officers and Principal Officers may be expected to be concerned with 'systematic service provision' (Stratum-3). Finally, the field social workers themselves, the residential workers, home helps, and other operational staff, will for the most part be dealing with individual cases one by one (Stratum-1 or 2).

Beyond this striking contrast in the basic form and kind of organization in the two services are further intrinsic difficulties arising from the different 'natural' scales of division at all levels within the two services. 'Natural' Health Districts, often grouped around one large general hospital, or an equivalent group of smaller hospitals are (as already noted) smaller than the size of some existing local authorities to which the SSD itself corresponds. On the other hand, with populations of around 250,000, Health Districts are of an order larger than the typical catchment area of a local Area Social Work office, which most conveniently and efficiently serves a population of about 40,000–80,000.[15] This in turn is of an order larger than the natural catchment area of a typical general medical practice (several thousand), or even a typical health centre (10,000–20,000).[16] Even in these larger SSDs that opted for a main substructure of major, all-purpose geographical Divisions headed by Stratum-4 Divisional Directors, such Divisions tend to be

[14] See Brunel Institute of Organization and Social Studies, Social Services Organization Research Unit (1974), *Social Services Departments*.

[15] See 'Seebohm' Report (1968), *Report of Committee on Local Authority and Allied Personal Social Services*, Chapter 19.

[16] See DHSS (1971), *The Organization of Group Practice*.

somewhat smaller than existing Health Districts. Nowhere are there ready equivalences.

Organizing for Collaboration in Individual Cases
It is within this difficult framework that collaborative arrangements have to be devised. As we have said, some of the problems, namely those to do with broader development and planning, are particularly influenced by the given legislative and administrative structure. To these we will return later. Others, however, stem more directly from both established patterns of actual professional practice in the two fields and from current uncertainties or conflicting ideas about what such patterns ought to be. We shall now consider some of these second kinds of issue, which bear chiefly upon the way in which individual cases are handled.

GENERAL STRATEGIES FOR IMPROVING COLLABORATION IN INDIVIDUAL CASES. How in general can better working links be established between various practitioners, for example doctors, nurses, and social workers, who are concerned in the same cases? How can better communication patterns be established; better co-ordination and continuity; more cross-fertilization of ideas; more opportunities for explaining and demonstrating the specific and different contributions of the various established and emerging professions? Very often it is claimed that the most important change needed is in the personal attitudes of many of the staff concerned. To the extent that this is true, there are obvious implications at least for a broadening of the content of basic professional training programmes, and perhaps for the establishment of specific further education programmes as well.

However, formal educative or re-educative programmes are not by any means the only strategies available for effecting improvement. Many different structural or organizational changes are also possible. For example, networks of interaction can be strengthened by such things as the appointment of liaison officers or of other 'contacts'; by the physical alignment of working premises and 'catchment areas'; or by the outposting of staff from one service into residential or day care institutions (hospitals, homes, centres, clinics) provided by the other. A further and quite distinctive step can be taken where a deliberate move is made not merely to establish a strengthened *network*, but a separate *team* involving staff of various disciplines from the two services.[17] In a team, a high degree of personal identification, commitment, and permanency is called for; new team members must be acceptable to pre-existing colleagues; and so on. There are pros and cons to both teams and networks.[18]

Let us look at some of these organizational strategies in more detail.

LINKING SOCIAL WORK TO HEALTH SERVICE INSTITUTIONS. Some of the alternative patterns of organization for creating better linkages of social work with *health service institutions* that have become identified in the course of the research described are as follows.[19]

(a) Arrangements can be made for all referrals for social services from a particular hospital, health centre, or group practice, to go to one particular area social work team, physically nearby, or with similar catchment area; what might be called straightforward *alignment* schemes.

(b) In addition, one of the social workers in the area team can be given a designated *liaison* role with the institution concerned.

(c) Alternatively, one or more social workers may be out-posted[20] full-time or part-time from an area team (that is, remaining still under the management of the Area Officer) or from a separate health or hospital social work team (remaining under the management of a separate

[17] For precise definitions of these, the contrasted conception of *network* and *team*, see Appendix B.

[18] See further discussion of this theme in Chapter 10, 'The Future of Child Guidance'.

[19] For further discussion, see A. Hey and R. Rowbottom (1974), 'The Organization of Social Work in Hospitals and Other Health Care Settings'.

[20, 21] For precise definitions of these specific terms, *outposting* and *attachment*, see Appendix B. Where social workers are *attached* to specific doctors, questions of the exact authority relation of the latter to the former inevitably arise. Whether or not doctors may in principle *prescribe to*, or *manage*, qualified social workers, is touched on in Chapter 5, 'Professionals in Health and Social Services Organizations'. The effect of any pronounced differences in the level-of-work capacities of doctors and social workers in such situations is touched on in Chapter 10, 'The Future of Child Guidance'.

principal health or hospital social work manager) to work in a particular health institution, where the volume of work justifies it.

(d) In effect, all the above represent varieties of attempts to establish stronger networks. Sometimes a deliberate decision may be made to establish still closer links by *attaching*[21] a specific social worker to a group medical practice, or to a specific medical 'firm' or team within a hospital.

Research has also revealed a whole range of factors (some pulling in different directions) which will influence choices of the best of these models to adopt in any given situation: such things as the volume of work; the desirability of maintaining strong integration with medical care in certain types of cases; the desirability of keeping continuity of social work with any one patient, both in and out of hospital; and so on. Discussions suggest that a variety of models may be called for within one SSD even within one large hospital, playing one factor against another in each situation. For example, the sheer number of group medical practices in the local authority area may allow for no more than alignment, liaison, or part-time outposting schemes. Larger hospitals or large health centres may justify full-time outposting or attachments.[22]

LINKING HEALTH CARE TO SOCIAL SERVICES INSTITUTIONS. We have been considering various organizational strategies for linking social work more effectively to established health care settings and institutions – to hospitals, health centres, and group practices. In principle, the same kinds of strategies must be available for the converse task of linking specific health services more effectively to various *social services settings* – to residential establishments and day centres.

Although we do not draw here on the same range or intensity of project-work or conference discussion, it is not difficult to identify examples in current practice of schemes for establishing stronger linkages of this kind. There are, for example, schemes which create 'visiting medical officers' to monitor hygiene and general health standards in residential or other establishments on a sessional basis. Then there is the frequent use of psychia-

---

[22] See A. Hey and R. Rowbottom (1974), op. cit.

trists and child psychotherapists on a sessional basis in certain children's homes, particularly in reception-assessment centres for children.

Beyond this, all sorts of further possibilities might at least be discussed in an exploratory way, for example the designation of certain community nurses as liaison officers for particular social services institutions where a high level of nursing work arises, as with the infirm elderly; or even possibly the actual attachment of such staff on a full-time or part-time basis. Or again, there is the possibility of the outposting or attachment on a part-time or full-time basis of occupational therapists or physiotherapists to specific social services institutions where the clientele suffer a high degree of handicap (this leaves aside possibilities of the direct employment of such paramedical staff by local authorities).

REFERRAL PATTERNS AND CASE RESPONSIBILITY. Looking more generally at cases which call for both health care and social services, discussions have often revealed that effective collaboration is undermined by lack of clarity in agreed referral patterns between the two services, and also as to who is supposed to be carrying prime responsibility at any time. Doctors, for example, often complain that cases referred by them to social services appear to get lost or forgotten, or that they are not kept informed of subsequent action by social services. Social workers, on the other hand, complain that they are expected to take on impossible case-loads. Residential, day care staff, and home helps often feel that they have in fact more contact with many clients than the field social workers who are nominally 'carrying' the case.

Within clear-cut health settings, and in respect of clear-cut health matters, the situation is tolerably clear in principle at least. Referrals for diagnosis, prognosis, and treatment are always to doctors. It is doctors who retain *prime responsibility*[23] for all such work, and where they 'refer' cases to other health professionals, for example nurses or physiotherapists, these are referrals for specific tasks to be undertaken within the

[23] See Chapter 5, 'Professionals in Health and Social Services'.

framework of a more-or-less broad medical prescription, and not referrals for suggested transfer of prime responsibility.[24]

When referrals are made by health services staff to social services, however, there is no one category of worker who invariably receives the referral or invariably carries prime responsibility. Many referrals go directly to social workers (that is to staff with this specific designation, whether or not they have a specific social work qualification). Many, however, go direct to home help organizers, or to occupational therapists employed by the local authority.

A number of questions arise here. Is it appropriate that referrals should go directly to social services staff other than social workers? Where a social worker and a home help organizer, for example, are both involved together, who takes prime responsibility? Does the doctor continue to carry prime responsibility in any sense in connection with the work of these social services staff? Our discussions revealed wide-scale uncertainty on many of these matters.

Considering the last question first it may be suggested as an underlying principle that there are always two distinct prime responsibilities to be assigned where health and social services staff work together, however closely integrated their mode of work. On the one hand, there is prime responsibility for the case seen as one of actual or potential 'social distress' and thus coming within the aegis of the local authority as the responsible body. On the other, there is prime responsibility for the case seen as one of actual or potential 'ill health'.

Clearly there is room for discussion about the exact borderline between 'ill health' and 'social distress', particularly in psychiatric work or child guidance. Nevertheless, each of the two agencies with which we are concerned here – health and social services – does have an independent role to play, and an independent accountability to observe. However closely his work is integrated with that of social services staff within a multidisciplinary team, it would appear to follow that the doctor will have an independent responsibility for the health needs of the client, even the client living within a residential home run by social services (although additional complexities will arise to

[24] But see further discussion in Chapter 9, 'Physiotherapy and Occupational Therapy'.

the extent that social workers are acting *in loco parentis*). Similarly the social worker will always have an independent responsibility for the social problems of the client, even the client in hospital (though social workers at present may not always have easy access to those who should be their clients).

So far as the location of prime responsibility for social care is concerned, several further guiding principles may perhaps be established in the effort to reduce or avoid uncertainty. First, there is the desirability of establishing which specific categories of social services staff as between, say, social workers, home help organizers, and heads of day or residential centres, can in practice assume prime responsibility for social services cases.

Second, there is the desirability that all such staff should be fully competent workers in their own field and capable of Stratum-2 work in that field, that is, of making independent assessments of need-in-depth. Thus, if any workers in any case were judged only to be able to work in Stratum-1, or still in process of developing full Stratum-2 competence, then the prime responsibility should be seen as resting with their Stratum-2 supervisors. (To strengthen this point we should observe that our own work has suggested that at the moment most social workers in the basic grade are *not* to be considered fully developed Stratum-2 workers.)[25]

Finally, it should be generally recognized that part of necessary competence to take prime responsibility is having a developed sense of when to involve professionals of other kinds. Thus, for example, if home help organizers are to receive direct referrals (from whatever source) and to carry prime responsibility, they must be competent to decide when expert social work intervention is called for, or the work of aids and adaptations specialists, or when (in some circumstances) a doctor should be called in.

Collaboration in Planning and Development
DIFFERENT LEVELS OF PLANNING. So far we have been concerned with the question of getting better understanding of the situations in which collaboration takes place in individual cases, and some ideas of the possibilities for better organization of work

[25] See Chapter 7 'The Stratification of Work and Organizational Design'.

at this level. We turn now to broader issues of planning and development.

Using ideas of work-strata it is apparent that the word 'planning' can be employed in three very different contexts:

(a) *planning in individual cases* (implying work levels not necessarily higher than Stratum-1 or 2),[26]

(b) *planning better systems* to deal with particular kinds of cases within given institutional settings (implying at least a Stratum-3 level of work);

(c) *comprehensive planning*, with a territory-wide focus, in some given range or field of service, involving extensive surveys of community need, the balanced provision of capital and manpower resources over extended periods of time (implying at least a Stratum-4 or 5 level of work).

Some of the issues in improving collaborative planning in the context of the individual case (a) have already been examined. We will now look at arrangements for collaborative planning in these further and broader contexts, (b) and (c) above, starting with the latter. Finally, we shall consider the role of liaison officers from both services in these broader planning and development activities.

COLLABORATION IN COMPREHENSIVE, TERRITORY-WIDE PLANNING OF SERVICES (STRATUM-4/5 WORK). Let us consider first, then, various arrangements for collaborative planning of comprehensive health and social services (Stratum-4/5) – comprehensive both in terms of range, however broad or narrow the particular field of interest concerned, and in terms of meeting social needs throughout the whole of some defined geographical area. Significant capital expenditure is often involved at these levels, and strong value or political considerations necessarily enter into questions of the allocation of resources to different and what are inevitably competing programmes; so that the sanction of the actual governing bodies of the various authorities concerned is invariably needed before plans can be put into action.

[26] It must be recognized that professional practitioners of higher than Stratum-2 capacity, e.g. many medical consultants, may sometimes be involved in individual cases (though at this level they are likely also to be involved in higher levels of planning of type (b) or (c) listed below).

On the health side a formal system for this sort of planning is being brought into existence at the time of writing, linking the planning of the AHA to regional and national plans.[27] On the social services side, not only comprehensive SSD planning is involved, but also any corporate planning systems which are being developed in local authorities.

Considering joint planning at this level, perhaps the most important thing to stress is the necessity of distinguishing *a range* of possible activities, each somewhat different in concept from the other, and each implying its own different working arrangements, thus:

1	2	3	4	5
Solely health planning	Health planning with formal social services liaison	Joint planning	Social services planning with formal health liaison	Solely social services planning

Where genuine joint planning is called for (the third zone in the figure above), and if work of the required level is to be done, it will be necessary to establish working groups of officers or senior practitioners of full Stratum-4 or 5 status from both services, whatever staff from lower levels may usefully contribute as well. Such joint officer and practitioner groups may well work under the aegis of the Joint Consultative Committee (see further discussion below).

On the other hand, as in the case of Health Care Planning Teams as they were originally constituted, there can be bodies which are concerned mainly with planning for one service, but which nevertheless demand regular, formalized liaison with the other service in order to undertake their work (the second and fourth zones in the figure above). Here, a core of officers or practitioners of Stratum-4 or 5 level will be called for from the prime service. By contrast, the liaison representatives from the second service could perhaps be Stratum-3-level on occasion. Such bodies on the health side (like the HCPTs) are established by Health Authorities; and any plans or proposals which they

[27] See DHSS (1976), *The NHS Planning System.*

produce are not binding on social services authorities. Conversely, plans produced by any bodies to promote social services, even with regular and formalized health liaison (that is in the fourth zone of the figure above), would not produce plans which were binding on Health Authorities.

Finally, of course, any working groups established by either authority purely to forward their own plans, even without any regular, formalized, representation from the other service (that is those in the first and fifth zones of the figure above), might nevertheless wish to keep some less formal contact with developing ideas and plans in the other service.

As to which of these five kinds of planning groups are needed for what kinds of topics, this has remained somewhat an open issue in our own explorations up to the time of writing. Where certain kinds of community needs call for major and separate contribution from both services in order to meet them at all adequately, as is the case for example with the elderly, then full-scale joint planning would seem to be indicated. It would also seem to be called for wherever in current circumstances there is a need for a major switch of effort and resources from health services to social services, as, again given current thinking, is the case in services for the mentally handicapped.

Beyond this, however, it is difficult to draw general conclusions. Any need – say, services for the acutely ill – may justify full-scale joint planning if the authorities concerned believe it does. Nor of course does the establishment of joint-planning arrangements necessarily imply that systematic arrangements for separate and more detailed planning in the two services are unnecessary. (What seems less likely is that genuine joint-planning teams – those in the third zone – as well as, say, health planning teams with formal social services liaison – those in the second zone – are both necessary on the same topic.)

What is to be avoided, however, is the confusion of one form with the other. In the first years of the new NHS we frequently encountered the assumption, for example, that Health Care Planning Teams could and should adequately tackle full-scale joint planning. But they were rarely, if ever, properly equipped to do this. Representation from social services was often thin, and, even where plentiful, at too low a level. Sometimes no more than one Stratum-3-level health services liaison officer was in attendance. Whereas such representation might be adequate for what is described above as 'health planning with formal social services liaison' (the second zone in the figure), it was quite inadequate for genuine joint planning (the central zone), as results tended to prove.

JOINT CONSULTATIVE COMMITTEES. There are two possible and contrasted views of the Joint Consultative Committee (JCC), the body which brings together elected members of the local authorities and the appointed members of AHAs. In the first view, the JCC is seen as an authority in its own right, desirably with full discretion to determine the use of funds allocated to it from whatever source, and dealing authoritatively with all services which are not clearly the separate responsibility of the AHA or the local authority. In the second view, the JCC is seen in effect as a negotiating forum, where representatives of a number of separate authorities, separately financed and with divergent styles, interests, and even political approaches, meet in order to see if agreements can be hammered out on matters of common concern, in the interests of the community at large.

The second view is surely the more realistic. JCCs do not in fact have power to employ their own staff and provide their own services. They are not spending authorities.[28] The very concept of 'joint planning' implies the existence of two or more independent entities or authorities. Moreover, such authorities may well have divergent aims and interests. Effective joint planning can only ever result if there is the political will and commitment in all parties to the discussion. The absence of this does not say that the joint-planning machinery itself is wrong or inadequate.

THE PROPER ROLE OF JOINT PLANNING TEAMS. Extending this last point, the complaint was frequently met in the discussions described that existing health care planning teams or the like often tended in practice to show little by way of solid achievement.

---

[28] There is at the time of writing a special provision by central government for jointly financed schemes, in which JCCs of course have a special concern. Nevertheless, this money is made available to, and spent by, the AHA, not the JCC. (See DHSS Circular HC(77)17.)

Should they therefore be given 'teeth', that is more executive powers?

Now there is a temptation to assume that whenever a group is given a name – a 'management team', 'a planning team', or a 'Joint Consultative Committee' – that it necessarily acquires powers of decision and action in its own name, like the Area Health Authority or the local authority. However, in the first place, as we have already pointed out, planning teams at this level – Strata-4 and 5 – are inevitably deliberative in function. All major proposals and recommendations will need to be submitted to higher authorities for sanction.[29]

In the second place it must be recognized that any joint-planning body is (like the JCC) primarily a negotiating consensus-forming or consensus-testing body. Any executive powers which do exist will be no more than the aggregate of the executive powers (such as they are) of individual members. Even if JCCs establish joint officer planning teams, give them their broad terms of reference, and receive their reports, individual members will continue to represent their own employees and continue to be accountable to them for what they propose or agree. Again, the outcome of joint planning can be no better than the common willingness and combined abilities of all parties to it.

COLLABORATION IN DEVELOPMENT OF SPECIFIC SYSTEMS AND PRO-CEDURES (STRATUM-3 WORK). Having examined the proper functions and limitations of various bodies concerned with collaboration in comprehensive planning at Stratum-4 or 5, it becomes easier to see what is needed or possible for collaboration in development at Stratum-3; that is the systematic development of the way in which individual cases are dealt with, broadly within given capital facilities and establishments of staff.

For a start, precisely because proposals for change at this level do not involve significant changes in capital or revenue expenditure or significant shifts in the allocation of public monies, there is not the same need for formality of procedure or of getting sanction for change from statutory governing bodies. On the contrary, it is a continuing part of the everyday job of any

[29] See Chapter 7, 'The Stratification of Work and Organizational Design'.

Stratum-3 manager or Stratum-3 professional practitioner to be initiating such developments, negotiating freely and frequently with his counterparts and colleagues in other units and agencies as he does so. The establishment of formalized teams will not be so necessary as for comprehensive planning. Many changes will be able to be negotiated directly through established networks on a one-by-one basis, or by getting together greater or smaller discussion groups, as needed.

It·is doubtful if collaborative Stratum-3 work of this kind should be added to the brief of Stratum-4/5 planning or joint-planning teams. It is likely that the attempt to create or improve specific systems and procedures (other than identifying needs for such work to be undertaken elsewhere) merely blurs the focus of comprehensive planning. There is a difference too in the mode of work required at Stratum-4 and 5 as opposed to Stratum-3. In Stratum-3 work, the direct participation of a whole range of practitioners, including many in Stratum-2, will be essential if proposed changes in specific systems are to be tested for their relevance and effectiveness to specific cases. The lively comments of the practising social worker, nurse, or health visitor will often be much to the point. On the other hand, the usefulness of contributions from individual Stratum-2 workers in comprehensive planning at Stratum-4 or 5 is more debatable. Assumptions about the incidence and range of social or health needs arrived at by one particular Stratum-2 practitioner, based solely upon the particular stream of cases which happens to come his way, may be a poor and indeed misleading basis for comprehensive planning at Stratum-4/5, however insightful his vision in each case. (A contrast must be drawn here between this sort of individual participation and the right of Stratum-2 workers, and indeed Stratum-1 workers, to comment *en bloc* on proposed plans at some point, either directly or through elected representatives.)[30]

POST WITH SPECIFIC LIAISON FUNCTIONS. We may now consider briefly the potential contribution of staff in either health or social services who have some special liaison responsibility. On the health side there are often at the moment, for example, specific posts for community physicians under the title 'Specialist

[30] See Chapter 16.

in Community Medicine (Social Services)'. On the social services side there are a variety of posts with designated health liaison duties. The first point to stress here is that the occupants of such posts can clearly not be expected to handle all the necessary interaction between health and social services at all levels, or even at any one given level of work. Interactions without number must take place between individual practitioners, or their immediate managers or principals, in respect of individual cases, or in respect of improvements in systems for handling individual cases (Stratum-1 to 3). Nor could these two officers possibly handle all the interactions necessary in Stratum-4 or 5 comprehensive planning discussions.

The prime function for those with specific liaison duties would seem to be that of dealing with unresolved issues of collaboration of all sorts, and at any level; at least by alerting those in their own agencies who are responsible for sorting out the matters concerned or for establishing machinery to do so. Beyond this there will be potential work in representing their own employers in various formal discussions with members of the other services, on the development of specific systems and procedures (Stratum-3 work), or in comprehensive planning (Stratum-4 or 5).

Here however we come to a second crucial point, which is the level at which any liaison post itself is established. In many SSDs the grading of special health liaison posts has been pitched at a level which usually corresponds to an expectation of Stratum-3 work. In some, existing Deputy, Assistant, or Divisional Directors have had additional duties in respect of collaboration added to their existing roles, which suggests recognition for the need for higher level work. Our discussions suggest that Specialist Health Service Liaison Officers of the first type usually have ready access to the Director of Social Services for the purpose of advising and briefing him on health service matters. However they are not, given their level, members of the top management group of SSDs, and cannot therefore hope to exert a prime influence of major SSD policy decisions from a health point of view, or hope to keep the full sense of developing ideas and possibilities which Stratum-4 status and membership of the top management group might allow.

It is difficult to judge whether in health services community medicine posts with liaison function, which are universally pitched at medical consultant grade, are expected to operate at Stratum-3 or higher. In some authorities it appears that these particular community physicians frequently attend SSD top management team meetings; in which cases they are sometimes better informed about developing policies within the SSD than the SSD's own Stratum-3 liaison officer.

The point to emphasize is that where comprehensive planning is concerned and particularly where joint planning is concerned, rather than health planning with social services liaison, or *vice versa*, it will be essential that officers representing each side are chosen from amongst those who are judged sufficiently capable to handle the level of work required. This would imply, for example, that chief officers and their immediate deputies and assistants from the local authority side need to be personally involved in 'Joint Care Planning Teams' and their main sub-groups.

Conclusion

In summary the main points that have been made are these.

Even leaving aside the problems of lack of conterminosity and of separate Area and District structure in health services, there are certain intrinsic difficulties in collaboration between health and social services which spring from fundamental differences in organizational forms within the two, and the different 'natural' sizes of subordinate divisions and units within the two services.

At the level of collaboration on specific cases, various possible strategies have been identified for building stronger linkages which can be divided into two main categories:

(a) building stronger networks through such things as alignment schemes, designated liaison posts and the part-time or full-time outposting of staff from one service into specific institutions of the other;

(b) forming distinct multi-disciplinary teams, for example by the attachment of specific social workers to pre-existing medical teams.

It has been suggested that even in the most closely integrated work two distinct responsibilities arise in principle; a prime responsibility for health care, and a prime responsibility for social care. It appears that prime responsibility for health care always rests with a doctor, even in social services settings (leaving aside at any rate the difficult field of mental health). It appears that prime responsibility for social care, however, might rest with one of several different occupational groups in social services, not just with professional social workers. Some of the implications and consequences of this have been explored.

At the level of collaboration in comprehensive, territory–wide, planning – work at Strata-4 and 5 – a prime distinction has been drawn between joint planning (which requires senior staff in comparable strength of representation from all the services involved), and the planning of separate agencies (which require some degree of formal participation from other agencies, but of a lower grade).

At the level of collaboration in the development of specific systems and procedures – work at Stratum-3 – it has been suggested that the main emphasis need not fall on the setting up of formal teams or committees. In the nature of things senior managers or practitioners working at this level should be continually involved in producing piecemeal change and improvement in systems at their own initiative, and in collaboration with counterpart staff in parallel units and agencies. Such work is probably best kept out of comprehensive planning processes, either those within one agency or across several.

Appendices

Appendix A

Organization of the NHS

Elliott Jaques

This Appendix reviews the main features of the reorganization of the National Health Service for those who are not familiar with the Service. The reorganization created one of the largest social institutions in the world, and arguably one of the most complex.

The objective of the reorganization was to bring together into one integrated system the three previously independent services into which health had been divided: the hospital service of 20 Regional Hospital Boards in charge of some 366 Hospital Management Committees; the general practitioner service controlled by 231 Executive Councils; and the local government public health services controlled by Medical Officers of Health in 175 local authorities.

A few simple statistics may serve to indicate the sheer scale of the exercise. A total of some 900,000 people are employed in the service – almost 1 in 25 of the total employed population in Britain. It includes 60,000 doctors and 380,000 nurses, and some 325,000 administrators and hospital workers, catering and laundry staff. Then, in addition, there were the 70,000 members of nearly 40 different professional and semi-professional groups giving diagnostic and therapeutic services – the radiographers, pathology technicians, biochemists, physiotherapists, psychologists, dental technicians, occupational therapists, etc.

All health services were affected: general practice, medicine, surgery, maternal and child care, psychiatry and mental handicap, child guidance, school health, preventive medicine and health education, and public health. These services were carried out in thousands of GP surgeries, group practices, and clinics, 2500 hospitals, 126 local authority public health departments, assisted by 30,000 community nurses and midwives.

Here then was an exercise in large-scale social change in complex organization. Some of the very important conditions within which the reorganization had to be achieved are worth recalling since they so profoundly influenced what was possible. And their clear understanding is essential for an evaluation of certain outlines of the reorganization and as a foundation for the assessment of any modifications which might be contemplated.

The general features of the NHS which need to be taken into account must take as a starting point the objective of providing the following services:

> clinics, school services, education, and other services for prevention and detection of disease;
> physical treatment (medical and surgical intervention) for physical and psychological illnesses and impairment;
> psychological treatment for psychological disturbances and related physical symptoms;
> educational procedures and provision of aids to enable the physically and mentally handicapped to use their abilities as fully as possible.

The general pattern of the Service, starting with the personal relation between patient and his clinically autonomous GP or consultant, is that it is the independent practitioner who carries prime responsibility for the patient, standing between him and the vast array of NHS services available for his care, and with the authority to prescribe the use of those services for his patient.

The organization of health services tends to be based on the model of the services required for the prevention and treatment of physical illness by means of physical intervention. Within this prevailing model the key figures are the doctors – and where diagnosis, treatment, and prognosis for individual patients are concerned it is the consultant or GP (or junior medical staff on their behalf) who have primacy; that is to say, they automatically carry responsibility for the care of the patient, determine referrals for second opinion or for treatment, and prescribe drugs and other requirements. Doctors are thus the 'gate-keepers' through whom individuals gain access to health services.

By contrast, all the other services can be organized largely into ordinary managerial hierarchies, and are on the whole so organized.[1] Those services comprise some 30 to 40 independently organized and managed professional, scientific, and technical services – nursing, pharmacy, remedial and other therapies, laboratory and other diagnostic services – any several of which might have to be mobilized in the interests of particular patients at any given time.

In effect, the National Health Service is not a single service but a conglomeration of many different services requiring effective co-ordination if they are to run properly. One thing which seemed sure, however, was that these services could not readily be structured within the NHS into one single all-encompassing managerial hierarchy with one manager at the top. They are too different in qualitative content because of their advanced professional development (as argued in the Chapter 5 on professionals). They function independently of one another, in the sense that their services are separately prescribed and mobilized on behalf of patients. But they do require overall monitoring and co-ordination in connection with resource planning and with ensuring that resource use is being kept within policy limits.

Conditions Setting Limits to the Reorganization
A number of conditions had been established by the government as terms of reference, before the reorganization structure was developed. These conditions set the limits within which the design of that structure could be carried out.

The first condition was that the reorganization had to be worked out, planned, and implemented within the normal life of the government, leaving about $3\frac{1}{2}$ years by the time the decision to carry through the reorganization had been taken.

A second condition was that two main organizational features had to be incorporated. There were to be two tiers of appointed political authority. One tier was to be composed of 15 Regional Authorities with members appointed by the Secretary of State and with boundaries similar to the boundaries of

[1] Emerging exceptions are the cases of the higher-level professional workers who are achieving independent practitioner status and who do not appear readily to fall into ordinary managerial hierarchies. These problems are discussed, for example, in the chapters on professionals, PT and OT, and child guidance (Chapters 5, 9 and 10).

the previous Regional Hospital Boards.[2] The second tier was to be composed of Area Health Authorities (AHAs) each of which would serve a locality conterminous with the counties and urban communities under local authorities created in the local government reorganization which had occurred during the previous few years. Part of the membership of these AHAs would be appointed by the Secretary of State and part by the conterminous local authority. A third condition was that the integrated planning and provision of health care services would be organized in Districts with populations optimally between 200,000 and 250,000. These communities were seen as of a size allowing for a full District General Hospital Service and a manageable number of a total of perhaps two to three hundred consultants and general practitioners who could organize themselves into appropriate committees for planning purposes. This particular condition meant that many Areas would have to be divided into two or more Districts.

The purpose of conterminosity was to provide for effective and close joint planning between the health services and the local authority services – in particular between health on the one hand and the social services, education, and housing with which they are so closely connected, on the other.

General Structure
It was against this background that the following organizational decisions were taken for the NHS structure in England and Wales, with an important variation in Scotland and Northern Ireland.

England was duly divided into fifteen Health Regions, each with an appointed Regional Authority supported by a Regional Team of Officers (RTO). The RTO comprised a Regional Administrator, a Regional Medical Officer, a Regional Nursing Officer, and a Regional Treasurer. There

[2] For reasons which are analysed in Chapter 2, it appeared at the time – and would appear now – that too much organization was provided for in having both Area and Regional Authorities. The picture might have been different if the Regional Authorities had been founded upon a true regional social and political base; that is to say, given a genuine regional devolution in England (of a kind being considered by the Crowther Committee at the time of the NHS reorganization), there might develop a foundation for a group of what would be true *regional* health services. But that time is not now.

were, in addition, a range of specialist Regional Officers concerned with new buildings, with scientific development, and
other functions. Each Region was accountable for the development of plans for submission to the Secretary of State, for monitoring the implementation of plans when agreed, and for the
provision of those special services best organized on a Region-
wide basis.

Each Region in turn was divided into a number of Areas,
in general conterminous with local government authorities.
Most of these Areas, however, were too large to carry the functions envisaged for the basic health service Districts, and were
sub-divided into between two and six Districts.

The problem then was how to manage and co-ordinate all
the various services in each District. No single chief executive
officer role could be established: GPs and consultants had to
be organized in committees without managers, since preservation of their clinical autonomy precluded their having
managers; and the independent diagnostic and treatment services required each to have its own managerial head. Due consideration led to a decision in favour of establishing a co-ordinative team for each Health Care District (the District Management Team – DMT), the principle of its composition being that
it would comprise the representatives or managers of all those
whose work was concerned with the *totality* of services. Without
going into the details of the background of the decision, those
selected as falling under this definition were: one representative
for the GPs and one for the consultants, elected by a District
Medical Committee (DMC) which represented all the doctors;
the District Community Physician (District-wide epidemiology
and health service planning); the District Administrator (District-wide monitoring and co-ordination); the District Nursing
Officer (nursing extending into all services); and the District
Finance Officer (District-wide financial policy).

The consultants and general practitioners were given the
opportunity to organize themselves into committees – the
general practitioners into a Local Medical Committee and the
consultants into a number of committees to represent each
major group of specialists. Those committees then elected
members to the District Medical Committee referred to in the
preceding paragraph. It is by means of this committee structure

that the consultants and GPs can work out a consensus view on what policies and priorities should be pursued with regard to District services and their modifications and development.

The heads of all the other services were directly appointed˙ by the AHA and accountable to it, and were not subordinate to the DMT. In effect there were 30 to 40 managerially free-standing professional services, monitored and co-ordinated by the DMT but accountable for remaining within the professional limits and keeping to the professional standards publicly established by their recognized professional bodies for their own work. This point is emphasized here, and is developed in several chapters. It is part of the argument that the extension of responsibility and independence to fully professional groups is one of the ways by which the personalization and individualization of large-scale bureaucracies may be achieved, and the sense of personal social responsibility generally enhanced and more widely spread throughout society – counteracting the present strong trends towards large-scale corporatism and reduction of individual independence and personal respect.

In single-district Areas, the AHA Chairman and members are able to have a direct and uncomplicated relationship with their co-ordinative team (in this case an Area Management Team). In the multi-District Areas, however, well-known complications have arisen. Because of the difficulties for any AHA to deal directly with more than one District, they were given the support of a specialist team – the Area Team of Officers (ATO) – composed of an Area Administrator (AA), Area Medical Officer (AMO), Area Nursing Officer (ANO), and Area Treasurer (AT).

The setting up of ATOs, however, also raised the vexed question of what the organization relation between ATO and DMT members ought to be. If each District Officer were made subordinate to his Area counterpart – as was decided in Scotland – then the two elected GP and consultant members of the DMT would be at one organization level removed from the AHA because of the managerially interposed ATO. It could be predicted, therefore, that the doctors would seek to by-pass the DEG (District Executive Group, as it is called in Scotland) and to express their views directly to the AHA. This prediction has by and large proved to be the case in Scotland, where the doctors use the Area Medical Advisory machinery through which they have direct access to the AHA, and the DEG is rendered less effective as a result. Alongside this practice there is an accompanying tendency for the doctors' representatives to get together with the District Executive Group and to try to achieve direct access to the AHA, pushing the Area Executive Group aside.

In England and Wales the ATO members were put in a monitoring and co-ordinative relationship with their DMT Officer counterparts. ATO members were placed at one grade higher than the District Team members, one of the main arguments being to provide a sort of career peak. (One of the consequences has been that nearly every other profession has sought to be organized on an Area basis, or at least to have an Area Officer appointed, in order also to achieve a higher graded career peak post.)

The contracts of the GPs are managed by a Family Practitioner Committee (FPC). This Committee determines how many practitioners shall be allowed in the Districts in its Area, allocates resources for GP surgeries, plans health centres, monitors GPs' expenditure, determines special payments, and handles complaints. The FPC receives its funds directly from the DHSS, but its activities are monitored by the AHA, and its executive officer is a subordinate of the Area Administrator.

Finally, there is a Community Health Council (CHC) in each District, appointed by the Regional Health Authority from among leading members of the main community organization concerned with health. The CHCs must report publicly each year their assessment of the quality of District health services. They have right of access to all health service facilities in their district, and must be consulted on any plans for the closure of hospitals or clinics.

The relationship between the Health Service and local government is mediated by a Joint Consultation Committee (JCC), made up of half each of members of the local authority and members of the AHA. The function of this body is to work out joint development projects and joint budgeting, so as to enable an effective interplay between health service planning and the social services, education, housing, and employment services with which they are so closely connected.

The general pattern of organization is illustrated in the accompanying diagram.

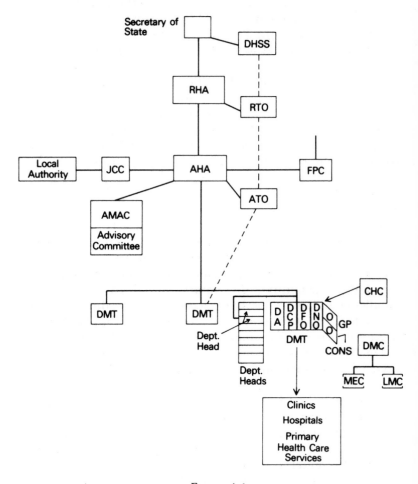

FIGURE A.1

A summary of the main abbreviations may be useful:

AHA   Area Health Authority
AMAC   Area Medical Advisory Committee
ATO   Area Team of Officers
        AA   Area Administrator

AMO   Area Medical Officer
ANO   Area Nursing Officer
AT   Area Treasurer
CHC   Community Health Council
DMC   District Medical Committee
DMT   District Management Team
       DA   District Administrator
       DCP   District Community Physician
       DFO   District Finance Officer
       DNO   District Nursing Officer
DHSS   Department of Health and Social Security
FPC   Family Practitioner Committee
HCPT   Health Care Planning Team
LA   Local Authority
LMC   Local Medical Committee
MEC   Medical Executive Committee
RHA   Regional Health Authority
PO   Principal Officer
RTO   Regional Team of Officers
   RA   Regional Administrator
   RMO   Regional Medical Officer
   RNO   Regional Nursing Officer
   RT   Regional Treasurer
SCM   Specialist in Community Medicine
SSD   Social Services Departments
SW   Social Worker

Appendix B

Definitions of Concepts

Attachment

1. Attachment arises where it is wished:

   (a) to supplement the work of A2 by allocating B from another occupation or specialism to work closely with him; whilst

   (b) maintaining managerial support and control from a superior A1, in the same occupation or discipline.

2. In all cases B must be personally acceptable to A2 at the time of attachment and continue to be so.

3. Thereafter, two distinct situations may arise.

   (i) *Attachment-with-Monitoring and Co-ordination*

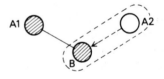

4. A2 may be given authority to *co-ordinate* B's work with his own and that of others, and to *monitor* such things as adherence to employment contract, minimal competence and basic standards of behaviour. (In addition, in some situations A2 might carry *prescribing* authority.)

5. A1 will continue to carry a full *managerial* relationship to B.

   (ii) *Attachment-with-Co-management*

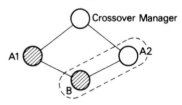

6. If, and only if, A1 and A2 themselves share a common manager it may be possible to establish a co-management situation, in which the exact division of managerial functions is as follows.

7. A1 is expected:

    (a) to induct B in technical matters, and to help him deal with technical problems;
    (b) to co-ordinate his work with that of similar participants in the field;
    (c) to appraise B's performance and abilities, to keep B informed of his assessments, to arrange or provide training, to arrange transfers or re-attachments (or dismissal);
    (d) to attempt to provide continuity of service where B is absent, or where a transfer or re-attachment is in hand.

8. A2 is expected:

    (a) to induct B into the local work situation, and to help him with operational problems;
    (b) to assign appropriate work to him;
    (c) to help A1 appraise his performance and abilities.

9. A1 should be able to give direct instructions to B provided they are within policies established by the 'crossover' manager, and provided they do not conflict with A2's policies or instructions. A1 must be able to see that B's special competence is being used in an appropriate way.

10. A2 needs to have authority of veto in the attachment of B, authority to join in official appraisals of B's performance and ability and authority to initiate his transfer elsewhere. (Note the distinction of *attachment* from either *outposting*, or *secondment*, or *functional monitoring and co-ordinating*.)

Binding Professional Standards

1. Binding professional standards are the necessary standards and norms of behaviour by which members of a professionally developing occupational group must abide. Beyond a certain degree of professional development, such standards become absolute and binding, and it is imperative that they

should not be abandoned out of deference to the judgment of a more highly qualified or experienced superior.

2. Binding professional standards thus stretch beyond the general limits set by law and social norms that constrain every member of society. However, although they curb the possible direction by superior officers and bodies, they do not in themselves make such managerial relationships impossible.

Collateral Relationship

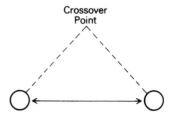

1. A collateral relationship may arise where the work of two people, ultimately subject to the authority of a common manager or superior body, interacts in such a way that mutual accommodation is needed in certain matters, and where it is not appropriate that either has authority over the other. (Their tasks may be complementary, or they may be supplementary, or they may be unrelated, apart from use of common resources.)

2. Each person in the collateral relationship is expected:

   (a) to accommodate to the other's needs as far as is reasonable;

   (b) to refer to the next higher level of authority any significant problem of mutual work which he has been unable to resolve.

3. Where collateral colleagues fail to reach agreement, ultimate resolution can only be found at the *crossover* point represented by the common manager or superior body.

Co-ordinating Role

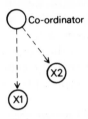

1. A co-ordinating role may arise where it is felt necessary to establish one person, with the function of co-ordinating the work of a number of others in some particular respects and where a *managerial, supervisory* or *staff* relationship is inappropriate. The activity to be co-ordinated might, for example, be:

    -- the production of reports, estimates, plans or proposals;
    – the implementation of agreed schemes or projects;
    – the overcoming of unforeseen problems affecting normal work.

2. The co-ordinator is expected:

    (a) to propose specific actions and programmes;
    (b) to keep himself and others informed of actual progress;
    (c) to help overcome setbacks and problems encountered in carrying out agreed programmes.

3. In carrying out these activities the co-ordinator needs authority to make firm proposals for action, to arrange meetings, to obtain first-hand knowledge of progress, etc., and to decide what shall be done in situations of uncertainty, but he should have no authority in case of sustained disagreements to issue overriding instructions. X1, X2, etc., have always the right to direct access to the higher authorities who are setting or sanctioning the work concerned.

Encompassing Profession
1. An encompassing profession is one whose knowledge is deeper and more embracing than that of other professions dealing within the same field of work. Two professions may have different areas of competence in such a situation, but

the one has *prescribing authority* over the other on the grounds that it has a broader theoretical base.

2. The case for *prescribing authority* is more obvious when a comparison is made between a 'craft' whose technicians have a special competence in the execution of certain tasks, and a 'profession' where there is a greater depth of understanding and penetration of complex problems.

Functional Monitoring and Co-ordinating

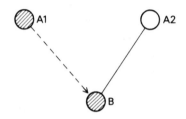

1. Functional monitoring and co-ordinating may arise where it is desired to *monitor* the work of B in occupational or technical respects, and to *co-ordinate* it with the work of other practitioners in the same function or field, whilst leaving intact in all its essential elements the managerial or directive relationship between A2 and B.
2. Specifically, A1 is expected:
   (a)   to help to select B (either in an advisory role or with the right to veto);
   (b)   to provide advice to him in the specialist field concerned, where such is needed;
   (c)   to *co-ordinate* his work with that of other similar participants in the field;
   (d)   to *monitor* the adherence of B to any established policies or practices in the specialist field concerned;
   (e)   to provide for B's technical training.
3. A1 should not have authority to provide official appraisals of B's work, or to initiate his transfer or dismissal. Such authority rests with A2.
4. A2 may be an individual manager of B, or a composite body to whom B is directly accountable.
   Note the distinction of *functional monitoring and co-ordinating* from either *attachment, secondment* or *outposting*.

Independent Practice

1. Independent practice is a situation where though the professional practitioner may be employed he has freedom to pursue his professional practice as he thinks best (within available resources) provided he stays within certain broad limits of professional ethics, contract, and accepted norms of behaviour. There is independent practice where it is deemed that there is a pre-eminent need to establish a voluntarily maintained relationship of trust and co-operation between a specifically identified professional practitioner and a specifically identified 'patient' or 'client'.

2. Through this relationship the patient/client is provided with a personalized service, through his personal practitioner who indicates the necessary treatment and makes NHS resources and services available to him. The degree of freedom required by the professional practitioner to facilitate such treatment implies tenure of employment and the exclusion of managerial control even from within the same profession; it also requires a capacity on the part of the practitioner to cope with work at both the *'systematic provision'* (Stratum-3) and *'situational response'* (Stratum-2) levels (see the chapter on work-strata, p. 119, and also *Agency Service*, p. 78).

Managerial Role

1. A managerial role may arise where it is wished to make a person A fully accountable for the work of another, or others, B.

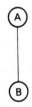

2. Specifically, A is expected:

   (a) to help to select B;
   (b) to induct him into his role;
   (c) to assign work to him and allocate resources;

   (d) to keep himself informed about B's work, and to help him deal with work problems;

   (e) to appraise B's general performance and ability, and in consequence keep B informed of his assessments, arrange or provide training, modify role, or arrange transfer or dismissal.

3. A needs the authority:

   (a) to veto the selection of B for the role;

   (b) to make an official appraisal of B's performance and ability;

   (c) to initiate transfer or dismissal.

Monitoring Role

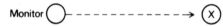

Monitor ○‒ ‒ ‒ ‒ ‒ ‒ ‒ ‒ ‒ ‒ → Ⓧ

1. A monitoring role may arise where it is felt necessary to ensure that the activities of X conform to satisfactory standards in some particular respect and where a managerial, supervisory, or staff relationship is impossible or needs supplementing. The aspect of activity being monitored might, for example, be:

   – adherence to contract of employment (attendance, hours of work, for example);

   – safety;

   – financial propriety and security;

   – level of expenditure;

   – technical standard of work;

   – adherence to personnel policies.

2. Specifically, the monitor is expected:

   (a) to ensure that he is adequately informed of the effects of X's activities;

   (b) to discuss possible improvements with X or with X's superiors;

   (c) to report to the manager or superior body to whom he is accountable sustained or significant deficiencies;

   (d) to recommend new policies or standards where required.

3. The monitor needs authority:

    (a) to obtain first-hand knowledge of X's activities and problems;

    (b) to persuade X to modify his performance, but not to instruct him.

He should not have authority to make or recommend official appraisals of X's work. He should not have authority himself to set new policies or new standards.

Outposting

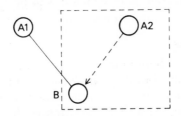

1. Outposting may arise where it is wished:

    (a) for B to work within a site for which A2 already carries some general responsibility; but

    (b) without B's manager A1 actually *attaching* him or *seconding* him to A2.

2. In this situation the role of A2 must be limited to:

    (a) inducting B into the local setting;

    (b) monitoring the adherence of B to local regulation and practice;

    (c) co-ordinating the activities of B so far as local problems or developments are concerned.

Prescribing Relationship

1. A prescribing relationship may arise where:

    (a) a person of one occupation needs the direct help of a person of another in achieving the goals of his own work; and

    (b) the knowledge base of the first occupation is accepted as encompassing that of the second.

2. The prescriber needs authority to determine particular tasks to be carried out, at an appropriate level of specificity.

3. He is expected:
   (a) to check that the person receiving the prescription performs the task adequately and, if not, to withdraw the task;
   (b) to monitor the general standard of work produced.

4. The person receiving the prescription is expected to refer back to the prescriber if he feels that either the objective of the task or the context in which it is to be carried out is unsuitable.

Prime Responsibility

1. In a situation where many members of a variety of professions are involved in the consideration of a particular case, the practitioner who has prime responsibility is ultimately in charge of the case. He co-ordinates the actions and decisions of all those practitioners brought into the case and ensures that all underlying needs are met. More specifically he has *co-ordinating* but not *managerial* authority to:

   (a) make a personal assessment of the general needs of the case at the time of assumption of prime responsibility;
   (b) undertake personally any action needed, or to initiate such action, through subordinate or ancillary staff;
   (c) refer, when and as necessary, to colleagues and other independent agencies for collaboration in further assessment or action, or for action in parallel;
   (d) keep continuous awareness of the progress of the case, and take further initiative as necessary.

2. Further, although it may not be true for *agency services*, where the practitioner with prime responsibility is in independent practice, he has the right and the duty to decide when to relinquish extended collaboration with colleagues, or when to terminate all further action on the case.

Profession

1. A profession is an organizational group which has a developed body of theoretical knowledge, the application of which must be within the bounds of an ethic or impartiality

and objectivity; it implies the exercise of insightful judgment to assess real needs appropriate responses in a variety of situations rather than the simple carrying out of prescribed tasks. Professional associations are usually formed to further the development of this specialized knowledge and practice (as well as to protect collective interests).

2. At a certain stage of development the possibility of managerial control of professional members by non-members must be excluded. This happens when the latter can no longer judge the competence of such professionals nor assess the technical problems encountered. Only monitoring and co-ordinating role relationships are possible in this context.

3. Parallel with the development of theoretical knowledge and practice is the evolution of specific professional standards and norms of behaviour. When such prescriptive and prohibitive/proscriptive limits are absolute and binding, the individual member must model his behaviour accordingly, irrespective of contrary direction by a superior. Maintenance of these standards is encouraged by the support of professional associations and the necessity of public registration, where such exist. (See *Binding Professional Standards* and *Independent Practice* (p. 77).)

Representative Role

1. Where any group wish to express the consensus of their views and feelings, or to negotiate with another body, they may choose to do so through the medium of an elected representative.

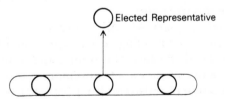
Elected Representative

2. The elected representative needs to carry some degree of discretion in presenting views or negotiating, even if he is specifically mandated. (A *delegate* is a representative who works only to a specific mandate.) He is accountable to the group for what he says and does, and if he is judged inadequate by them they must be able to replace him.

3. Elected representatives must be distinguished from individuals who are appointed by some external agency to advisory or executive bodies because they are typical of the group from which they come.

Secondment

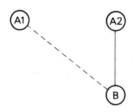

1. Secondment may arise where it is desired to transfer B from his original manager A1 to some other manager A2 for some limited period, such as the time to complete a particular project or the time for B to gain some desired training or experience.
2. In this situation the new manager A2 will be expected:
   (a) to induct B into his new position, and assign work and allocate resources to him;
   (b) to review B's work, and to provide A1 with appraisals of his performance;
   (c) to help B's personal development in his work during the time of his secondment.
3. A2 needs to have authority to veto B's secondment in the first instance, and to initiate his return should his performance prove unsatisfactory.
4. The original manager A1 will be expected:
   (a) to provide a continuing official appraisal of B's work;
   (b) to provide for B's formal training, and to make appropriate plans for his career-development.
(note the distinction of *secondment* from both *attachment* and *outposting*.)

Service-giving Relationship
1. A service-giving relationship may arise where a person needs to be able to request from others, whom he does not manage, the provision of resources or facilities to be used in his own work.

2. The service-giver is expected to provide an appropriate service to meet each request, or to notify the service-seeker if this is impossible, and to discuss alternatives.
3. The service-receiver is expected to draw any deficiencies in services to the attention of the service-giver, to negotiate improvements if possible, and, if not, to report sustained or significant deficiencies to the attention of superior authorities.

Staff-officer Role
1. A staff-officer role may arise where a manager A needs assistance in managing the activities of his subordinates B1, B2, in some particular dimension of work such as personnel and organizational matters, or the detailed programming of activities and services.

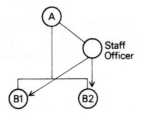

2. Specifically, the staff officer is expected:

   (a) to help to formulate policies or schemes in the field concerned, taking into account the experience and views of A's other subordinates;
   (b) to see that agreed policies or schemes in the field concerned are implemented by A's other subordinates: issuing detailed procedures and programmes; ensuring adherence to these programmes; and interpreting agreed policy.
   (c) to deal with the daily flow of communications and problems coming to A in the field concerned: sorting, filtering, exploring, and initiating, and co-ordinating appropriate response wherever possible.

3. In carrying out these activities the staff officer needs to have authority to issue instructions. If B1 does not agree with the staff officer's instructions he cannot disregard them, but must take the matter up with A. The staff officer should have no authority to make official appraisals of the performance and ability of B1.

Supervisory Role

1. A supervisory role may arise where a manager A needs help
   in managing the work of his subordinates B1, B2, etc., in
   all its aspects.

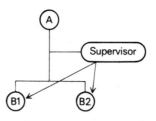

2. The supervisor is expected to help A in inducting new staff,
   assigning specific work, and dealing with specific work problems.
3. The supervisor needs the authority to give instructions to
   B1. If B1 does not agree with the supervisor's instructions
   he cannot disregard them, but must take the matter up with
   A, his manager.

Work-strata and Grades

1. The five-level system of work-strata is a classifactory scheme
   for deploying staff in the most effective way for the
   attainment of organizational goals. Each stratum specifies
   the tasks to be done and the amount of discretion and responsibility required to accomplish them effectively. As one
   moves from a lower to a higher stratum, responsibility and
   discretion increase.
2. Within each work-stratum there is a grading system which
   creates subdivisions according to special experience and
   competence, and for career planning and progression. Being
   in a higher grade in the same stratum allows for *monitoring*
   and *co-ordination* but not for *managerial* responsibility and
   authority. An effective manager of a subordinate must be
   in the next higher work-stratum. In this way the work-strata
   provide a clarification of a person's accountability and authority and can be applied to all types of organizations.

Bibliography

BALINT, M. (1957) *The Doctor, His Patient and the Illness:* London, Pitman Medical Publishers.

BARBER, J. and WALLIS, J. (1976) 'Assessment of the Elderly in General Practice': *The Journal of the Royal College of General Practitioners*, Vol. 26, No. 163: London, Longman.

BLAU, P. M. and SCOTT, R. (1963) *Formal Organisations:* London, a Preliminary Measurement': *Sociology*, Vol. 3, No. 1, 37–53.

BROWN, W. and JAQUES, E. (1965) *Glacier Project Papers:* London, Heinemann Educational Books.

BROWN, W. (1971) *Organization:* London, Heinemann Educational Books.

BUTLER, J. R. and PEARSON, M. (1970) 'Who Goes Home?' Occasional Paper on Social Administration, No. 34: London, G. Bell & Sons.

BUTLER, J. R. (1973) *Family Doctor and Public Policy:* London, Routledge & Kegan Paul.

CAMERON, K. (1956) 'Past and Present Trends in Child Psychiatry': *J. Ment. Sci.*, No. 102, pp. 599–603.

CANG, S. A. (1976/7) 'Why not a hospital-at-home here?': *Age Concern Today*, No. 20.

(1977) 'An Alternative to Hospital': *The Lancet*, April 1977.

CANG, S. A. and CLARKE, F. (1978) 'Home Care of the Sick—an emerging general analysis based on schemes in France': *Community Health*, Vol. 9, No. 3.

CARLSON, R. (1975) *The End of Medicine:* London, Wiley & Sons.

CLYNE, M. (1961) *Night Calls:* London, Tavistock Publications.

ETZIONI, A. (1964) *Modern Organisations:* Englewood Cliffs, N.J., Prentice-Hall.

(1969) *The Semi-Professions and Their Organisation:* New York, The Free Press.

FOOT, M. (1962) *Aneurin Bevan: A Biography:* London, MacGibbon & Kee.

FREIDSON, E. (1970) *Professional Dominance, The Social Structure of Medical Care:* New York, Atherton Press.

GOODE, W. J. (1969) *The Theoretical Limits of Professionalisation*, in Etzioni (Ed.).

GRECO, R. S. and PITTENGER, R. A. (1966) *One Man's Practice:* London, Tavistock Publications.

GREEN, M. (1975) 'Services for the Elderly', in *Specialised Futures:* Nuffield Provincial Hospital Trust.

HALLAS, J. (1976) *CHCs in Action:* Nuffield Provincial Hospitals Trust.

HARBERT, W. (1977) 'The Hospital Anachronism': *Health and Social Services Journal*, April 22.

HAYEK, F. A. (1960) *The Constitution of Liberty:* London, Routledge & Kegan Paul.

(1973) *Law, Legislation and Liberty*, Vol. I: Rules and Order: London, Routledge and Kegan Paul.

HEALTH SERVICES ORGANIZATION RESEARCH UNIT, BRUNEL UNIVERSITY (1976) (with Social Services Organisation Research Unit): 'Future Organisation in Child Guidance and Allied Work': Working Paper.

(1976) (with Social Services Organisation Research Unit): 'Professionals in Health and Social Services Organisation': Working Paper.

(1977) 'Organisation of Physiotherapy and Occupational Therapy in the NHS': Working Paper.

HEY, A. and ROWBOTTOM R. W. (1974) 'The Organisation of Social Work in Hospitals and Other Health Care Settings': *Health and Social Service Journal*, LXXXIV, 4374, 352–5.

HICKSON, D. J. and THOMAS, M. W. (1969) 'Professionalisation in Britain, tain, a Preliminary Measurement': *Sociology*, Vol. 3, No. 1, 37–53.

HOLLAND, W. and GILDERDALE, S. (1976) 'Principles & Policies'. *British Journal of Hospital Medicine*, Vol. 16, No. 6.

ILLICH, I. (1973) *Medical Nemesis:* London, Calder & Boyars.

JACOBS, J. (1971) 'Perplexity, Confusion and Suspicion': *Social Science and Medicine*, Vol. 5, 151.

JAQUES, E. (1961) *Equitable Payment:* London, Heinemann Educational Books.

(1964) *Time-Span Handbook:* London, Heinemann Educational Books.

(1965) 'Social-Analysis and the Glacier Project', in *Glacier Project Papers:* London, Heinemann Educational Books.

(1968) *Progession Handbook:* London, Heinemann Educational Books.

(1976) *A General Theory of Bureaucracy:* London, Heinemann Educational Books.

(1978) *Levels of Abstraction in Logic and Human Action:* London, Heinemann Educational Books.

JEFFREYS, M. (1976) 'Measuring the Quality of GP Care': *Science and Public Policy*, Vol. 3, No. 1, pp. 40–5.

JOHNSON, T. J. (1972) *Professions and Power:* London, Macmillan.

JONES, K. (1972) *A History of the Mental Health Service:* London, Routledge and Kegan Paul.

(1975) *Opening the Door:* London, Routledge and Kegan Paul.

KENSINGTON & CHELSEA & WESTMINSTER (S) CHC (1977) *The Family Doctor in Central London.*

KESSEL, N. and SHEPHERD, M. (1965) 'The Health & Attitudes of Persons who Seldom Consult a Doctor': *Medical Care*, Vol. 3, No. 1.

KLEIN, R. and LEWIS, J. (1976) *The Politics of Consumer Representation:* London, Centre for Studies in Social Policy.

PACKWOOD, T. and MACDONALD, I. (1976) 'The Organisation of Care for the Severely Mentally Handicapped': *Journal of Social and Economic Administration*, Vol. 10, No. 3.

PACKWOOD, T. (1977) 'Rehabilitating these departments back to the front line': *Health and Social Service Journal*, 25 March.

PARSONS, T. (1952) *The Social System:* London, Tavistock Publications.

Rehin, G. (1972) 'Child Guidance at the end of the Road': *Social Work Today*, March, 21–4.

Rhodes, P. (1976) *The Value of Medicine:* London, Allen and Unwin.

Rice, A. K. (1949) 'The Role of the Specialist in the Community': *Human Relations*, Vol. 11, No. 2, 177–84.

Rowbottom, R. W. *et al.* (1973) *Hospital Organization:* London, Heinemann.

Rowbottom, R. W. (1977) *Social Analysis:* London, Heinemann.

Royal College of General Practitioners (1973) 'Present State and Future Needs of General Practice': report from *General Practice* No. 16, R.C.G.P.

Sharman, E. M. (1972) 'Problems of a Rehabilitating Service': *Physiotherapy*, January.

Social Services Organisation Research Unit, Brunel University (1974) *Social Services Department, Developing Patterns of Work and Organization:* London, Heinemann.

Sorensen, J. R. (1974/5) 'Biomedical Innovation, Uncertainty, and Doctor–Patient Interaction': *Journal Health & Social Behaviour*, Vols 15–16, 366–74.

Speller, S. R. (1971) *Law Relating to Hospitals and Kindred Institutions*, 5th Edn: London, H. K. Lewis.

Stamp, G. (1978) 'Assessment of Individual Capacity', in E. Jaques (Ed.) *Levels of Abstraction in Logic and Human Action:* London, Heinemann.

Stimson, G. (1974) 'Obeying Doctor's Orders: a view from the other side': *Social Science and Medicine*, Vol. 8, 97.

Stimson, G. and Webb, B. (1975) *Going to See the Doctor:* London, Routledge and Kegan Paul.

Strauss, A. *et al.* 'The Hospital and its Negotiated Order', in E. Friedson (Ed.), *The Hospital in Modern Society:* London, Macmillan.

The Labour Party (1973) *Health Care: Report of a Working Party.*

Townsend, P. (1976) 'Local Authority Plans for Social Services for Old People in 1963', in *Sociology and Social Policy:* Harmondsworth, Penguin Books.

Virgil *Georgics*, 2.

Warren, W. (1971) 'The Development of Child and Adolescent Psychiatry in England and Wales': *The Journal of Child Psychology & Psychiatry*, Vol. II, 241–57.

Whitmore, K. *The Contribution of Child Guidance to the Community:* London, MIND.

Wilensky, H. L. (1964) 'The Professionalisation of Everyone': *Amer. J. Sociol*, Vol. 70, No. 2, 137–58.

Wilson, M. (1975) *Health is for People:* Darton, Longman & Todd.

Official Reports

1955   Report of the Committee on Maladjusted Children (Underwood Report) (Ministry of Education), London, HMSO.

1959   Mental Health Act of 1959 (DHSS). London, HMSO.

1966   Report of the Committee on Senior Nursing Staff Structure (Salmon Report) (MoH and SHHD). London, HMSO.

1966/   Committee on the Civil Service (Fulton Report). London, HMSO.
1968

1967 &   Organisation of Medical Work in Hospitals (Cogwheel),
1972   HM(68)67, HM(72)43 (DHSS). London, HMSO.

1968   Report of the Committee on Local Authority and Allied Personal Social Services (Seebohm Report). London, HMSO.

1968   Report of the Royal Commissioners on the Care and Control of the Feeble Minded, Cmnd. 4202. London, HMSO.

1971   The Organisation of Group Practice. Central Health Services Council Standing Medical Advisory Committee. London, HMSO.

1971   Better Services for the Mentally Handicapped, Cmnd. 4683 (DHSS). London, HMSO.

1972   Management Arrangements for the Reorganised National Health Service (DHSS). London, HMSO.

1972   Management Arrangements for the Reorganised National Health Service (DHSS). London, HMSO.

1972   National Health Service Reorganisation: England, Secretary of State for Social Services, Cmnd. 5055. London, HMSO.

1972   Report of the Committee on Nursing (Briggs Report) Cmnd. 5115. London, HMSO.

1973   The Remedial Professions (DHSS). London, HMSO.

1973   Management Arrangements for Reorganised NHS–Defining Districts, HRC(73)4 (DHSS). London, HMSO.

1973   Social Work Support for the Health Service. DHSS Circular, LASSL(73)47.

1973   Report from the Working Party on Collaboration between the National Health Service and Local Government on its activities to the end of 1972 (DHSS). London, HMSO.

1973   Report from the Working Party on Collaboration between the National Health Service and Local Government on its activities from January to July 1973 (DHSS). London, HMSO.

1974   'Social Trends', Central Statistical Office. London, HMSO.

1974   NHS Reorganisation Circular HRC(74)35 (DHSS). London, HMSO.

1974   Child Guidance. Joint circular from Department of Education and Science. 3/74.

1974   Report of the Committee of Inquiry into South Ockendon Hospital (DHSS). London, HMSO.

1974   Community Medicine in the Reorganised Health Service, HSC(1S)13 (DHSS). London, HMSO.

1974   Social Work Support for the Health Service (DHSS). London, HMSO.

1975   Report of the Committee of Inquiry into the Regulation of the Medical Profession. Secretary of State for Social Services. London, HMSO.

1975   Facilities and Services for Mental Illness and Mental Handicap Hospitals (DHSS). London, HMSO.

1976   The Organisation of the In-Patient's Day (DHSS and Welsh Office). London, HMSO.

1976   Fit for the Future the Report of the Committee on Child Health Services (Court Report), Vol. II, Cmnd. 6684–1. London, HMSO.

1976   Report of the Hospital In-Patient Enquiry for 1973, Preliminary Tables (DHSS). London, HMSO.

1976   Health and Personal Social Services Statistics for England 1975 (DHSS). London, HMSO.

1976   Priorities for Health and Personal Social Services in England (DHSS). London, HMSO.

1976   The NHS Planning System (DHSS). London, HMSO.

1977   Professional Conduct and Discipline. General Medical Council.

1977   The Way Forward (DHSS). London, HMSO.

1977   Joint Care Planning: Health and Local Authorities, HC(77)17. DHSS.

Author Index

The authors of the various chapters in the book are indexed in the General Subject Index. Titles for the authors listed here will be found by reference to the footnote given; where there is an issue of two or more reports in the same year by the same author, the title is also given here, though it is sometimes abbreviated.

General Subject Index

On staff matters, the entries are confined to Administration; Consultants; Doctors; Employee; Managerial and Managers; Nurses; and certain medical specialists by title, *as* Physiotherapist.

For matters concerning the population at large consult: CHC; Community; Patient; Public; *and* Relationships.

Extensive use is made of ACRONYMS, *such as* DCP, DHSS, *and* RTO, *the keys to which will be found on page 318. The letter-by-letter system of alphabetization has been adopted throughout and this determines the position of acronyms; thus* AHA *will be found after 'Agency' and not as if it were spelled in full under 'Area'.*

'n' *indicates a footnote;* 123 & n *indicates main text and footnote. There is a separate index of authors starting at page 338.*